KLEMER'S
Counseling in Marital and Sexual Problems

SECOND EDITION

KLEMER'S

Counseling in Marital and Sexual Problems

A Clinician's Handbook

SECOND EDITION

edited by

Robert F. Stahmann, Ph.D.,

Professor, Department of Child Development and Family Relationships,
and Director, Marriage and Family Counseling Clinic,
Brigham Young University, Provo, Utah.

and

William J. Hiebert, S.T.M.,

Director of Educational Services and Training,
Marriage and Family Counseling Service,
Rock Island, Illinois.

with 25 contributors

The Williams & Wilkins Company
Baltimore

Made in the United States of America

Library of Congress Cataloging in Publication Data

Klemer, Richard H ed.
  Klemer's Counseling in marital and sexual problems.

  Includes bibliographies.
  1. Marriage counseling. 2. Marriage. I. Stahmann, Robert F. II. Hiebert, William J. III. Title.
HQ10.K55   1977   362.8'2   76-50142
ISBN 0-683-07898-4

Composed and printed at the Waverly Press, Inc.
Mt. Royal and Guilford Aves.
Baltimore, Md. 21202, U.S.A.

Foreword

As stated by Dr. Klemer in his preface to the first edition, "This book has been written by its many contributors to provide sound, clinically tested suggestions for helping . . . . patients who have very real and urgent marital and sexual problems." The co-editors of this second edition, Stahmann and Hiebert, have faithfully carried forward this fundamental commitment to professional practicality inaugurated by the late Dr. Klemer.

The level of distinguished contributors on which the reputation of the first edition was based has remained largely intact. Moreover, an impressive team of new authors has been recruited to enhance both the depth and coverage of this complex field. More than a decade has passed since the original publication of this volume. In that time our understanding of marital and sexual problems has experienced an explosive growth!

Hence the need for new experts and new emphases. As indicated in the subtitle for the first edition, "A Physician's Handbook," this volume was originally aimed primarily at the physician who wished to become more knowledgeable in the special field of marital and sexual counseling. For, as Ethel Nash put it in her chapter on "Marital Counseling Instruction in the Medical Curriculum," the physician functioned at that time "even if unwillingly, in a social climate in which a majority assumed him to be the best source of help for problems related to sex." Yet in the half-generation since the writing of the first edition, a new profession has come of age in the clinical health sciences field — the marriage and family counselor — who deals with the complete gamut of marital, sexual, and family relationships. It is this more emergent profession to which the second edition of COUNSELING IN MARITAL AND SEXUAL PROBLEMS is addressed.

Consequently, the proportion of medical doctors represented

among the contributors has decreased considerably, while nonmedical specialists with backgrounds in psychology, sociology, family relations, and pastoral counseling have greatly increased. Those contributors to the first edition, including Dr. Klemer, who were members of the American Association of Marriage and Family Counselors represented a minority. Whereas, in the present edition the overwhelming majority of contributors hold membership in the AAMFC.

Included are such nationally and internationally known authorities as Whitaker, Mace, Vincent, Clinebell, Nichols, and others. Carl A. Whitaker, M.D., and David V. Keith, M.D., contribute a chapter on "Counseling the Dissolving Marriage." This is a recognition — not well-developed a decade ago — that the dissolution of a marriage may be undertaken as a positive process with counseling rather than as a desperate act of impotent frustration. William C. Nichols, Jr., Ed.D., contributes a chapter on "Counseling the Childless Couple," another recognition of an emerging marital style in contemporary American culture. David R. Mace, Ph.D., co-founder with his wife, Vera, of the Association of Couples for Marriage Enrichment (ACME) contributes a chapter on "Resources for Couple Growth and Enrichment." Again, the leading authority in a major new development in the field of marital and sexual relationships provides the reader with the latest comprehensive information and advice.

Clark E. Vincent, Ph.D., contributed an outstanding chapter to the first edition on the subject of "Counseling Involving Premarital and Extramarital Pregnancies." His significant contribution to our knowledge in this special area is retained and updated for the second edition. Howard J. Clinebell, Jr., Ph.D., one of the nation's leading pastoral counselors contributes a major chapter in the section on premarital counseling regarding its religious dimensions. Perhaps it may seem unfair to single out these representative chapters for special mention. However, it is not in any sense to suggest that these are the best of the book. It is merely to suggest by reference to the contributions of these widely known authorities that the entire volume represents the finest available expertise on COUNSELING IN MARITAL AND SEXUAL PROBLEMS.

A final special word of credit is deserved by the co-editors of this second edition, Robert F. Stahmann, Ph.D. and William J. Hiebert, S.T.M. These co-editors are probably the ideal successors to the original editor, Dr. Klemer. For they admirably carry forward another of his objectives as he stated them in his original Preface to the first edition, "Conciseness and clarity of expression, for quick idea absorption and immediate use, have been stressed throughout the book."

This second edition is concluded with an appendix which appropriately includes the core professional information needed for the clinical marriage and family counselor—information about the AAMFC including its Code of Ethics and Membership Standards. The enlarged and updated INDEX will be of inestimable utility to professional readers.

Claremont, California   C. RAY FOWLER, PH.D.
Executive Director,
American Association of Marriage and Family
Counselors

Preface

The primary goal of this book is to bring together in one source information, ideas, and guidelines of use to the practicing marriage counselor. The emphasis is on couple counseling. The approach is dyadic and interactional. Individually, the chapters provide relevant information on specific topics. In combination, the chapters systematically cover the major considerations in marital, premarital, and sexual counseling.

Klemer's first edition was directed to the physician as marriage counselor. Our scope is broader, purposefully expanding the focus to the interdisciplinary practice of marriage counseling. The content is intended for persons engaged in the practice of marriage counseling or for students in graduate training in the field. Thus, those in the fields of marriage counseling, psychology, pastoral counseling, psychiatry, social work, and related professions, as well as medicine, will find the content to be useful. The authors contributing the chapters represent those professions. All chapters were written specifically for this book.

We express special acknowledgement to our contributing authors and to our advisory editor, G. James Gallagher. This volume is truly the outcome of an interdisciplinary and interpersonal effort.

We acknowledge the support and encouragement of J. Joel Moss, Ph.D., Chairman of the Department of Child Development and Family Relationships and Blaine R. Porter, Ph.D., Dean of the College of Family Living, both at Brigham Young University, Provo, Utah, and C. Bruce Grossman, M.S.S.A., Executive Director of the Marriage and Family Counseling Service, Rock Island, Illinois. Secretarial matters were well attended to by Verlene Haws, Betty Kovich, and Joan Peterson. And, from the Stahmann point of view, the strength and reassurance of my wife Kathy and children, Ben, John, and Paul have been the sustaining element.

—ROBERT F. STAHMANN, PH.D.
—WILLIAM J. HIEBERT, S.T.M.

Contributors

G. HUGH ALLRED, Ed.D.
Professor, Department of Child Development and Family Relationships, Brigham Young University, Provo, Utah.

NANCY C. ANDREASEN, M.D.
Assistant Professor, Department of Psychiatry, University of Iowa Medical School, Iowa City, Iowa.

BILL H. ARBES, Ph.D.
Associate Professor, Department of Psychiatry, University of South Dakota School of Medicine, Sioux Falls, South Dakota.

ANNE BARCLAY-COPE, M.S.
Marriage and Family Therapy Training Program, Brigham Young University, Provo, Utah.

LEMON CLARK, M.D.
Fayetteville, Arkansas.

HOWARD J. CLINEBELL, JR., Ph.D.
Professor of Pastoral Counseling, School of Theology at Claremont, Claremont, California, and Director, Pomona Valley Pastoral and Growth Centers.

E. LEE DOYLE, Ph.D.
Sexual, Marital, and Individual Therapist, Dallas, Texas, and Texas Woman's University, Denton, Texas.

VINCENT D. FOLEY, Ph.D.
Associate Professor, Department of Counselor Education, St. Johns University, Jamaica, New York.

JOSEPH A. GILLESPIE, M.Th.
Department of Pastoral Counseling, Aquinas Institute, Dubuque, Iowa.

WILLIAM J. HIEBERT, S.T.M.
Director of Educational Services and Training, Marriage and

Family Counseling Service, Rock Island, Illinois.

JOHN B. JOSIMOVICH, M.D.

Professor of Obstetrics and Gynecology, The University of Pittsburg, Magee-Women's Hospital, Pittsburg, Pennsylvania.

DAVID V. KEITH, M.D.

Clinical Assistant Professor of Child Psychiatry, University of Wisconsin Medical School, Madison, Wisconsin.

DAVID R. MACE, Ph.D.

Professor of Family Sociology, Bowman-Gray Medical School, Winston-Salem, North Carolina.

WILLIAM C. NICHOLS, JR., Ed.D.

Consulting Psychologist and Marriage Counselor, Birmingham, Michigan.

DAVID A. REED, Ph.D.

Clinical Professor, Obstetrics and Gynecology (Psychology), Jefferson Medical College, Philadelphia, Pennsylvania.

JEAN J. RUTHERFORD

Seattle, Washington.

ROBERT N. RUTHERFORD, M.D.

Associate Clinical Professor of Obstetrics and Gynecology, University of Washington School of Medicine, Seattle, Washington.

A. LYNN SCORESBY, Ph.D.

Associate Professor, Department of Child Development and Family Relationships, Brigham Young University, Provo, Utah.

MAX J. SPENCER, M.D.

Gynecology and Infertility Counseling, Provo, Utah.

ROBERT F. STAHMANN, Ph.D.

Professor, Department of Child Development and Family Relationships, and Director, Marriage and Family Counseling Clinic, Brigham Young University, Provo, Utah.

MORRIS TAGGART, Ph.D.

Marriage and Family Consultation Center, Houston, Texas.

ALEXANDER B. TAYLOR, Ph.D.

Marriage and Family Therapist, Beverly Hills, California.

CLARK E. VINCENT, Ph.D.

Professor, Department of Medical Social Science and Marital Health, and Director of Marital Health Clinic, The Bowman-Gray School of Medicine, Winston-Salem, North Carolina.

CARL A. WHITAKER, M.D.

Professor of Psychiatry, University of Wisconsin Medical School, Madison, Wisconsin.

DONALD S. WILLIAMSON, Ph.D.

Family Therapist and Clinical Director, Marriage and Family Consultation Center, Houston, Texas.

Contents

Foreword v
Preface viii
Contributors ix

PART I

Counseling in Marital Problems

1.   **Treatment Forms for Marital Counseling** 1
     Robert F. Stahmann, Ph.D.
2.   **Commonly Recurring Couple Interaction Patterns** 17
     William J. Hiebert, S.T.M. and Robert F. Stahmann,
     Ph.D.
3.   **The Initial Interview** 34
     William J. Hiebert, S.T.M. and Joseph Gillespie, M.Th.
4.   **Extramarital Involvements in Couple Interaction** 50
     Donald S. Williamson, Ph.D.
5.   **Counseling the Dissolving Marriage** 65
     Carl A. Whitaker, M.D. and David V. Keith, M.D.

PART II

Special Issues/Dimensions in Marital Counseling

6.   **Counseling in Parent-Child Relationships** 81
     G. Hugh Allred, Ed.D.
7.   **Counseling in Parent-Adolescent Relationships** 105

A. Lynn Scoresby, Ph.D.
8.   Counseling Couples in the Middle Years 117
      Alexander B. Taylor, Ph.D.
9.   Counseling the Childless Couple 134
      William C. Nichols, Jr., Ed.D.
10.   Alcoholism and Couple Counseling.................... 146
      Vincent D. Foley, Ph.D.
11.   Medical Aspects of Marital Conflict 160
      Morris Taggart, Ph.D.
12.   Resources for Couple Growth and Enrichment 173
      David R. Mace, Ph.D.
13.   Deciding Who Must See a Psychiatrist 184
      Nancy C. Andreasen, M.D.

PART III
Counseling in Sexual Problems

14.   Male Sexual Conditioning 205
      David M. Reed, Ph.D.
15.   Female Sexual Conditioning 221
      E. Lee Doyle, Ph.D.
16.   Talking with Clients about Sexual Problems 240
      William J. Hiebert, S.T.M.
17.   Counseling the Sexually Dysfunctioning Couple 250
      Bill H. Arbes, Ph.D.
18.   Counseling Involving Premarital and Extramarital Preg-
      nancies 264
      Clark E. Vincent, Ph.D.
19.   The Climacteric Years in the Woman, Man, and Family .. 283
      Robert N. Rutherford, M.D. and Jean J. Rutherford

PART IV
Premarital Counseling

20.   Premarital Counseling: An Overview 295
      Robert F. Stahmann, Ph.D. and Anne Barclay-Cope, M.S.
21.   Premarital Counseling: Process and Content 303
      Robert F. Stahmann, Ph.D., and William J. Hiebert,
      S.T.M.
22.   Premarital Counseling: Religious Dimensions 315
      Howard J. Clinebell, Jr., Ph.D.
23.   Premarital Counseling: Sexuality 330
      Max J. Spencer, M.D., Robert F. Stahmann, Ph.D., and

William J. Hiebert, S.T.M.
24. **Medical Aspects of Contraception and Family Planning** ... 340
John B. Josimovich, M.D.
25. **The Premarital Physical Examination: A Physicians Guide** . 351
LeMon Clark, M.D.

Appendix

AAMFC: What It Is and What It Does 361
AAMFC: Code Of Professional Ethics 363
AAMFC: Membership Standards 368

Index 371

Part I

Counseling in Marital Problems

ROBERT F. STAHMANN, Ph.D.

1

Treatment Forms for Marital Counseling

Marriage counseling or therapy refers to the systematic application of techniques or interventions which are intended to modify the maladaptive and/or maladjustive relationships of married couples (after Gurman, 1975). The marriage counselor, regardless of discipline (physician, psychiatrist, psychologist, pastoral counselor, social worker, marriage and family counselor, etc.), serves as a counselor-consultant to the marriage relationship, not to one spouse or the other. Thus, the focus of change is with the marital relationship. Usually, both partners are actively involved in the counseling sessions, and since the marital relationship or system is the focus, both partners are the objects of the therapy and behavior change. Current clinical practice of marriage counseling, across the multitude of specific marital and sexual problems, is developed in the various chapters in this volume.

Those professionals working with and treating marital relationships have been and are closely identified with family therapy. "Therapy" has been associated with the medical model, the context in which the family therapy movement originated. "Counseling" with couples was the term used in nonmedical settings and has become a term to indicate growth and development apart from the implication of pathological illness. The reader will find the terms "counselor," "therapist," and "consultant" used throughout the chapters by the various authors. These terms can be used interchangeably.

This chapter presents a review of various models and forms used in marital counseling, introduces and discusses a diagrammatic model for the conceptualization of the five primary forms of marital counseling, discusses data related to outcomes of marital counseling, and discusses a number of issues that are related to the treatment of marital problems.

3

Forms for Marital Counseling

There has not been clear agreement as to the conceptualization and limitation of the various forms or models used in marital counseling. This is due primarily to the fact that marital counseling is a relatively "new" field with an emerging and rapidly growing literature. Also, because of the interdisciplinary nature of the study and practice of marital counseling, there is a diversity of opinion and practice. However, in recent years, there have been a number of excellent reviews published which have helped to reach concensus as to preferred or common forms in practice in marriage counseling. Forms for marital counseling as reported in four such reviews are summarized here in Table 1.1 (Cookerly, 1976; Greene, 1970; Gurman, 1975; and Olson, 1974).

J. Richard Cookerly, in evaluating different approaches to marital counseling, has identified six major forms of marriage counseling (Cookerly, 1976). They are:

"1. Individual marriage counseling, wherein only one spouse is treated for the purpose of resolving marital difficulties.

2. Individual group marriage counseling, wherein one spouse but not the other is treated in group counseling sessions for the purpose of resolving marital difficulties.

3. Concurrent marriage counseling, wherein both spouses are

TABLE 1.1
Forms of marital counseling identified by four writers

Author	Cookerly (1976)	Greene (1970)	Gurman (1975)	Olson (1974)
Marital coun- seling form	Individual	Classical psycho- analysis	Individual	
	Individual group			
	Concurrent	Concurrent	Concurrent	Concurrent
	Concurrent group			
	Conjoint	Conjoint	Conjoint	Conjoint
	Conjoint group		Group*	Marital group
		Collaborative		Collaborative
		Combined		
		Crisis counseling		
				Conjugal Marital behav- ior modifica- tion

* Group treatment involving both partners discussed, although whether conjoint or concurrent was not specified in studies reviewed.

treated in separate individual interview sessions for the purpose of resolving marital difficulties.

4. Concurrent group marriage counseling, wherein both spouses are treated in separate group sessions for the purpose of resolving marital difficulties.

5. Conjoint marriage counseling, wherein a couple is treated together in the same interview sessions for the purpose of resolving marital difficulties.

6. Conjoint group marital counseling, wherein a couple is treated together in the same group sessions for the purpose of resolving marital difficulties." (Cookerly, 1976, p. 481.)

Cookerly (1976) discussed three approaches to marital counseling—individual, concurrent, and conjoint. He combined each of the three approaches with each of the two common treatment modalities—individual interview sessions and group counseling sessions and thus arrived at the six forms.

Bernard L. Greene (1970) has proposed the "'six C' classification of therapeutic modalities" in marital counseling as:

"I. Supportive therapy.
   A. Crisis counseling—an orientation stressing sociocultural forces and explicitly acknowledging the implications of the "here and now" situation.
II. Intensive therapy.
   A. Classical psychoanalysis—an individually oriented approach.
   B. Collaborative therapy—the marital partners are treated by different therapists, who communicate with the permission of the spouses, for the purpose of maintaining the marriage.
   C. Concurrent therapy—both spouses are treated individually but synchronously by the same therapist.
   D. Conjoint marital therapy—both partners are seen together in the same session by the same therapist.
   E. Combined therapy.
      1. Simple—a combination of individual, concurrent, and conjoint sessions in various purposeful combinations.
      2. Conjoint family therapy.
      3. Combined-collaborative therapy.
      4. Marital group psychotherapy." (Greene, 1970, pp. 257–259.)

It can be seen that in Greene's discussion he moves from the simple to complex interactions; from the single person in therapy to the marital and family system. He stated: "Treatment can thus be visualized, in terms of a spectrum of therapeutic settings, with the dyadic approaches of classical and collaborative techniques at one end, the triadic approaches of concurrent, conjoint marital, and combined therapies in the middle, and conjoint family therapy and marital group therapy at the other end." (Greene, 1970, p. 259). As shown in Table 1.1 Greene expanded on the individual, concurrent, and conjoint approaches introduced by Cookerly to also include collaborative, combined (which included group counseling), and crisis approaches.

Gurman (1975) in a review paper evaluating the outcomes of marriage counseling, identified four therapy types or forms. They are: (1) individual, (2) concurrent, (3) conjoint, and (4) group, all of which were also discussed by both Cookerly (1976) and Greene (1970). Gurman (1975) additionally reported that the following combinations of therapy forms have been reported in the marriage counseling literature: (1) conjoint + group, (2) conjoint + concurrent + group, (3) concurrent + individual, and (4) conjoint + individual.

Six approaches to marital therapy were identified by David Olson (1974). As shown in Table 1.1, Olson (1974) did not include an "individual" category in his discussion, rather focused directly on the marital dyad. Thus, he defined marital therapy as "any therapeutic intervention technique which has as its major focus the alteration of (the) marital dyad." (Olson, 1974, p. 23). The six approaches he discussed were: (1) concurrent marital therapy, (2) conjoint marital therapy, (3) marital group therapy, (4) collaborative marital therapy, (5) conjugal therapy, and (6) marital behavior modification.

Of the four studies reviewed, there was agreement among all that concurrent and conjoint forms exist and are widely used forms of marital counseling. Individual counseling was identified by three of the writers and collaborative by two. These four forms of marital counseling, along with the tandem approach, to be discussed, are the five major forms of marriage counseling discussed in this chapter. See Fig. 1.1.

Fig. 1.1 shows the forms of marriage counseling: (I) conjoint, (II) tandem, (III) concurrent, (IV) collaborative, and (V) individual. In addition, three client configuration possibilities are shown: (1) a person, (2) a couple, or (3) a group. The third dimension shown in Fig. 1.1, and indicated by the splitting of the cube, is the dimension of the number of counselor(s) present in the session, either one counselor or two co-counselors.

It should be noted that theoretical orientation such as gestalt, symbolic interactionist, behavior modification, systems, transactional analysis, psychodynamic, etc. are not a part of Fig. 1.1. Similarly, specific techniques such as game analysis, script analysis, attending, flooding, minimal encourages, empty chair, etc. are not presented. Such topics, while somewhat related to the marital counseling forms, are not crucial to them and thus are beyond the scope of this chapter. Many of the other chapters in the book deal with these topics.

The shaded cells in Fig. 1.1 indicate whether the particular compo-

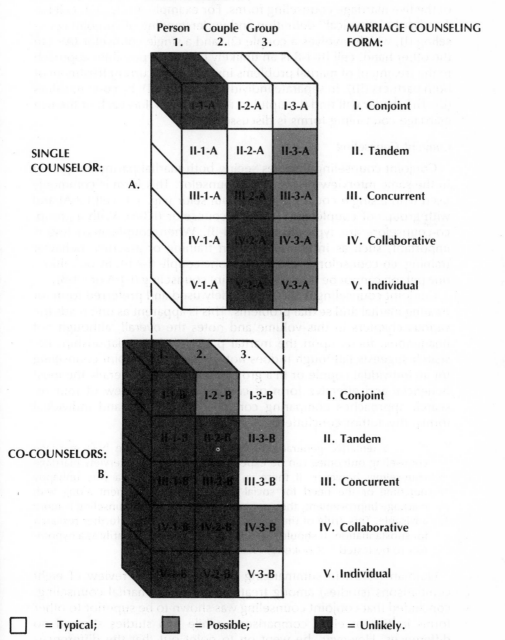

CLIENT CONFIGURATION
DURING SESSION:

	Person 1.	Couple 2.	Group 3.	MARRIAGE COUNSELING FORM:

SINGLE COUNSELOR:

A.

I-1-A	I-2-A	I-3-A	I. Conjoint
II-1-A	II-2-A	II-3-A	II. Tandem
III-1-A	III-2-A	III-3-A	III. Concurrent
IV-1-A	IV-2-A	IV-3-A	IV. Collaborative
V-1-A	V-2-A	V-3-A	V. Individual

CO-COUNSELORS:

B.

1.	2.	3.	
I-1-B	I-2-B	I-3-B	I. Conjoint
II-1-B	II-2-B	II-3-B	II. Tandem
III-1-B	III-2-B	III-3-B	III. Concurrent
IV-1-B	IV-2-B	IV-3-B	IV. Collaborative
V-1-B	V-2-B	V-3-B	V. Individual

☐ = Typical;   ▨ = Possible;   ■ = Unlikely.

FIG. 1.1. Marriage counseling forms with typical, possible, and unlikely client configurations for single counselor and co-counselor combinations.

nents of the cell (client and counselor) result in the typical, possible, or an unlikely combination. This helps to define and conceptualize each of the five marriage counseling forms. For example, in Fig. 1.1, cell I-2-A indicates a "typical" definition and understanding of conjoint counseling (I), which involves a couple (2), and a single counselor (A). On the other hand, cell III-1-B is an unlikely (although possible) approach to the treatment of marital problems involving concurrent treatment of both partners (III), in separate individual sessions (1), by co-counselors (B). The reader will find it helpful to refer to Fig. 1.1 as each of the five marriage counseling forms is discussed.

Conjoint Counseling

Conjoint counseling involves seeing both marital partners together in the same interview by the same counselor. This form is commonly used with a single couple and one counselor (Fig. 1.1, cell I-2-A) and with groups of couples and a single counselor (I-3-A). With a group, co-counselors are typically used (I-3-B). When couple modeling is important, such as in communication training or assertive behavior training, co-counselors are used with one couple (I-2-B). By definition, one person cannot be treated in conjoint counseling (I-1-A or I-1-B).

Conjoint counseling is the most widely used and preferred form for treating marital and sexual problems. This is apparent as one reads the various chapters in this volume and notes the overall, although not unanimous, focus upon the marital pair and their relationship. Research suggests (although it does not prove) that conjoint counseling for an individual couple or in a group of couples is generally the most beneficial and effective form of counseling. In a review of four research approaches comparing conjoint, concurrent, and individual forms, the author concluded:

> " . . . a tentative general rule emerges: Normally, the best marriage counseling outcomes can be expected from conjoint interview marriage counseling; however, if there is a high likelihood of a very unhappy outcome or the need for social adjustment improvement along with marriage improvement, then conjoint group marriage counseling is more advisable. This "rule of thumb" is, of course, in need of further research for substantiation. It should, therefore, be regarded primarily as a hypothesis to be tested." (Cookerly, 1976, pp. 493–494.)

Gurman (1975), in summarizing the results of his review of eight comparisons (studies) among treatment forms in marital counseling, concluded that conjoint counseling was shown to be superior to other forms in five of eight comparisons, while two studies showed no differences. However, he went on to point out that the differences among conjoint, concurrent, and group treatments were not great. What was striking was the superiority of these treatments over individual treatment for marital problems. What did matter and was related to positive outcome was that both partners were involved in counseling!

Tandem Counseling

Recently a form of marriage counseling which combines the individual and conjoint forms — the "tandem approach" — has been discussed (Murphy, 1976). James M. Murphy defined the tandem approach as a form of combined treatment in which "individual sessions and conjoint marriage counseling sessions are held *alternately* by the same professional" (Murphy, 1976, p.13). The tandem approach emphasizes the separation between the two kinds of sessions (individual and conjoint) by scheduling them on different days. Also for separation, the "couple is not to rehash the conjoint sessions during the individual sessions. If one spouse (in an individual session) refers to a conjoint session, as happens frequently in the beginning, the therapist encourages him to talk about his own behavior during the conjoint session and not to analyze the absent spouse." (Murphy, 1976, p.17.)

Murphy (1976) indicated that while the two forms of therapy are worked at in tandem, the two processes are very different because of the different systems involved — individual therapy with one person and conjoint therapy with two or more persons. Looking at Fig. 1.1, the tandem form is defined in cells II-1-A and II-2-A, indicating the individual session with each partner in combination with (tandem), although separated from, the conjoint session. Although Murphy (1976) did not discuss group approaches with the tandem form, it would seem that the single counselor could meet the couples in conjoint group sessions (II-3-A) or even bring in a co-therapist for the conjoint group sessions (II-3-B) and still be operating within the tandem format. Because of the high investment of professional time needed and questionable payoff, it seems unlikely that the tandem model would employ co-counselors in working with an individual couple (II-1-B and II-2-B). For example, with co-counselors, 6 h of counselor time (two counselors times three sessions) would be required for 4 h of client time (two clients times two sessions)!

The tandem approach appears to be most appropriate for working with couples where there are intrapsychic components that can best be treated individually, but at the same time maintaining a focus on the marital relationship through the conjoint sessions. Many individually trained counselors might prefer this form, particularly during the stage of their training and experience when they are moving from the individual orientation to the interactional orientation in marital therapy. As Murphy (1976) indicated, the tandem approach should not be used with symbiotic couples, those not distinguishing themselves from each other and thereby unable to distinguish conjoint from individual purposes, or when one or both partners are paranoid.

Concurrent Counseling

In the concurrent form of marital counseling, both partners are seen individually and concurrently by the same counselor. The four review studies cited earlier and shown in Table 1.1 all included the concurrent category in their listings. Greene (1970) has traced the introduction of the concurrent technique to 1948 and an article by Bela Mittlemann on the "concurrent analysis of married couples."

The concurrent approach assumes that the counselor wishes to work with both marital partners simultaneously, but for some reason(s), does not work with them conjointly. Thus, in effect, the counselor is doing individual therapy with both spouses. The usual guidelines for individual therapy would be in effect, particularly stressing the confidential nature of the information from each person and the individual or intrapersonal focus of the therapy. The counselor does not divulge information gained from one spouse to the other spouse. The primary advantage of the concurrent approach in marital counseling is that it provides the counselor with a therapeutic relationship with both spouses. At the same time, the disadvantage is that the spouses are seen apart from one another, thus out of their marital context. Obviously, first hand observational data on the relationship and marital interaction are missing in the concurrent form.

The typical practice for the concurrent form of marital counseling is shown in Fig. 1.1 in cell III-1-A for individual therapy and in cell III-3-B for group therapy. These cells indicate that the client is seen without their marital partner in individual therapy by a single therapist or in a group of individual clients by co-therapists. The practice of a single therapist working with a group (III-3-A) is possible and undoubtedly done, although not commonly. The practice of co-therapists working concurrently with the spouses (III-1-B) is possible, although I know of no instances of this in practice. By definition of concurrent therapy, both spouses cannot be present during the same counseling session (III-2-A and III-2-B).

The concurrent form may be the treatment of choice when there is a severe psychiatirc disorder and, for example, one partner is hospitalized. See Andreasen's discussion in Chap. 13. Other reasons for electing the concurrent form of therapy would be based either on the client's unwillingness to participate in conjoint therapy (and the therapist's willingness to accept that structure!) or the therapist's noninteractional point of view.

Collaborative Counseling

In the collaborative form of marital counseling, both partners are seen individually and within the same time span, but by different counselors. The fact that both partners are in therapy is known to each other, as is the fact that the separate therapists will "collaborate" or communicate with the awareness and permission of both marital partners. The collaboration by the therapists is presumably to enable each therapist to work more effectively in the individual therapy that he or she is engaged in with each spouse. Thus, the collaboration should be at regular intervals.

Most therapists do not consider the collaborative form to be a choice of preference for marital counseling because of the inability to deal directly with the marital relationship. All that can be done is to infer the relationship from the individual spouse in therapy and through the eyes of the "other" therapist for the absent spouse. The advantage of the collaborative form is that both partners are in therapy at the same time, which can be an important step. Collaborative counseling may be indicated when the spouse(s) are opposed to being in therapy with the same therapist or where there is an inability or nonacceptance of the interactional point of view by the therapist. The collaborative form can also help the counselor(s) and client(s) move from the individual orientation to the interactional orientation in therapy. In fact, it is my preference, when working with the collaborative form, to move from it into conjoint sessions involving both partners and both therapists (cell 1-2-B, Fig. 1.1).

The typical counselor-client configuration for the collaborative form is shown in cell IV-1-A, Fig. 1.1, indicating the single client with the individual therapist. Group forms of collaborative counseling, with an individual or co-counselors, are possible, although not common. (See cells IV-3-A and IV-3-B in Fig. 1.1). The possibility of using co-counselors in the individual collaborative sessions exists (cell IV-1-B), but seems unlikely. As indicated previously, the movement from the collaborative sessions into sessions involving the two counselors and clients is desirable, but also changes the format into conjoint (cell 1-2-B).

Individual Counseling

Individual counseling involves one client and one counselor in a one-to-one counseling relationship. The focus is intrapersonal and does not involve the spouse or the marital relationship. Most marriage counselors do not consider individual counseling to be marital counseling because of the single partner involved and the absence of the marital relationship in treatment. If both partners were in individual counseling at the same time, the therapists would not communicate or the counseling form would change to collaborative. In individual counseling the counselor-client relationship is absolutely confidential.

Recently there has been some research evidence that points to the ineffectiveness of individual counseling for the treatment of marital problems. Cookerly (1976), quoted earlier, concluded from a number of studies that the conjoint forms (both individual and group) were preferable to individual and concurrent forms of treatment in achieving satisfactory counseling outcomes. Similarly, after reviewing a series of studies, Gurman (1975) concluded:

> "Still, the comparative *in*effectiveness of *individual* therapy for marital problems seems striking. In conjunction with the data I've presented earlier, it can be tentatively concluded that the following generalizations about individual treatment of marital problems hold: (1) that individual therapy has failed to be shown superior to any other modality in controlled studies; (2) that individual therapy achieves a significantly lower success rate than other approaches; and (3) that the frequency of deterioration in individual "marital" therapy is roughly *twice* that of other approaches as a group. The clinical implications of these findings would seem to generally be in accord with the many theoretical arguments *against* the treatment of marital problems in an individual therapy context." (Gurman, 1975, p. 8.)

Individual counseling is illustrated in Fig. 1.1, with the one-to-one counselor-client format (V-1-A) and the co-counselor group format (V-3-B) the most common configurations for clinical practice. An individual counselor working with a group is shown in cell V-3-A, although practice is to use co-therapists in a group setting. Co-counselors working with an individual client is possible but uncommon (cell V-1-B). By definition, the couple cannot be seen together in individual counseling (cells V-2-A and V-2-B).

Marital Counseling Outcome

What can be expected as a general improvement rate for outcome in marital counseling? While the data to answer such a question are very limited, there are some useful data available. Beck (1976) and Gurman (1975) both found that the improvement rate for clients in marital counseling was approximately 62 to 66%. These data are based on a wide variety of studies, including virtually all available studies done in the field of marital therapy. Such an improvement rate should be encouraging to the marriage counselor in that it is comparable with the rate for client improvement in individual therapy, where the spontaneous remission (natural improvement with no therapy) is 43% (Lambert, 1976), while the spontaneous remission rate for marital problems has been estimated at approximately 17% (Gurman, 1975).

In discussing marital outcome Beck (1976) pointed to a close agreement between descriptions by clinicians and research findings. She said.

> "Changes cited by both include increased satisfaction with the marriage, improved attitudes of the spouses toward each other, modifications in

communication patterns, reduced hostility and conflict, and increased frequency of positive references to the mate, plus such positive changes in the characteristics of each spouse separately as less nervousness, defensiveness, depression, and preoccupation with self; and more responsiveness, openness, and readiness for self-exploration, and an improved self-image. Areas in which counselors reported little change, like patterns of dominance, similarly showed no significant change in these more formal assessments. Thus, one finds a convergence not only among a number of different research studies, but also among research findings as a whole and the observations of practitioners." (Beck, 1976, p. 463.)

Treatment Considerations

In order for the counselor to work with marital or sexual problems, there are a number of issues which must be dealt with regardless of the therapy form, theoretical orientation, or techniques used by the counselor. (See a discussion of similar issues related to the initial interview in Chap. 3). These treatment considerations are presented here because they should be consciously considered by the therapist, along with the treatment form, in marriage counseling.

Relationship Focus

The first consideration relates to the point already made that the counselor in marital counseling is identifying the relationship as the "problem" or "patient," and thus, that marital relationship is the focus of intervention and change. Typically clients do not see it that way and tend to identify one or the other as the focus of counseling (see Hiebert and Gillespie, Chap. 3). The counselor must orient or reorient the clients to this relationship focus. For example, the counselor will serve as a consultant to the relationship and both partners as they work toward the goals which are set and emerge in the counseling-therapy process. The process and outcomes are the creation and result of the marital and counseling relationships and their interaction.

Structure/Control

A second issue facing the counselor is that of structure with the clients. The basic issue is "Who is in charge of therapy?" Simply because the clients have sought out therapy is not enough to assume that they have, in fact, relinquished control to the therapist. The therapist must appropriately assert control from the first contact with the client(s). Structuring for the clients will likely begin before the first contact because of the reputation of the therapist. The clients may have expectations relating to both process and outcome. Structuring certainly begins with the first contact with the counseling process, whether with a receptionist or therapist, whether in person or via telephone. At that point, the message is given to the prospective clients regarding format (*i.e.*, conjoint or individual interview, etc.)

and procedure (*i.e.*, length of sessions, pretesting or assessment instruments, fee payment, etc.).

Therapy Triangle

Third, even though the focus of the intervention and marital counseling is the marital dyad, with the inclusion of the counselor, there must be the realization that the therapy unit is a triad. The triangle is a basic unit of human interaction. The basic dynamic of the triangle is that two persons will be involved in the main current of interaction and one person will be an observer. The observer can have power in the triangle and thus intervene in the system (Satir, 1967).

The triangle yields at least three interactional combinations of which the counselor needs to be cognizant. In *mediation* one person (usually the counselor) serves to balance and arbitrate the relationship between the two other persons. In an *alliance*, two persons are going to help the third. Such could be the situation with the counselor and a spouse if the idea of an "identified patient" is accepted by the counselor. In *collusion* there is the dynamic of two persons going against the third. Although it is usually not the intent of the couple to collude against the counselor when they enter counseling, the skillful counselor can use this dynamic as a powerful change agent on behalf of the clients.

Contracting

A fourth issue for the counselor is that of contracting which is the process of setting limits and building expectations with the clients. (Some counselors use written statements or contracts, although the majority apparently do not). Contracting is a way of letting client(s) know that the counselor expects a change and will work with them for it. The clients will generate the type and extent of change desired and commit themselves to that objective. Obviously, the techniques used and emphasis placed on contracting will vary for therapists, but the counseling process itself and the clients imply change, whether overt or covert, in behavior or feeling. Structure is articulated through contracting. For example, in setting the number of counseling sessions with the clients the counselor is providing information that is useful to the clients as they attempt change. By defining the limits of or parameters of therapy, the counselor can avoid getting into problems that are not central to the focus of therapy and/or that he or she cannot solve.

Session Length

The length of the counseling or therapy session is another factor that must be considered. It is probably true that most counselors treating marital problems tend to see clients in the "50-min h" which derives from individual therapy. However, in marital counseling, particularly when the two partners are seen together in a conjoint interview, many counselors prefer to see them for longer sessions, frequently 70 to 90 min. The professional setting, orientation of the counselor, and client expectation are also factors in determining the length of the counseling session(s). For example, it would appear that the physician would spend less time in "marital consultation" with a couple (see Clark, Chap. 25) than the clergy in "prewedding counseling" (see Clinebell, Chap. 22).

Session Frequency

The time interval between counseling sessions is also a consideration. It appears that the typical interval is approximately 1 week. However, there are many exceptions. Crisis counseling is a notable exception, where the length of sessions may be longer than regular sessions and often the sessions will be daily or several per week. Also the "tandem" form of marriage counseling (Murphy, 1976) discussed earlier in the chapter may involve three sessions per week – an individual session for each partner and one conjoint session. The interval between sessions may change as therapy progresses. It is common for sessions to be held weekly for most of the course of therapy and then to increase the interval as termination approaches.

Conclusion

The literature in the field of marital counseling was reviewed and five major forms of counseling were identified and discussed: (1) conjoint, (2) tandem, (3) concurrent, (4) collaborative, and (5) individual. A model (Fig. 1.1) was presented as an aid in conceptualizing the marital counseling forms and to aid in specifying the three dimensions of counseling form, client configuration, and number of counselors for practice and research.

Regardless of the counseling form used, the following treatment considerations are important for the counselor to recognize: (1) relationship focus, (2) structure, (3) the therapy triangle, (4) contracting, (5) session length, and (6) session frequency.

Conjoint counseling and the related tandem form are the preferred and most successful forms for use in working with marital problems.

REFERENCES

Beck, D. F.: Research findings on the outcomes of marital counseling. In *Treating Relationships*, (Olson, D. H. L., ed) Graphic Publishing Co., Lake Mills, Iowa, 1976.

Cookerly, J. R.: Evaluating different approaches to marriage counseling. In *Treating Relationships* (Olson, D. H. L., ed) Graphic Publishing Co., Lake Mills, Iowa, 1976.

Greene, B. L.: *A Clinical Approach to Marital Problems.* Charles C Thomas, Springfield, Illinois, 1970.

Gurman, A. S.: *Evaluating Outcomes in Couples Therapy.* Paper presented at the Annual Meeting of the American Association of Marriage and Family Counselors, Toronto, November 7, 1975.

Lambert, M. J.: Spontaneous remission in adult neurotic disorders: a revision and summary. *Psychol. Bull.* **83:** 107–119, 1976.

Murphy, J. M.: A tandem approach: marriage counseling as process in tandem with individual psychotherapy. J. Marriage Family Counseling, **2:** 13–22, 1976

Olson, D. H.: Marital and family therapy: integrative review and critique. In *Marriage and Family Therapy* (Nichols, W. C., Jr., ed) National Council on Family Relations, Minneapolis, 1974.

Satir, V.: *Conjoint Family Therapy.* Science and Behavior Books, Palo Alto, California, 1967.

WILLIAM J. HIEBERT, S.T.M., AND
ROBERT F. STAHMANN, Ph.D.

2

Commonly Recurring Couple Interaction Patterns

Many professionals, and lay people alike, believe that marriage is beyond definition—a complex and mysterious process in human life. That idea is bolstered by the belief that each marriage is unique. The belief in the uniqueness is founded on an underlying belief in the individuality of human beings. To put it in blunt terms, each human being is different from every other human being. The celebration of the experience and concept of differentness runs through psychological literature. It has been ably expressed by Virginia Satir in a chapter devoted to that subject in her landmark book *Conjoint Family Therapy* (Satir, 1967, pp.11–19).

Appearing in counterpoint fashion to the belief in the uniqueness of the human being and the uniqueness of marriage is the belief, a la Gertrude Stein, that marriage is marriage is marriage. Or, to echo an even older source, "There is nothing new under the sun." (Ecclesiastes 1:9). The idea that marriages have much in common with each other rests on the belief of similarity that we human beings have much in common with each other, especially our human-ness.

The struggles between those who believe that human beings and marriages are unique and those who believe that people and marriages share much similarity have taken many forms. A vivid portrayal of that struggle was experienced by the authors while attending a national convention. The occasion was a live demonstration of therapy being conducted by Dr. Albert Ellis. In the follow-up discussion an individual in the audience challenged Dr. Ellis, criticizing him for moving in too quickly, making assumptions regarding the similarity of human beings, and violating the concept of uniqueness. Dr. Ellis retorted "People are nauseatingly similar." (American Association of Marriage and Family Counselors National Convention, Dallas, Texas, 1972.)

Our contention is that the beliefs about uniqueness and similarity must be held in tension. That, held together and in tension, these two concepts or beliefs form a composite which approaches wholeness.

To believe only in the concept of uniqueness would mean that a therapist could not learn from his/her previous counseling experiences and couples. Training would have questionable value. The very concept of therapy, driven to its ultimate conclusion, would be impossible. Those who find themselves in this school of thought frequently resist all attempts to make sense out of life, seeing the traditional work of diagnosticians as a menace to their belief.

Those who believe only in the concept of similarity are often given to over-generalizations. Learning and training, within this context, means to know one's self. Therapy becomes "what works for me."

Our contention is that uniqueness and similarity must be held in tension. While it is true that each individual is different from every other individual, it is also true that we share similarity in our humanness. This chapter, therefore, is written with this tension in mind. While at one point in the chapter we may be stressing concepts or dynamics related to differentness, we are doing so with a backrop and awareness of the equicontribution of the concept of similarity. At another point we may be stressing the similarity between spouses and/or marriages, but it is done with an appreciation and backdrop of the equicontribution of the concept of differentness.

Modalities

In years past marriage counseling was essentially a process of treating individuals. The therapist looked at the marital conflict as a result of one individual's respective neurosis. When treatment was beneficial, the change was regarded as coming about as a result of the improved adjustment of the neurotic individual. To put it in a sentence, the therapist was treating an individual who had a marriage problem.

This chapter follows a different model and makes different assumptions.

This chapter defines marriage counseling to be a process which focuses on the marital relationship. Rather than being individually oriented, this chapter is relationship oriented.

Behind our definition of marriage counseling is an assumption about marriage. We assume that marriage has some purpose, that it makes sense. We assume that people marry to meet needs. When the needs of both partners are met the marriage could be described as functional. When the needs are not met, when the relationship is out of balance, the relationship becomes dysfunctional.

Marriage counseling with a relationship focus has different goals than marriage counseling with an individual focus. Rather than being a process of resolving individual conflicts, marriage counseling with a relationship focus is a process of awareness. Marriage counseling, then, becomes an invitation: an invitation to see, experience, and become aware of what the partners do to each other, a searching for links to their mutual involvement and responsibilities.

This chapter assumes that marriage counseling is not so much a search for *why* but for *what* marital partners do for and/or to each other. If couples can be helped to see that, they will be helped immeasurably toward health. If couples not only see what they do to each other but choose to change it, they'll be helped even more into a new level of growth and satisfaction.

Development of Patterns

This chapter did not have its development upon the invitation to write this book. Rather, the content of this chapter evolved over several years in a two-fold way: a result of our clinical practice in marriage counseling and our involvement in training programs for marriage counselors.

First, the clinical setting. Both authors were involved in growing marriage counseling programs in the late 1960's. Independently of each other, both noted what seemed to be patterns or similarities in marital systems. Our interest in recurring marital interactional patterns was further heightened by the pioneering work of Dr. Paul D. Arnold in his research with couples using the Minnesota Multiphasic Personality Inventory (Arnold, 1970). As a result of Dr. Arnold's (1970) research, he was able to corroborate the idea that not only do marital couples have recurring patterns of interaction, but that marriage counseling populations have profiles which are different from couples in general and persons appearing for individual treatment at psychiatric centers.

Second, our training experiences. In the late 1960's and the early 1970's both authors were involved in carving out a training program for senior doctoral candidates in marriage counseling and family therapy. All of the trainees were well-trained in individually oriented concepts and techniques of counseling, but had no exposure to general systems theory nor the organismic model of therapy. (For more on the organismic model see Chap. 10 by Foley.) As such, the trainees had difficulty "seeing" what couples did to each other. For example, the trainees would have difficulty "seeing" how Helen would help George with his drinking and how George would help Helen to have her affair. In order to prepare the trainees to "see" systems more quickly and to get some handles on systems, the following patterns were devised as teaching tools.

Lest the reader skim over the above too quickly, we repeat it again.

The patterns which we will discuss below were designed as *teaching tools*. As such, the patterns evolved with input from several sources: clients, trainees, supervisors, research, psychological assessment, and the literature in the field.

Not only did the patterns evolve with input from several sources, but the use of patterns as teaching tools had several benefits. First, the trainees were enabled to "see" marital systems more quickly and more expeditiously. Second, by being able to spot clues of a particular pattern during the initial interviews, the trainee was enabled to pursue the evaluation process during the initial interviews with a greater sense of direction. In other words, the trainee was able to shape the questions during the initial interview to either flesh out the existence of a subtle pattern or to establish its nonexistence. (See Chap. 3 by Hiebert and Gillespie on the relationship of patterns to the initial interviews.) Third, trainees whose eyesight had been sharpened to see systems had a greater sense of confidence in working with couples and families and a sense of direction in regard to treatment and treatment choices.

Before discussing the patterns, we would like to caution the reader regarding four issues.

First, the patterns listed below are presented in highlight fashion. To use an analogy from art, we are sketching on the canvas the basic outline. Your task is to flesh it in and to paint it. Our task is to highlight and emphasize the basic shape. In order to do that we will at times make use of stereotypes.

Second, the patterns are designed to be descriptive. Space will not be taken to raise conceptual issues regarding the nature of the human personality, nor the ideology and conceptual frameworks regarding various emotions and behaviors.

Third, the patterns have their value in flexibility. The authors caution the reader against seeing them as rigid categories, inflexible bins in which to dump marriages. They are not to be viewed as static categories, rather with the realization that some marital interactions will more closely resemble one style, while others will have bits and pieces from various styles and still others will nowhere be found among the styles. Remember, use them flexibly.

Fourth, the various patterns have little to do with gender. While we will characterize each style with given behavior for the male and female, it is important to remember that in most of the styles the behavior can be reversed. While in many of the patterns it will be more common to see the male behave in one way and the female in another, in most of the patterns practitioners will also see the reverse. Obviously cultural conditioning has a great deal to do with the roles males and females play in these various marital patterns.

The Half Marriage

Description—We begin our list of patterns by talking about the "Half Marriage" because it is perhaps the easiest of all patterns to see and because it occurs commonly in marriage counseling populations. In fact, bits and pieces of this particular style/pattern can be found in the other styles.

The male/female dynamics and behaviors are reversible.

When this particular couple enters the counseling room for the initial session, their behaviors usually appear quite different and are easily identifiable. The husband appears as a retiring, retreating, non-verbal person, while the wife appears as a verbal and forward person. The husband retires from confrontation in the interaction, generally avoiding the direct expression of negativity and anger. His passive style is in contrast to the wife's, who with greater ease reports he negativeness and anger regarding the marriage. The wife's confrontive and attacking style of dealing with her disappointments and pain can be characterized as aggression.

While the husband's passive style and the wife's aggressive style appear in marked contrast and differentness on the outside, they are rather similar human beings on the inside. Both of these people could be described as having marked dependency needs. Both of them want very much to lean on the other person, both want to be taken care of, and both want the other to be strong.

At the same time, both of these individuals experience their dependency with a great deal of pain. Each feels helpless and small in contrast to the spouse or to other people. Both experience dependency with a great deal of distaste. They despise that quality of their personality.

In an attempt for both to appear to be the strong partner that the spouse wants and to prevent the spouse and other people from seeing their sense of smallness and helplessness, each goes about to build an elaborate protection of that vulnerable side of their personality. The wife covers her dependency needs in two ways. First, she frequently behaves in a pseudoindependent style. That is, she involves herself in various community activities in an attempt to appear as though she doesn't need him, as though she can do things on her own. If one examines her community activities, however, one would see that while she is active, she is isolated and lonely. Second, the wife covers her marked dependency needs with a veil of anger. By being angry she protects herself from being seen as dependent or weak, and at the same time manages to convince herself and other people that her unhappiness is the fault of her husband who is really weak. The husband, on the other hand, covers his dependency needs by a sense of reserve and blahness. He layers over his vulnerableness by a none-motionalness, by retreating into himself.

As the conflict in this marriage mounts, as each person feels that they are not being taken care of and becomes suspicious that the other person isn't as strong as they thought he/she was, nor is doing the job of taking care of them, the conflict escalates. As the wife becomes more aggressive in attempting both to convince him that he is not doing the job of taking care of her and attempting to get taken care of, he becomes more and more removed from the interaction, withdrawing more and more into himself.

While they look so different on the outside, both of these individuals share a similarity in another dimension. Both of them have poor self-concepts; their self-esteem is suffering. Each feels in some way unattractive, and their nonverbal behavior often reflects their low self-esteem.

Sexually this couple often experiences difficulty. The struggle that takes place in other areas of the marriage carries itself out in the sexual relationship. She, in her aggressive style, emanating anger, frequently complains about their sexual relationship, with the result being that the husband becomes less and less initiatory in the relationship and interested in it. As the relationship cools sexually, the wife becomes more and more angry about the husband's retreat. Typical of this pattern, while she complains about his lack of assertiveness, his difficulty maintaining erection, or his difficulty with premature ejaculation, she too has her difficulties, frequently being nonorgasmic. Thus, a sense of apathy overtakes the sexual aspect of the relationship.

The male's behavior as described above is equally as visible, although not with as much flair. He is a withdrawn, isolated, and lonely male who could best be characterized as inexpressive.

Cameo of the Half Marriage — There are a number of behaviors which are typical of this particular marital pattern and which may help the counselor spot it more quickly. For one thing, this couple experiences frequent ups and downs. While this relationship often survives many years, it does so with many arguments and separations. Frequently, this couple will separate and come back together many times during their lifetime. At other times this couple will separate and get a pseudodivorce, but the relationship will perpetuate itself after the divorce, occasionally with some improvement in the relationship.

The behavior which we have described as typical of the wife, although the male could just as easily be in that position and the wife in the other position, can be easily spotted. This is the kind of person who when seeing you will say, "How come you didn't wave to me when I was downtown yesterday?" or "How come you never visit me?" In each case, the question is so designed to put the receiver on the defensive. It makes the subtle assumption that the receiver is responsible for the other's health and happiness, while also protecting the sender from disclosing the fact that they were hurt or upset because the receiver didn't wave, say hello, or come over to visit.

Treatment of the Half Marriage—The treatment of this particular interactional style involves dealing both with the relationship and how each individual approaches the relationship and what he/she expects to get out of it.

Some attention will need to be spent with the wife helping her to see that her aggressive style is really an attempt to control the relationship, an attempt to fulfill her own dependency needs by attempting to require the husband to be stronger and take care of her. At the same time, because she dislikes the quality of her personality which wants to be taken care of, she cannot allow that behavior to take place. Clarification of that conflict and its resultant request adds to confusion on the part of the husband and his backing off of what appears to him to be a double bind situation in which he loses both ways.

The husband's low self-esteem means that he is very uncertain in the marital interaction, that he has a great deal of difficulty understanding what is going on, and that he often feels very inadequate in the realtionship. The process of working with this couple involves the husband clarifying and often reidentifying what he thinks and feels and allowing him to express it, building his sense of esteem and his ability to not only communicate within the relationship, but have the right to his own thoughts and feelings. In other words, the husband needs to get in touch with and relearn the expression of feelings. As the process proceeds with the husband functioning with greater surety, he will begin to move into the relationship and take a more active role. If the wife learns to express her dependency needs without covering them with anger or attacking, the husband will become more active in the relationship and will move away from his withdrawn style.

Both of these individuals have a great deal of difficulty accepting the dependent portion of their personality. Because they dislike it so much, the wife can't own up to it and needs to cover it by attacking and projection, while the husband needs to withdraw and pretend he doesn't have such dependency needs. Being able to accept their dependency needs will not only help them to be less dependent but will also aid them in being more effective in seeing to it that their own needs are being met.

This particular couple benefits greatly from going over various incidents that happen in their life together. Trouble will occur over and over again when one partner does not clarify what he/she wants of the other partner, makes assumptions, and then becomes angry or withdrawn to cover the hurt when the other did not behave in the desired way.

This particular couple has been characterized as a half marriage as a way of saying that both of these people on the one hand want so much to be taken care of but at the same time dislike it greatly and experience a great deal of pain about whether they really want to be in that relationship. It's a way of saying that they are struggling with their investment, wanting it and not wanting it at one and the same time.

Attaching-Detaching Marriage

Description — This particular couple's appearance in the counseling room is often initially met with surprise by the counselor. On the surface they appear to be a charming couple. Often both partners appear to be very adequate people. She seems to function well as a mother and he seems to function well as a father. When it comes to vocations, both of them appear to function well in their own respective jobs/career. Both of them appear to be adequate and capable when it comes to managing the financial aspects of the family. In other words, both seem to be successful people.

This couple, however, very much like the couple in the half marriage, have a great deal of similarity under the surface. Both of them want to be taken care of by each other which contributes to ineffective relationship dependency needs. But in contrast to the couple in the half marriage, this particular couple experiences difficulty in regard to dependency needs on a slighty different dimension. They deal with it in terms of a struggle for intimacy. As the relationship begins to develop, the wife begins to attempt to heat up the marriage, attempting to get closer to her husband and attempting to get him to fulfill her various needs. Thus, the wife begins to accelerate her demands on him. She wants to know that he loves her, that he accepts her. She is looking for proof. As the wife accelerates her demands, attempting to get closer to her husband (attaching), he begins to back away (detaching). The closer the wife pushes, the more she attempts to attach, the farther away the husband moves, attempting to detach himself from her.

As the therapist observes this couple it is not difficult to see that the wife is determined that she is somehow going to penetrate through his particular shell. In a very persistent manner she struggles to attempt to win his love, to maneuver him into some statement, proving in some way that he does love her. The more she accelerates her pressure, the more she attempts to move in to the husband, the further away he gets, the more he builds his protective shell. The husband becomes very blah on the surface, watching very carefully that he does not give his wife any clue to what he is really thinking and feeling on the inside.

As the relationship draws into greater conflict, the wife will frequently become very disillusioned with the relationship, giving way to hysterical outbursts of anger and rage. The more the wife rages, the more the husband withdraws.

This marital relationship frequently has a kind of cycle about it. First, the wife will attempt to get closer to the husband, to do things and say things that are designed to please him and win from him some statement of approval or acceptance. The wife does this because she thinks she needs to earn his love. After this has gone on for a while the second stage comes about during which she decides that she shouldn't have to win his love and affection, that it ought to just be there. When she finally decides that she should not need to win his love and affection, she becomes angry and explodes. Following the explosion and a period of time the cycle begins over again with the wife going back to stage one.

While this couple on the outside appears to be very different, she dynamic and generally pleasant, he appearing reserved and cool, they are really both very sensitive people and easily hurt.

Cameo of the Attaching-Detaching Marriage — There are several aspects of this relationship which provide excellent clues to its existence. When looking at the courtship history, for example, this couple is often easy to spot. First, there is frequently a marked contrast in their behavior. The wife during the early dating experiences appears as a very vivacious, fun, strong, and independent woman. The husband was attracted to this because she lent a sense of ease and comfortableness to the dating and frequently facilitated their social life. The husband, on the other hand, appeared during their early dating process to be the strong, silent, and reliable type. The wife was attracted to this personality because she saw him as the kind of guy who could take care of her and who would give her a sense of purpose and direction in life.

Another interesting dynamic of the courtship experience with this couple is that the one who is the attaching personality (the wife in the case we have described) was often unusually active in attempting to cement the relationship. Sometimes this takes the shape of the wife becoming pregnant before marriage plans are firmed up, or it takes the shape of the wife initiating plans to live together.

When in the counseling room with this couple, the interaction is often very clear. Several analogies come to mind. Often it appears as though the husband is some kind of great sphinx sitting on the sands of Egypt. The wife appears to be an exotic dancer dancing round and around the great stone sphinx, convinced that somehow if she can only dance creatively and exotically enough the great stone sphinx might at least wink. Thus, the wife keeps attempting to light some kind of fire under the husband, wondering if he really is alive on the inside, if there really is something in that body. At points in the marriage she will attempt to jab a pin inside him and pull it out to see if there is blood on the end, to see if he really is alive. She will make use of all kinds of exotic tactics in an attempt to get closer to him, to attach, to up the temperature of the marriage. Each time she steals downstairs to turn the thermostat higher, he sneaks in when she goes away and turns it back down to 50°.

Treatment of the Attaching-Detaching Marriage — As indicated in the above commentary, this particular marriage has a great deal of struggle over the issues of both dependency and intimacy. The husband experiences a great deal of difficulty between giving too much emotional investment versus being lonely. When he experiences tension in that regard, he backs away from meeting his wife's demands because he has a fear that they will not end. It is as though he feels that if he once starts pleasing her then all he'll have time to do is please her and he'll never be able to take care of himself or get his own needs met.

At the same time that the husband is experiencing a conflict between giving too much and not giving, the wife also feels undeserving about satisfactions. While on the one hand the wife feels that she needs to be loved and accepted for who she is, she also feels that she should not be loved and accepted just because she is or because she deserves to be loved. Rather, she feels she needs to earn love. On the other hand, she becomes angry with that, feeling that she should be loved just because she is.

The depencency/intimacy struggle is over the issue of the meeting of needs. The husband feels that if he begins to satisfy his wife's demands, she'll keep on demanding and demanding; the wife feels the husband should be meeting all her needs. These two together form the system.

The counseling process is usually very helpful for this couple. During the process, taking the time to find out what each thinks and feels has the effect of improving the relationship. For the first time the wife finds out the husband really does think and feel, and as counseling helps to improve communication, the couple begins to relax as each gets to know more about the other. Through this exchange of thoughts and feelings the couple can safely begin to meet some of each other's dependency needs. The counseling process is a way of regulating communication, a way of helping them to achieve a somewhat satisfactory emotional exchange which in turn begins to help the conflict over dependency needs and communication.

Sado-Masochistic Marriage

Description — When this couple first comes into the counseling room, their behavior will be very clear. The husband will be behaving in a rather aggressive fashion, being openly angry, perhaps hostile. The wife, on the other hand, will be behaving in a rather passive style.

As their interaction develops, greater differences in their behavior will be evident. The husband will not only be aggressive in style, being confrontive about his angry and negative feelings, but his style will turn to attacking. As the interaction develops, he will become sadistic in his anger, attacking his wife in a belittling style or manner.

In contrast to the attacking behavior of the husband, the wife appears to be exceedingly submissive and dependent. She takes all of his barbs, accepts them as though she thinks she deserves them. The more he attacks, the more she give in; the more she gives in, the more he attacks.

While this couple looks very different on the outside, they too share many similarities on the inside. Both of these individuals are exceedingly dependent, both needing to lean, both wanting to be taken care of, and both wanting very much to have the other be a good "parent." While they are both very dependent, they both deal with their dependency rather differently. He deals with his by attempting to hide it, by behaving as the supramasculine male. He behaves with great macho. She, on the other hand, more openly acknowledges her dependency, acting as if she knows she really doesn't have much of a husband but that's the best she really deserves and she's going to make the best of it.

In addition to their mutual dependency, both of these individuals suffer from low self-esteem. As such, both are insecure, although their insecurity is handled in a different way.

As the marriage continues the interaction takes a characteristic style. The husband becomes more and more attacking as the years go on, while the wife becomes more and more helpless. The more he attacks, the more helpless she becomes; the more helpless she becomes, the more he attacks.

Cameo of the Sado-Masochistic Marriage — This couple has several clues to its style which are generally easy to spot. First, this couple usually has great difficulty with the housework. Invariably the husband attempts to supervise the wife and regularly interferes with her housework. The wife responds by being exceedingly disorganized in domestic affairs. She appears totally incapable, as a very disheveled and disorganized person.

Another clue to this particular couple is their sexual behavior. Frequently the wife complains about his abusiveness and roughness in their sexual relationship. While the husband is frequently physically violent in their sexual relationship, the wife is nonorgasmic.

In terms of their behavior in counseling, the style will be repeated over and over again. The husband will blame his wife for difficulties in the marriage and her ineptness. The more he blames, the more she seems to accept the blame. After this goes on for a period of time, however, the wife will become frustrated with the needling of her husband and react by exploding. The hysterical outburst will come at the point where the wife has reached her masochistic limits. It's at this point that this couple usually comes for help.

Treatment of the Sado-Masochistic Marriage — There is something especially telling about this particular couple in terms of their behavior with the counselor. First, the couple will bring its struggle in the marriage into the counseling room. The husband is already frustrated and angry that he has not been able to control his wife and now looks for help from the counselor. Second, both of these individuals look at counseling not as an experience where they can learn about themselves and each other, but as a kind of courtroom where they each want to hire the counselor to help them in their attack against the other person. This particular behavior is easily spotted because this couple keeps insisting on dredging up situations from the past and getting into heated arguments about them in the counselor's presence.

In treating this couple the point of intervention is crucial. On the surface it appears that this husband is in control of this relationship, that he calls the shots. On more careful examination, however, the counselor will discover that the point of intervention is more effectively taken by dealing with the wife. She is not as passive as she appears and, in fact, in a very subtle way is exceedingly skillful in maneuvering the husband. In spite of how angry and hurtful he becomes, he can never quite control her. If the counselor looks carefully he/she will see how the wife goes about to set up the situations which provoke her punishment. The kernel in this system relates to the wife's difficulty with her own self-esteem and her own needs to feel that she is not a deserving person.

If the counselor has difficulty coming to grips with this particular style or pattern, we suggest reading the children's story of Cinderella. As it is generally interpreted, people believe that the ogre in the story is the stepmother. Think about that carefully and discover that there is something very annoying in Cinderella's manner, the way in which she behaves in a nicer fashion, making the stepmother and the two stepsisters appear all the worse in the contrast. It's rather similar to an experience you may have had where you become angry with an individual and inform them of your anger and they smile nicely, thank you for telling them, and urge you to say angrier things about them.

While this couple, even with treatment, will probably not be the kind that will be written about in *Redbook,* they do have a possibility of improvement in terms of the satisfaction of their relationship. If the counselor can get at how the wife sets up her own punishment, at the power she has in that relationship, treatment will have the effect of lessening the pattern, which will allow room for greater satisfaction for both of them.

This particular couple needs each other and frequently while living in continual conflict, stay together during the duration of their life-times. Nonetheless, with careful and specific treatment, this couple's satisfaction can be improved. They are, however, a challenging couple because of the struggle for power that they bring into the counseling situation. As such, it is not helpful for the therapist to be nondirective or unstructured. The more structured and directive the therapist, the more effective the treatment.

Child Marriage

Description — The child marriage contains two individuals who are really quite similar in basic dynamics and behaviors. Both of them are essentially children and as such their behavior can be characterized in terms of how one would characterize children. Both of these individuals are quite dependent, each wants the other to be a good "parent." At the same time, each person wants to behave in childish ways, wants childish gratification, and is prone to temper tantrums or violence when they do not get their way.

Both of the individuals in this child marriage usually experience themselves as little and empty. They very rarely see themselves as having anything to offer the other person. Rather, they experience themselves in need of receiving from the other person.

Both usually experience life with loneliness and desire affection from the other person. At the same time neither is very capable of giving affection and does so rarely. This can also be seen in the area of health. Each wants to be taken care of when sick but each experiences the other's illness as an inconvenience and a pain. They both want to be taken care of when sick but neither wants to take care of the other.

Both of these individuals are very rarely separated from their parents and thus are still very tied to the family of origin. As such, the parents frequently interfere in the marital relationship, and a general state of bedlam exists as this couple is buffeted from side to side in a multigenerational struggle.

Cameo of the Child Marriage — One important clue to this particular marital interaction is the way in which it structures the marriage. Frequently, this couple spends little time together, each person being very active with friends from the same sex. The husband wants to spend time with the boys, but expects the wife to take care of the house and be responsible. She wants to spend time with the girls, but expects the husband to take care of the house and be responsible. Each becomes jealous over the other's friends and tries to limit the other's involvement with friends.

Another telling clue of this particular interactional style has to do with how the marriage deals with conflict. The most usual way of dealing with conflict is flight. When the husband and wife disagree, when each tries to get the other to do what he/she wants and fails, the battle is carried out by leaving. One or the other leaves the marriage to go to mother, to father, to friends, or simply run away.

A third striking clue of this particular marriage is the manner in which they deal with each other when they disagree. Generally speaking, this couple has a great deal of action. They fight, they hit each other, they tear up each other's clothes, they throw things out the window, they behave like children. In fact, this couple has a penchant for involving other people in the community in their marital struggle. The police, the courts, the pastor, the parents, the neighbors all get involved in trying to settle this couple. They are very much like two children, a brother and sister who get into a fight and when the fight gets dirty the parents step in and try to separate them.

Treatment of the Child Marriage — Most counselors are in the counseling profession because they want to help people. This particular couple will strain a counselor's patience. Generally speaking, treatment of this marriage will not produce any change.

When this particular couple comes for counseling they are not requesting what we generally associate with counseling. Rather, they are simply requesting the re-establishment of a tranquil balance in the marital relationship. If the counselor thinks that he/she is going to change these individuals, treatment difficulties will result. Neither is coming to change; each would like the other changed. If the contract for therapy isn't clear, all that will result is counselor frustration and lack of client change.

If treatment is undertaken with this couple, several recommendations are made. First, the treatment contract should be short. Second, the contract should be designed to re-establish a sense of balance. Third, the goal for treatment should include helping this couple become aware of how they are intimate with each other by their fighting. Fourth, help the couple not take themselves so seriously.

Neurotic Marriage

Description — This particular marriage could be characterized as a complementary relationship (Lederer and Jackson, 1968). One person takes on the role of caretaker, while the other person takes on the role of patient, expecting the mate to relieve the patient's suffering.

As the years begin to tell in this relationship, both caretaker and patient become more and more irritated and angry with the pain and disappointment that takes place in this rigidly constructed complementary relationship. The caretaker begins to become angry at the sense of failing to be a good caretaker, to get the job done. In like manner the patient begins to suffer, begins to experience a sense of disappointment in the kind and nature of care being given by the caretaker.

As resentment sets in, the caretaker begins to experience a loss of confidence and a sense of failure in getting the job done. The patient, in like manner, becomes depressed and experiences a sense of helplessness.

Cameo of the Neurotic Marriage — This particular couple can be characterized as having a highly unsatisfactory marriage, one that is easily visible because upon entry into counseling it is very clearly established that one spouse is in the role of caretaker and the other spouse is in the role of patient. It is a lopsided marriage and appears so very obviously (Fisher, 1968).

Treatment of the Neurotic Marriage — This marriage relationship usually appears after years of interaction in the caretaker-patient style. As such, its pattern is exceedingly chronic and beyond the scope of successful treatment in marriage counseling.

Therapeutic Marriage

Description — The therapeutic marriage is a relationship in which both persons try to behave as if he/she is the doctor and the other is the patient. It is a relationship which can be characterized as one in which he tries to help her and in which she tries to help him.

The difficulty with this relationship is that each person becomes a member of the older generation while simultaneously becoming a member of the younger generation. In order for the husband to help the wife, he becomes a member of the older generation, while she becomes a member of the younger generation, a child. And in order for the wife to help the husband she becomes a member of the older generation (her mother), while he becomes a member of the younger generation (a child).

This couple very rarely functions as adults with each other. They most often function as a parent to the other, each taking responsibility for and charge of the other person.

Cameo of the Therapeutic Marriage — When beginning a history of this relationship this particular couple will frequently stand out in the early courtship process. At the time this couple was courting each of them was usually experiencing some difficulty in life. Perhaps he was having difficulty holding a job, perhaps she was having difficulty separating from her parents. Thus, at the point of dating, each person began to take responsibility for improving the other person's situation in life. Each became the other's doctor, trying to treat the other person's problems.

The difficulty in the relationship is that each person becomes confined to his/her role. Thus, the doctor becomes frustrated either because the patient won't get well or is getting well too fast. Or, the patient becomes distressed because the doctor won't treat him/her or is angry that the other person still tries to treat him/her.

Treatment of the Therapeutic Marriage — If the counselor wants to work effectively with this couple, the first thing necessary is that the counselor becomes the parent to these two individuals and cuts the attempt of the partners to be helpful to each other. This accomplishes several purposes. First, it allows each client to take the marriage counselor on and thus shift responsibility for their life to the therapist. Second, this then allows the couple to be adults together with each other, releasing themselves from this peculiar role where each becomes the other's parent. Third, by moving in with this couple in this fashion, the counselor helps the couple to become kids together, to learn to develop a sense of playfulness in their relationship.

In becoming the "parent," the counselor does not take responsibility for the clients or the relationship in any real sense. Rather, the counselor can become the "parent" by very actively promoting growth in each of the partners, stimulating those areas where growth is needed. Then, the couple can learn to deal with solutions to their joint living, each having taken care of their own separate areas that needed growth.

Pseudomarriage

Description — The pseudomarriage is a marriage in which the couple essentially is in a relationship that is not a marriage. To put it in other terms, some people have a wedding but never get married. It is a relationship that lacks a kind of intimacy, a relationship in which the bonding process never quite took place.

Bonding problems in marital relationships have many origins. Perhaps one of the most common problems relates to the issue of pregnancy prior to marriage. There are some couples in which a pregnancy occurs and the couple goes ahead and has the wedding, but the couple never really gets married. Perhaps this could be thought of as the child having the wedding. In any case, sometimes the couple moves ahead with the wedding but never really become married to each other. Even though the couple may live together for years, a careful examination of the relationship will indicate that the temperature in the relationship is very cool.

Some marriages begin for convenience sake, with the marriage serving another purpose. This marriage, too, can be a pseudomarriage, each being involved with the marriage for some other reason or purpose.

Similar to the above convenience marriage is the marriage in which each person is already married to somebody or something else, but gets involved in the marriage for appearances sake. An example of this kind of marriage would be the situation in which one or both spouses is primarily and exceedingly heavily invested in their own career, and the marriage is purely secondary and of less importance than their primary investments in careers.

Cameo of the Pseudomarriage—The best way for the counselor to experience this "marriage" is to explore the nature of the intimacy in the relationship. This can be best gotten at through the use of a structured evaluation process outlined in the next chapter. This will give the counselor some sense of the nature of this relationship, and its looseness or lack of bonding will become apparent.

Primary investments outside of the marital relationship will also be easily identified through the use of a structured evaluation and it will be determined that this couple is in fact really married each to something or somebody else.

Treatment of the Pseudomarriage—Treatment of the pseudomarriage is a process of making use of the structured evaluation (see Chap. 3) whereby the counselor can help the couple come to terms with the nature of this relationship. It's a way of saying that this couple is not in need of marriage counseling; there is no marraige. This couple needs to decide whether they want to get married.

Conclusion

This chapter has focused on commonly recurring patterns of marital interaction. The purpose was to help the reader "see" more quickly and efficiently some marital systems and give direction to interventions and treatments.

While the reader will identify some of the patterns discussed here in other chapters in this book, marital interaction patterns not discussed as part of our conceptualization will also appear. This is the way it should be. We have highlighted and identified seven common patterns. The reader "fleshes in" the highlights as well as creates his/her own patterns of marital interaction.

REFERENCES

Arnold, P. D.: *Marriage Counselee MMPI Profile Characteristics with Objective Signs that Discriminate Them from Married Couples in General.* Unpublished Ph.D. dissertation, University of Minnesota, 1970.

Fisher, E. O.: *Help for Today's Troubled Marriages.* Hawthorne Books, New York, 1968.

Lederer, W. J., and Jackson, D. D.: *The Mirages of Marriage.* W. W. Norton, New York, 1968.

Satir, V.: *Conjoint Family Therapy.* Science and Behavior Books, Palo Alto, California, 1967.

WILLIAM J. HIEBERT, S. T. M., AND
JOSEPH P. GILLESPIE, M. Th.

3

The Initial Interview

Marriage counselors *and* clients, at the onset of marriage counseling, oftentimes feel directionless. The marriage counselor is trying to figure out where to begin and where to go. The couple wonders where to start, what to mention, and what to skip.

This chapter focuses on the initial marriage counseling interview(s), developing a model or instrument that will provide direction for both the marriage counselor and the couple.

On Making Sense

Not everything makes sense. Sometimes we labor through marital interviews with pains not unlike those accompanying a very difficult birth. Oftentimes, however, the material brought forth is less than joyful, more often than not it is enigmatic and, in many instances, just downright nonsensical. Perhaps we, like the King of Hearts in Alice in Wonderland (after reading the nonsensical poem of the White Rabbit) can lament: "If there is no meaning in it, that saves a world of trouble, you know, as we needn't try to find any."

On second thought, if we know what we are looking for, that is, if we understand that each marital interaction has an exciting history and a vibrant rhythm all its own, then we can begin to ferret out a dynamic interactional pattern that does make sense.

Definition

The *structured initial interview* (SII) is parallel to a social history but different in some respects. It is informational in orientation but rhythmic in its conclusions. The SII seeks concrete facts about the family of origin, personal idiosyncrasies, courtship maneuvers, and marital experiences. The SII also sets up a framework for diagnosis and treatment planning. The SII, in effect, is a way of initiating therapy without labeling it therapy. In effect, it is a technique to: (1) bind anxiety; (2) structure information; and (3) pinpoint the marital and interactional pattern.

History

The SII is really nothing new. Other clinicians in the field of marriage and family counseling have developed techniques similar to ours. From the clinical and didactic expertise of our colleagues in the field of marriage and family counseling, the authors have learned much about how other clinicians approach their couples. We have translated hundreds of our own cases into a model, developing a theoretical framework which, in effect, works for us.

Practitioners such as Virginia Satir (1964), Bernard Greene (1970), and Arthur Williams (1974) have noted that the initial conjoint marital interview is a crucial step in the process of therapy. We have developed our own instrument for probing the interactional systems of marriage and family relationships as a way of trying to help the couple as well as ourselves to understand and make sense out of the history that will unfold in the subsequent counceling sessions.

Rationale for Structured Interviews

One of the most important lessons for a marriage counselor to learn is the art of structuring the initial interview. We say it is an art simply because it requires a great deal of experience as well as experimentation, feeling, and technique. It also requires an element of scientific methodology to ensure some consistency and reasonable predictability.

Oftentimes couples coming for marriage counseling do so with very vague complaints about what is wrong with their marriage. In using the SII evaluation, the counselor will be able to help the couple clarify as well as take ownership of the difficulties and vagueness of their relationship. The SII will help them to experience the history of their courtship and marriage in a unique way.

In effect, the couple is asked to make a specific contract to look at their courtship and marital history in a way which will allow them to begin with information to which they both have access. If the couple agrees to a contract to look at their courtship and marital history, counseling begins by doing just that. By presenting the couples with an invitation to spend one to three sessions looking at their own history, the counselor begins to structure a framework which will not only reduce anxiety but postpone any need to make a decision about the dysfuction and/or health of the relationship.

In actuality, the rationale for the SII can be summarized in the following points.

1. It provides a sense of direction for the therapist and the couple in therapy.

2. It helps the therapist understand that he/she "needs" the couples for information about them.

3. It helps to unravel the tapestry of the courtship and marital histories in a safe setting.

4. It changes the agenda from crisis counseling to an evaluation.

5. It creates a sense of movement and participation (healthy collusion) on the part of the couple.

6. It gives the couple a model for asking questions.

Healthy Collusion

With much skill and some luck, the cooperative adventure between the therapist and the clients brings with it a movement away from "scapegoating" and the "identified patient" syndromes. The introduction of looking at the clients' marital interaction from an historical point of view moves the focus of attention from the individuals to their joint marital experience. At this point there is a shift from individual responsibility or faultfinding to an exploration of mutual decisions, dreams and goals, and successes and failures.

In this context the counselor can avoid the self-congratulatory impulses of the "good guy" or the "all-knowing expert" in the relationship. The dramatic point to be emphasized and understood is that there are two people involved in this marital system and that they are both necessary to maintain the health or sickness of the relationship.

Dismantling the Totems and Taboos

The anxiety level of all of us increases when our "secrets" are talked about. In some ways our "secrets" can become a source of embarrassment as well as a source of change. When we are able to take ownership of our "secrets," then we are able to take responsibility for either talking about them or continuing to try to hide them. The marriage counselor through the SII is able to take the couple through their own shared "secrets" and to help them to talk about "secrets" in a way that makes them less threatening. Oftentimes much information comes out in the initial interview that was never talked about by the couple before this time. Sometimes this can be a very frightening experience for the couple, inasmuch as they claim that they never knew that fact about the other person or that they really felt that way about some particular event. Oftentimes the areas of sex, in-laws, and unfulfilled dreams are experienced as sources of buried anger and real frustration. When the counselor can, through his/her questions, create an atmosphere in which the old "totems and taboos" are talked about and viewed objectively, then the couple can begin to release themselves from the clutches of these binding memories.

Healthy Questions

We have discovered that asking the right questions gives us the right answers. While this may sound rather simplistic, it is our experience that when we are able to ask questions that make sense the couple is able to respond in a joint effort with answers that make sense.

We have found that through the use of "right questions" we have been able to: (1) begin to ask questions that are answerable, that is, questions related to factual experiences (e.g., In what year did you meet?); (2) begin to create a model for dealing with taboo or touchy issues by bringing them up in a clinical setting (e.g., Does your wife's obesity make it difficult for you to get close to her?); (3) begin to formulate hunches about who is in charge of this relationship; (4) begin to understand the key areas of resistance in the marital dynamic; and (5) begin helping to create a tentative diagnosis of the interactional model operating with this couple (See Chap. 2).

The Time Factor

All therapists are "bound by time" and, as such, require techniques to help them quickly and efficiently get to the root of problems in therapy. Oftentimes, however, the major complaint of couples who drop out of therapy revolves around the "timelessness approach" of the therapist. This approach borders on the unendurable even for the most dependent of clients and in many ways bespeaks the needs of the therapist rather than the clients. Marriage counselors need to come to grips with the fact that, while time is a healing factor, it can be structured in such a way as to promote awareness, confrontation, healing, and change in a matter of a few structured interviews. Much of the therapy of Milton H. Erickson, as recounted by J. Haley in *Uncommon Therapy* (1973), revolves around the attitude that the long-term goal of therapy should be viewed as the immediate goal of therapy. In this sense we too have come to view the SII as a way of implementing therapy immediately without really having to call it therapy. Milton Erickson was good at creating change in a rather oblique way. Oftentimes his method was so indirect that people were unaware that he was presenting them with alternatives to look at their behavior and to change it. In the same way we have discovered that using the SII helps couples to look at their history as well as the possibility of their future together.

Commitment and Contracting

We have discovered that it is absolutely crucial to try to clarify from the very beginning the level of commitment the clients have to each other and to looking at their relationship. We have discovered that if the following factors are present in the relationship, then it is possible to move through the SII with a sense of commitment and clarity. Therefore, when we have a sense of (1) a bonding and/or "glue" in the relationship, then we can (2) begin to look for a sense of agreement to do the SII which allows us to (3) look at the material with a sense of objectivity and finally (4) to postpone the need to make any decisions about staying married or getting a divorce at this point. We are well aware of the fact that it is not always easy to determine where the couple is having a problem during the first session. The SII, therefore, can be postponed until the counselor has some sense of direction and/ or feeling of commitment from the couple. We are well aware of the fact that it is the client's decision about their marriage that is at stake. We do feel, however, that we must have some sense of agreement and commitment if we are to proceed with the SII.

Contraindications

There are couples, however, whose goals are so divergent, or, whose conflict is so chronic, that any real change in the relationship is unlikely. If the counselor tunes in to that early in the first session, perhaps the SII should not be begun nor therapy continued. In any case, we have discovered that there are at least four factors that contraindicate the use of the SII. They are as follows.

1. One party wants out of the relationship and it is quite clear.

2. There is a real hesitancy on the part of one party to participate in the SII.

3. The couple is in the wrong office, *e.g.*, they really have a physical problem.

4. The immaturity level of this couple or the chronicity of the couple precludes any real climate for change and seriousness in therapy.

In these instances we have found it helpful for ourselves and for the couple to confront them with our observations and/or our unwillingness to keep them in therapy. At this point, too, we are willing to refer them to other professionals according to the situation and circumstances.

Technique and Style

Creating a model for an SII is not difficult. However, it has been our experience that it is important not to rush to the end of the history and want to deal with only "real issues." Each partner has their story to tell. The marriage counselor has much to learn. Conclusions can be arrived at at the expense of confusing and discouraging clients. Getting at the "real issues" and identifying them too soon can scare clients away. By using a casual but attentive style the counselor can set a pace which will allow the counselor to act as a chronicler of the couple's courtship and marital history. Moving slowly *and* efficiently can help to paint a realistic picture of their lives. In some ways, it is like asking a couple to sit for a portrait and at the same time to actively help in the painting of it. Before we begin to deal with the exact technique itself, it would be helpful to discuss visual aids.

Use of Visual Aids

What might be of use to the counselor at this point is a visual aid such as a blackboard or paper that can be hung with Scotch tape on the wall. We have found that the externalization of the history helps the couple to visualize their own time line and sense of historical development. In many instances, we have found that simply illustrating the key dates and movements in the relationship has helped the couple to relax and talk together about this experience. A sense of involvement heightens itself when there is disagreement upon key dates or events. The therapist as well as the couple can focalize on the visual aid as a way of creating a joint experience in therapy. Oftentimes, too, the therapist has a chance to observe how people relate to their history and can begin to sense the affect level of the couple when talking about the past. In any event, the use of the visual aid has helped us in therapy to create a sense of activity and involvement in the couple's history.

Use of a blackboard has the advantage of ease in erasing. It requires the counselor, however, to keep notes on significant events and experiences. The use of newsprint has the advantage of being saved for use in later sessions.

Sometimes couples are asked to take the chalk or pen in hand themselves and to sketch significant dates, events, or interactional diagrams on the board or paper.

More On The Contract

When the counselor has been assured that there are no contraindications for doing the SII, when all of the verbal and nonverbal signals appear to be "go," the counselor's next task is to propose an evaluation of the marital relationship. This evaluation process is the SII.

Before going ahead it is important to remark that the SII in our conceptualization can be anywhere from one to four sessions, each 1½ h in length. It is important, therefore, in making the contract with the couple to give them an estimation of the time it will take to accomplish the SII. We have found this rule of thumb helpful: if the couple has been married from 1 to 5 years, one to two sessions would be needed (including the first session); if the couple has been married 5 to 10 years, two to three sessions (including the first session); and if they have been married more than 10 years, three to four sessions (including the first session).

In regard to the contracting, we have found it helpful to give the counselor some leeway, such as saying one to two sessions, two to three sessions, etc. On the other hand, we have found it helpful to indicate that we will not go beyond the predicted number of sessions without doing so by the mutual agreement of all three parties in the counseling room.

Some comment about time is also helpful in the contracting process. By that we mean that some people are taken aback that the counselor would want to spend that much time evaluating. This can be handled easily by making use of the analogy that few people would go to a physician who would prescribe pills without taking the time to figure out what the pills were for. In addition, we have found it helpful to indicate that it is possible that we will use less time than we have predicted, or more time, depending upon how much living the couple has done in those years. For some couples 1 year of marriage is like 10 years in another marriage.

We also make it a point during the contracting process to indicate that we will share with the couple what we as marriage counselors and outsiders to this relationship see, think, and feel about this particular marriage. That is a way of saying that the SII is not exclusively for the private benefit of the counselor. What the marriage counselor thinks, sees, and feels will be in fact shared with the couple either as the sessions go along or at the last session.

The SII is predicated on the idea that counselors have a tendency to either become too involved with a couple or remain too distant from the couple. Counselors who get too involved with a couple and become part of their marriage often do so because they jump immediately into the dynamics and interaction without holding back enough to gain some perspective on the nature of the marital system and then deciding where in fact they are going to intervene in this system in order to change it. Counselors who remain too cool and distant often do so by virtue of the fact that they become a nonperson in the sessions, providing little or no feedback about what they see, think, and feel about the interactions of the couple before them. The SII, therefore, is a useful tool in trying to steer between these two poles, providing enough interaction that the couple experiences the therapist as a person who in fact gives feedback and helps them gain perspective and information from outside their system, but at the same time provides an appropriate amount of distance to facilitate the determination of how and where to intervene in the system.

The last comment we make to couples before beginning the SII may come as a surprise to some. We have found it useful to indicate that the SII is not therapy or counseling. Rather, we say that this will be an opportunity for us to get to know what it's like to be in this marriage and for them to have an opportunity to know whether they would like to work with us. When we complete the SII, we comment, we will then make a new contract, which may be to do marriage counseling, which may be to work on a specific aspect of their relationship (e.g., their sexual relationship, communication, etc.), or we may contract to do no further counseling because there is no need for it for a variety of reasons. Now this comment of ours about the evaluation not being therapy may seem strange to you. We do so because we think it important that clients not try to change before they have really decided they want to change. Williamson states it well: "Probably one of the most common causes of unsuccessful marital therapy is simply therapeutic interventions being made before people have decided to change....A sensitive therapist will restrain clients from changing before they have decided to change." (Chap. 4, pp. 630.)

Areas of Focus

What the counselor looks for when conducting the SII will depend upon the counselor's perspective on marriage. If the reader has some doubt that the perspective of the therapist makes a difference in how he/she organizes the material that is presented by the couple, choosing what to highlight or what to neglect, we suggest you read Vincent D. Foley's Chap. 10 on Alcoholism and Couple Counseling with this issue in mind.

The areas we will be outlining below will tell a great deal about how we perceive marital interaction and what our perspective is on marriage. Because of space, we will not take time at this point to refer to our perspective directly. The careful reader will note, however, that our perspective is similar to the perspective enunciated by Carl A. Whitaker and David V. Keith in Chap. 5.

While the areas of focus we list below indicate how we have organized the material according to our perspective, the SII is not to be viewed as ours. It is a tool which can be shaped by any counselor, adding or subtracting areas of focus depending upon the counselor's own perspective.

It is important to remember that as we view the SII it is multiphasic. On the one hand the SII allows the couple to relate their marriage to the counselor in terms that they know and in ways that they understand it. On the other hand, it allows the counselor to think on another level, to be looking at the material with his/her own special eyes (perspective).

Now we are going to outline some of our major areas of focus, some sample questions, and what we are looking for. Obviously, this is a rather difficult task. It is difficult to put in static written form the flexibility and fluidity of the SII.

Courtship

Rationale — You may find it rather unusual that we give such careful attention to the dating relationship of a couple. At times, in fact, we spend more time on the dating relationship proportionately speaking to what is actually spent on the years of marriage.

The reason we spend so much time on the dating experiences relates to one of our basic assumptions. We assume that at the point of marriage the partners needed each other. That's a way of saying that we believe that marriage is not accidental. The question running through our minds is, "Why did this woman (man) pick this person out of all the millions of men (women) in the world?" Our search for the answer has a two-fold purpose: (1) to give the couple some awareness of their special relationship (system) and how they carved it out; and (2) to give the counselor some understanding of its scope and nature.

The reason, therefore, that much time is spent trying to understand the relationship during the courtship phase is that this is when the marital system began and was in fact carved out. Often it can readily be seen in the courtship interaction.

Sample Questions — When did you meet? What year? Who introduced you to each other? Who initiated further dates? Were you dating other people at the time? When did this relationship become exclusive? What did they like about each other? What did they discover? What was different about each other? What didn't they like? How did their families react to each other during their dating? When did each say on the inside, "You're for me?" When did each say to the other, "You're for me?" When did they get engaged? How did this happen? Did the relationship change after the engagement? How did they determine the wedding date? How did they determine who was to be in the wedding? Were they sexually involved prior to marriage? Were they able to talk about sex? Did they have any serious disagreements before marriage? How did he (she) know that she (he) was angry?

All these questions and many more are part of the exploration of the dating relationship. The reader may be wondering whether all of these questions are necessary. It has been our experience that these questions are necessary in giving us clues to understand the sense of rhythm in the couple's relationship and its consequences for their present marriage.

Clues to Systems and Patterns —

Commitment Process — We make an assumption that marriage is a unique relationship, and that it involves a particular kind of bonding that we refer to as a commitment. That commitment takes place on many levels, involves the whole person, and involves a lengthy span of time.

During the courtship evaluation, we are concerned about the nature of the bonding process within the couple. Generally speaking, the commitment process takes a usual form. By that we mean that the commitment process begins in privacy, when each person in the relationship says, "You are for me." The second step in a usual commitment process is a dyadic one in which each person *says* to the other, verbally and nonverbally, "You are for me." The third step in the commitment process is a public one, when the couple announces their bonding or commitment to each other to the world.

Some marital struggles have their origin in a faulty or fradulent bonding process. Briefly they are these. (1) Some couples in the process of having the wedding never have a marriage. From the very beginning their relationship is cool. Rather than having a marriage they have a pseudomarriage or a nonmarriage. Not to discover the lack of bonding and proceed with marriage counseling would lead to a rather fruitless experience. (2) Some couples have difficulty with the bonding process in regard to becoming exclusive. This can be related to many factors, including the inability to deal openly and overtly with differences, negativity, and anger. The bonding thus occurs in a peculiar way and may continue as a struggle after the wedding. (3) By examining the bonding process the counselor will also receive some clues as to peculiar kinds of bonding such as in the caretaker marriage mentioned by Hiebert and Stahmann in Chap. 2.

Dependency—It has been our experience that certain themes appear over and over again in marriage counseling populations. One of these themes has to do with dependency needs and the inability of partners to fulfill them.

By careful examination of the courtship process a counselor can get hints and clues about the dependency needs of both partners and how they handled them.

For example, the speed with which the bonding takes place may have something to do with the dependency levels of the various partners. Sometimes very dependent people meet and move together very quickly, talking about marriage on the first date and living together by the end of the 1st week.

How individuals handle their dependency needs also can be seen during the courtship experience. People who experience their dependency needs as significant very rarely can talk about them. Usually they despise that part of their personality and thus avoid talking about them or cover their dependency needs with a quality of rebelliousness, irritation, or anger. Silence and aloofness is another favorite technique for people who want to appear strong even though they feel weak on the inside.

Self-esteem—Another theme that appears over and over again in marriage counseling populations has to do with self-esteem.

Couples who have difficulties with self-esteem and enter a dating relationship for the purpose of building their own self-esteem have a great deal of difficulty handling differences of opinion. During the courtship process they usually act very similar, as though they think, feel, believe, and fantasize in exactly the same manner. Disagreements or arguments are avoided at all costs, each feeling the need to be loved by the other and thus not wishing to threaten the prospect of being loved by a disagreement or an argument. Thus, the courtship experiences of couples of low self-esteem are often remarkably calm and peaceful. Couples with good self-esteem deal with differences of opinion and have disagreements and arguments in an attempt to arrive at mutually satisfying solutions.

Even though couples with low self-esteem do experience differences, they usually camouflage them. It is important, therefore, when looking at the dating relationship to not only ask each partner what they found out about the other that they felt was different, strange, or unusual, but how they went about to plan a program to change that other person.

All of this is a way of saying that couples with low-esteem often have a great deal of difficulty with fusion. These couples believe that marriage should be a state of perfect togetherness where they see, think, feel, and fastasize alike. When they discover differences, they attempt to obliterate the other person to bring them to a state of oneness and togetherness. A further exploration of the concepts of fusion or symbiosis can be found in Chap. 5 by Whitaker and Keith.

Power/Shape — An exploration of the courting relationship will also give the counselor an opportunity to get some sense about how the relationship was set up and who accepted it. The counselor will be able to get some clues regarding the complementary or symmetrical quality of the relationship.

In addition, careful questioning of the couple will enable the counselor to get some sense about the struggle for power in this relationship. Who is in charge? And what are the covert and overt rules for power and the inflicting of pain?

Marriage

Rationale — Our basic concern in exploring the years of the marriage, which we usually do on a year by year basis, is to develop some sense of the rhythm of the relationship.

Rhythms — Some marriages change and shift over the years. We are interested in noting the movement. This can be most clearly conceptualized in terms of intimacy or closeness. Sometimes couples are working on getting closer, heating up the relationship so to speak, making a bid for greater intimacy. On the other hand, some couples are attempting to increase the distance, attempting to cool the relationship, working on other agendas. This is described in Chap. 4 by Williamson.

Some couples develop a kind of lock in the relationship. It is as though the relationship has become dead; they can neither come closer nor get away from each other. This state of symbiosis is also described by Williamson in Chap. 4.

Year by Year—Once again we want to remind you that the SII is a flexible tool. You can add or delete areas based on your own perspectives of marriage and your own perceptivity.

While we conduct the SII generally on a year by year basis, we do so always with a concern to avoid minutia, to avoid getting bogged down. If the counselor enters an area of unresolved conflict, he/she should briefly examine the parameters of the conflict and move on. Don't think the conflict can be solved in this portion of the contract.

To put it simply, keep moving. Search for themes and rhythms.

Generally speaking, we use the themes or areas of focus in a chronological fashion, looking at each of the themes or areas of focus in a year by year fashion.

Sometimes, however, we telescope the years. Some couples have little going on; it stays the same year by year. At other times we form composites, looking at specific areas of focus during the whole duration of the marriage. In other words, we handle it schematically. For example, one might look at all of the pregnancies, comparing them and contrasting them in terms of how they were experienced by the wife and the husband, and the effect of each child on the relationship.

In the case of a marriage of long duration, we assign homework after the first session, familiarizing the couple with what we are looking for and assigning them the task of preparing themselves for the next session by going over the material in advance.

Systems—As we see it, couples carve out systems, maintain, and defend them. The purpose of examining the years of the marriage is to help give the couple some sense of the bilateral quality of their relationship, the manner in which each of them helped carve out and develop the patterns. While we are attempting to give them some sense of how they each participated in getting where they are, we are looking for the clues to systems and the dynamics outlined by Hiebert and Stahmann in Chap. 2.

Areas of Question—In order to give you some flavor of the kinds of themes we explore in the marriage, we list the following. Keep in mind the year by year progression. Similar areas are discussed by Stahmann and Hiebert in Chap. 21 relating to premarital counseling.

Wedding and Honeymoon—How did the wedding go? What were your expectations? How did the honeymoon go? What kinds of expectations did you have? When did the first difference of opinion come about?

Social Life — What kind of social life did the two of you have at the beginning of this relationship? Who initiated it? How were decisions arrived at in regard to what you would do? Who were your friends? His, hers, both?

Finances — How did the two of you decide to handle your money? Who decided that? Did anybody have veto power? How much could each of you spend without asking the other?

Sexuality — When did the two of you first begin your sexual experiences? Did you discuss it before it happened? How did you each experience the first time? Who initiates now?

Children — How did the two of you go about deciding whether to have children? Did you talk about contraception and family planning? What were your different attitudes and ideas about it? How did wife experience husband reacting to the pregnancy? How did husband experience the wife responding to the pregnancy? How did the pregnancy go? How was the delivery? What kind of changes took place after the coming of the child?

Vocation — Year by year each person is asked, "Are you satisfied with your job?" Are you getting where you want to go? How does the job affect the marriage? Does the job take too much of you?

The Purchase of House(s) and Moves — Moving makes an impact on people, sometimes changing the way they relate to the world and thus affecting how they relate to the family. Each move is explored, how it came about, how each person responsed to the move. The purchase of a home is also explored, this representing a particular kind of commitment to the relationship in some individual's mind.

In-Laws — Periodically during the course of the SII the counselor evaluates the relationship with the in-laws, the frequency, the ongoing contact, ongoing difficulties between spouses, illness among the parents, or divorces.

Emotions — During the course of the SII the counselor checks out how the couple handles anger, the giving and receiving of affection, the manner in which each can or does manipulate the other, how they experience their closensss and/or distance.

Parents — During the SII we generally survey the parental family. This is done briefly rather than in a thorough fashion and can be done at various points in the SII. Sometimes we do it at the beginning, other times we do it in the middle, and sometimes we do it at the end. In general, however, we save extensive work with the parental family for the first contract following the contract to do the SII.

Again you will notice that we ask many questions, but with a sense of timing in the historical development. Many of the questions are raised again and again. The basic themes of decision making, power plays, intimacy, and distancing factors are searched for. In fact, we can best describe our experience of the SII as that of weaving a tapestry. We are concerned to weave together how the couple carved out their relationship, how they each helped it along, and how they each helped build the system. Thus, we want to know how Helen helped Al with his drinking, how Al helped Helen with her affair, etc . . .

Sometimes couples experience the SII as very therapeutic even though we have mentioned that it is not therapy. Sometimes, though, it gets the job done by itself. Nonetheless, the counselor is setting the stage for a drama, the cast of characters of which has already been screen tested, properly cued regarding the script, and in some ways immune from stage fright.

Clues to Systems and Patterns — During the SII we are essentially in search of the marital system, trying to get some sense of the couple's interaction. In the back of our mind is a grid provided by Hiebert and Stahmann in Chap. 2. We do not try to fit the couples into the grid, but rather use the grid to get some handles on the marital system.

Again we will list some of the themes we are searching for, some of the themes we think important in understanding the marital relationship. Since many of the themes are similar to the themes searched for during the courtship, we will note them briefly.

Fusion/Symbiosis — As outlined in the courtship section, we continue to be alert for difficulties in dealing with differences of opinion. Fused couples relate with a right/wrong perspective, seeking to attain oneness and agreement.

Dependency/Anger — Can the couple talk about how each needs the other? Or, do they need to attack the other or cover their dependency with psuedoindependence or anger?

Self-esteem — As outlined in the courtship section, we attempt to delineate how each partner attempts to maintain and build his/her own self-esteem, robbing from the other's esteem.

Bonding — We continue to watch for the dynamics outlined in the courtship section.

Affairs — Careful attention is paid to the amount of closeness or distance in the relationship. Extramarital affairs (with people or activities) are often related to the nature of the marriage. Williamson describes this in greater detail in Chap. 4.

Dissolution — Sometimes couples come in for marriage counseling when they are already along the path to a dissolution. The exploration of the marital years, therefore, provides us some clue as to where they are along the dissolution line and whether someone has secretly made a decision about the marital relationship. This is further described by Whitaker and Keith in Chap. 5.

Readiness for Therapy — All the time the counselor is involved in conducting the SII the counselor has an opportunity to get some sense as to whether this couple is ready for therapy. Are the couple interested in seeing how each can change and how each contributes to the system? Or, are they there because they want the counselor to choose, to determine who is right and who is wrong in the relationship? Or, do they want the counselor to babysit while one goes ahead and gets a divorce?

The use of the contract to evaluate the relationship allows the counselor an opportunity to get out. Sometime, in fact, couples are not ready for therapy, are not coming for good reasons. To determine that a couple is not ready for therapy is in fact helpful, both to the couple and for the counselor.

Closing the SII

As we said earlier, sometimes comments and observations are made at each session as the evaluation proceeds, and at other times they are made at the end. Whichever way it is done it is important that couples get some sense out of how the counselor experiences their marriage. To us that means helping the couple get some sense out of what the counselor sees and experiences about their relationship. It may be a description of how the counselor experiences the intimacy or distance in the marriage, the low self-esteem and how they each tend to build their own self-esteem by robbing from the other, the anger, pain, and dependency which is experienced but cannot be described or talked about, or the sense of struggle for power that takes place in the relationship. What is described has to be what attracts the counselor, where the counselor is in regard to marriage, what strikes a chord in the therapist. If the couple is to get some sense out of how they behave, some sense of their system, the counselor needs to describe how he/she sees and experiences the marriage functioning.

Always the choice is there as to whether the counselor wants to work with this particular couple and whether they are ready for work. By contracting to evaluate the marriage the counselor and the couple both have an opportunity to get out, either because they have gotten what they needed or it isn't the right scene for one, the other, or both.

Conclusion

By now you may be wondering whether or not the couple has been inundated by the amount of material that has been evoked. We hope that it is so! By getting into the SII the counselor can raise all kinds of issues, bring up all kinds of concerns that have never been verbalized, probably never even conceived. By doing so it has the effect of shuffling the pain around, evening it up, so that no one person stands as the problem, no one person stands cleaner than the others.

We think that the SII also provides for a more total view of human beings. By going through the experience of looking at their marriage couples get some sense out of how their own marital history is a unique lending of both pain and pleasure, that they are not in fact one big blob of pain.

The SII also allows couples to develop a sense of awareness about their mutual responsibilities for growth, interaction, and pain.

Not only does the SII allow the couples to come to some sense of their own unique relationship and their own responsbility for marital growth and interaction, but it allows the counselor to participate in a special way, sharing his/her knowledge, information, creative imagination, and stirring responses.

If nothing else, the counselor and the couple have challenged the mystery of the marital relationship, have examined its health and dissatisfactions, and without magic are able to talk about "real therapy" and the possibility of continued movement and change. The nineteenth century social analyst Walter Bagehut once commented in regard to royalty that "its mystery is its life. We dare not let daylight in upon the magic." We have come to believe, however, that the SII allows us to talk about the mysterious life and/or death of a marital relationship and are able to allow daylight in upon its magical aspects. The real mystery and difficulty in marriage counseling oftentimes does not revolve around the couple's unwillingness to talk about their marital relationship, but rather the counselor's inability to find a structure in which they can do so easily. It is our hope that the SII will preserve the beauty and the mystery of the marital relationship and at the same time introduce sufficient reality to dispel the myths and magic which might be preserving its pathology.

REFERENCES

Greene, B. L.: *A Clinical Approach to Marital Problems: Evaluation and Management.* Charles C Thomas, Springfield, Illinois, 1970.

Haley, J.: *Uncommon Therapy: The Psychiatric Techniques of Milton H. Erickson, M.D.* Norton, New York, 1973.

Satir, V: *Conjoint Family Therapy.* Science and Behavior Books, Inc., Palo Alto, California, 1964.

Williams, A. R.: The initial conjoint marital interview: one procedure, *Family Coordinator.* Vol. 23, No. 4, pp. 391–395, October, 1974.

DONALD S. WILLIAMSON, Ph.D.

4

Extramarital Involvements in Couple Interaction

There may or may not be more extramarital affairs today than there were 10 or 100 years ago. How could we know? But unquestionably the occurrence is frequent enough to merit some reflection.

Today, with mass education and a higher standard of living in the Western World, there is consequently less fear of transcendental moral sanctions on the one hand and more money and leisure time to get into mischief with on the other hand. It is then hardly unexpected that there is greater sexual freedom than ever before and widespread emphasis on sexual experience as a pleasant and adequate end in and of itself.

This psychologically sophisticated era puts more emphasis on the right of the individual to personal emotional satisfaction and to a sense of fulfillment in life. A more widely disillusioned world after two World Wars nourishes a common belief that the good times are to be had in the here and now, if they are to be had at all. So it would not be surprising if this were shown to be an age with an unusual flair for complicating numerous marriages by the enmeshment of equally numerous "third parties" into an ancient three character drama with a well-known script. But yet a script which carries at least the possibility of a different epilogue, given enough playful imagination and appreciation for the absurd in human behavior.

With this in mind then, one of the more interesting ways to conceptualize an extramarital affair is to see it as "amateur psychotherapy."

The Affair as Amateur Psychotherapy

The extramarital affair has been dubbed "amateur psychotherapy." (Whitaker, 1973.) It is an attempt to drag in, use, triangulate, and most

50

often "victimize" some third party by enmeshing him or her in the dynamics of the conflicted and distressed marital interaction between the original couple. The hope, at whatever level of awareness, is somehow to use the third person to bring change and, therefore, maybe resolution in some form to the painful marriage in which both parties are being hurt about equally, since two parties to the same marriage cannot in honesty be experiencing it very differently. Hence, the term "amateur psychotherapy."

Of course the third party, that is the "victim," is very often engaged in a similar process with a spouse or lover and, therefore, in consort with his or her new associate is simultaneously both "victimizer" and "victim." Sometimes the third party to the marital relationship in question is not married nor ever has been. In this case, the third party is frequently still resolving the grief issues of the original love affair, namely, the unsatisfactory but lingering courtship with the opposite sex parent. Once again the victim is simultaneously also victimizer. That is, he or she is using the new relationship with the married associate in an attempt to resolve another prior and conflicted relationship.

One implication of this is that each of the two players in the affair is likely to think of himself or herself as being involved in two distinct and different dyadic relationships, one usually sweet and the other sour. But it would be more accurate for each to recognize that he or she is involved in a very intense and complex emotional triangle, in which any movement toward or away from one of the other two actors is simultaneously a complimentary move toward or away from the second. More than this, such a move in relationship to the first, which has implications for the second, is at the same time reactive to an earlier initiative by the second, who was at that time the first. Except that that initiative was a response to a prior move by ----. And so on and so on through an unending circular process in which any particular piece of behavior which is isolated is at one and the same time an initiative, a stimulus, and a reaction. Although commonly the actor sees it only as a reaction for which someone else should take part or full responsibility. (This is why the marital therapist is little concerned with blame or even causality in any "true" sense, but searches rather for the most available point of intervention or the angle with some leverage in order to initiate change.)

Amateur psychotherapy of this sort through the medium of an affair is most likely to occur when one or both of two conditions exist within the marriage. First, when it has the character of a therapeutic marriage. (Warkentin, 1966.) Second when there is an extreme measure (that is, more than the usual large amount) of psychological fusion of the man and woman who are married.

The Therapeutic Marriage

The therapeutic marriage, put bluntly, is the situation where two people marry each other with a view to healing each other, or at the very least to raising each other, and to doing a better job of it than the original "mother-father" managed to do. It is likely to be a very intimate, dependent, and turbulent marriage. Man and woman take turns at playing parent to child, doctor to patient, and strong to weak. The big problem of course is with the timing. When both want at the same time to be on the up end of the marital seesaw, there's nobody left to push the marriage off the ground. But somebody must be on the low end weeping if the other is to be high and dry. So one (or both) may leave the seesaw and become swingers instead.

When the therapeutic marriage is a "success," that is when one or both are healed, then ironically there may be great pressure upon the marriage to end. For the healed spouse wants to terminate the therapy, which means the therapist. The newly strong individual wants to terminate any unduly dependent relationship. Extremely dependent marriages make both parties angry. To be very dependent upon another humiliates and enrages the one taking his or her turn at being very dependent. To be heavily depended upon bows the shoulders and provokes resentful anger in the person taking his or her turn at being the strong one. The only alternative to a mutually clinging dependency may appear to be termination of the "therapy," that is the marriage.

Surprisingly often, rather than renegotiation or termination of the therapeutic marriage, that is the "therapy", one partner may seek or take a referral or be encouraged to seek or take a referral to another therapeutic love relationship. This then is the affair which in turn picks up on and continues the amateur psychotherapy begun in the therapeutic marriage.

The therapeutic marriage is heavily laced with "transference." That is to say each partner is held to be not only wholly responsible for the important regrettable behavior in the family of origin of the other, but is also at the same time expected to make it right. Second, each is expected to turn out to be in fact the exact composite picture existing in the fantasies of the partner built from expectations, projections, and infantile wishes. This is indeed a tall order, usually impossible to reach, even from the top of a seesaw.

With the passage of time this hurricane-style transference tends to blow itself out. The resolute determination of a marriage partner to find and see whatever and whoever it is that he or she wants to find and see in the other is doomed sooner or later to dissolve in the face of the relentless and repetitive reality of the person and the behavior of the spouse. While both may play with equal enthusiasm, it is always in the end an inevitably one-sided contest. This is not to deny that it is moving occasionally to hear one partner sigh to the other even as the curtain has begun to drop, which is to say, when the divorce is due to be final the day after tomorrow, "If only you had remained the person you were when I married you."

The Fused Relationship

While the therapeutic marriage is characterized not simply by transference but also by "fusion," yet the *fused relationship* so frequently leads to an extramarital affair that it merits some further attention on its own. This affair need not necessarily be with another person, although that is more often the case. But variations devised on the theme and readily available to observation include an affair with a child, a pet, a job, sports, the church, clothes, money, study, automobiles, family of origin, and such like.

There is obviously some degree of fusion in every marriage or else two people would never be able to agree on anything. But when the quantitative difference reaches a certain level, the psychological fusion becomes the dominant characteristic of the marital interaction. So we can speak of a *fused relationship*.

Psychological fusion occurs when two people are so overidentified with and overinvested in each other emotionally, within a closed and restricted relationship, that neither one is able to be aware of or to take a separate individualistic "I position" on any significant thought or issue which involves both of them. Each of these persons will rather tend habitually to make "we" statements. Fusion here means the ready sacrifice, denial, negation, or obscuring of the psychological boundaries of the self with regard to thought, impulse, and feeling in the context of an emotionally intense relationship with an intimate.

Each will resolutely include the other in any statement, attitude, or position. Each may attribute almost any statement to the other rather than own it alone. There will be many covert processes and a chronic pattern of collusion, both conscious and unconscious, between the two parties on significant issues. The fusion can spread to the point where neither one any longer knows for sure whether he (or she) is speaking for self or the partner, or part of the self and part of the partner, or part of the partner and part of the self, and so on. It becomes reminiscent of Charlie McCarthy and Edgar Bergen, with each taking turns to be the doll, but also being uncertain at times as to which one is the doll. Rather than saying "I think . . . " the partner speaking might more accurately begin, "One or another of us thinks . . . " or "Part of each of us thinks . . . " [(Indeed this can be useful and a chastening verbal exercise to suggest in marital therapy. It may also be effective for the therapist to read the lips of the speaker and then respond directly to the other spouse as if he (or she) was a ventrilo-quist throwing his (or her) voice. It is unnerving to see how naturally the second party will pick up and continue the play. The therapist may feel outnumbered.)]

In the fused relationship each partner eventually will appear to lose the capacity for individual thought and action. Each may become unable to exercise even simple acts of will or make even minor deci-sions in an autonomous way if in the presence of the partner. (To anyone who has listened to couples discuss what movie they should see, or what each is going to order from the menu in the restaurant, or discuss new clothes for "one or another" of them in the store, or consider buying a particular art object the point is clear.)

Laing captures the mood magnificently if in a painfully funny way. (Laing, 1970.)

> He can't be happy
> when there is so much suffering in the world,
> She can't be happy
> if he is unhappy.
>
> She wants to be happy
> He does not feel entitled to be happy.
>
> She wants him to be happy
> and he wants her to be happy.
>
> He feels guilty if he is happy
> and guilty, if she is not happy.
>
> She wants both to be happy
>
> He wants her to be happy.
>
> So they are both unhappy.
>
> He accuses her of being selfish
> because she is trying to get him to be happy,
> so that she can be happy.
>
> She accuses him of being selfish,
> because he is only thinking of himself.
>
> He thinks he is thinking of the whole cosmos.
>
> She thinks she is mainly thinking of him,
> because she loves him.
>
> How can she be happy
> When the man she loves is unhappy.
>
> He feels she is blackmailing him
> by making him feel quilty
> because she is unhappy that he is unhappy.

She feels he is trying to destroy her love for him
by accusing her of being selfish,
when the trouble is
that she can't be so selfish as to be happy
when the man she loves is unhappy . . . . . .

This same kind of experience between intimates has been conceptualized as an addictive relationship or as addictive love by Peele and Brodsky (1974). They suggest that people can become addicted to each other in the same way that they become addicted to drugs and so they use the term "addiction" not in a metaphorical sense but quite literally. When a person requires larger and larger doses of a substance in order to obtain the desired effect, he has built up a tolerance to it. Withdrawal is the body's traumatic adjustment to a body's drugless state. (Peele and Brodsky, 1974.)

"Most agonizing to the addict is an intangible feeling that something central is missing from his body and his existence. As a person becomes hooked on a drug he becomes more dependent upon the reassurance it brings and less able to deal with the problems and uncertainties that made the drug desirable in the first place. Eventually he cannot be deprived of this reassurance without trauma. This is addiction! The addict not only feels more helpless facing the world at large, he also feels helpless facing the drug he needs. He believes that he can neither live without it nor free himself from its grasp."

We see many people in marital consultation who feel this way about each other and about their relationship.

Why Seek Change Through an Affair?

In the case of the therapeutic marriage, the outside third party is dynamically necessary to create movement or momentum because such is the intensity of the mutual dependency that neither one has the psychological freedom or strength to move back or away from or achieve some greater measure of social distance from the other. Unless of course he or she has an alternative love object to use as a psychological anchor point, and to whom to transfer some of the love and the dependency, and with whom it can at least be fantasized that intimate needs will be met.

As for the fused relationship, the third party is necessary because such is the character and consequence of extreme psychological fusion between two people that neither one can step in any direction without the other moving at the same time and in a complimentary way so as to maintain the high degree of intimacy and engagement. There is no dynamic leverage or power within the relationship itself to use to change the relationship, since all of the resources and energy are being used to maintain it as it is on the one hand and to deny the unhappiness with this arrangement on the other hand.

Since sameness, agreement, and, therefore, nonindividuation is the goal, then neither one of them is able to make any conscious or self-conscious move away from the other or take any such unilateral initiative in order to bring about change.

One implication of this is that since in the case of either the therapeutic marriage or the fused relationship the purpose of the extramarital affair is to do something about what has become an emotionally intolerable situation, therefore, the decision to have an affair is routinely a decision of the marriage itself. In other words, both partners are involved in complex ways in the decision, through a process of collusion. This will be true whether the decision is conscious or unconscious, overt or covert, explicit or implicit, made, or simply allowed to happen.

Nor will it matter whether the affair includes sexual relations or is "just emotional." Nor, for that matter, will it matter if it is described as being "just sex" and does not include any apparent emotional engagement or investment. Nor will it matter whether the one having the affair (whereas the partner is actively "not having an affair") takes the initiative toward the third party, is simply seduced or responds passively by merely letting it happen, or just does not stop it sooner. Whatever the nuances of the script (and whatever the varying ethical considerations) the collusion and involvement of both partners in the scene frequently have a very similar psychological reality and impact.

The Collusive Affair

In clinical work, it is not unusual to consult with a couple who can easily recreate the fantasies each has had about the self and/or the partner having an affair. Very often over a period of time it has been discussed repeatedly, if playfully, between them. Sometimes the agreement has been explicit and includes even the decision as to who should be "the one to do it," although the decision is suitably disguised or coded so that one or both can later disclaim any responsibility for a role in the process, as may seem desirable.

Often in the planning stage, the language of disavowal is used by "one or another to the other," but the music doesn't jive with the words. So the affirmative decision and agreement are adequately read by both parties. The collusion has finesse and style. This kind of negotiating communication takes place at multiple levels within and between people. Perhaps "conscious" and "unconscious" are the further poles, with several stops or levels of awareness in between. And probably the two persons involved are not necessarily operating on the same level of awareness and intention at the same time. One spouse may be up on deck waving flags, while the other is in a darkened room below absentmindedly scanning the radar. And so it is that the partners frequently each remember what it was that was said, or how it was said, or what was really meant by what was said so very differently, and this happens with regard to almost any issue, provided it's a hot one.

Or later "one or another" invariably wishes that the other had made it clear "that that was what you meant at the time." Or had made it plain that he or she wasn't "only joking." Probably the affair in this regard is not exceptional, but rather illustrative of the ways in which most intimate negotiations or decision-making goes on between people. There is a multiplicity of messages passing back and forth at multiple levels, through a series of media, and all at the same time. There is instant decoding and response–in code of course. In the same person, one eye might be watching the flags while the other is simultaneously scanning the radar. In intimate relationships of any duration, there are very few, if any, truly unilateral decisions made on important issues which involve both parties, and, therefore, the relationship. While this sounds mystical and even magical, perhaps at this point in our knowledge of human communication it takes poetry to do justice to the richness and the absurdity of human behavior, especially between intimates.

Where the purpose of an affair in a therapeutic marriage or fused relationship is to create crisis in order to bring about change, then the biggest reason for chagrin utlimately rests in the fact that so seldom is it used imaginatively to that end. Rather, the affair and resulting crisis tend either to lead to divorce, or at least to a chronically forfeited sense of trust and intimacy, or to "more of the same," as defined by Watzlawick. (Watzlawick et al., 1974.) That is to say, the most common response to the crisis caused by the affair is a panicked attempt to increase therapy in the therapeutic marriage or to achieve even more fusion in the fused relationship. If one hoped for goal of the affair is more individuation and selfhood on the part of one or both partners, then this is indeed an unsuccessful outcome and is forboding of more distractions ahead.

While the phenomena of the therapeutic marriage and the fused relationship are perhaps the most intriguing, yet there are obviously many other occasions when a married person decides to have an extramarital involvement.

Other Patterns of Motivation for an Affair

An affair may be a way of achieving some measure of emotional separation, without the discomfort and inconvenience of going through the necessary social and legal processes of divorce. Or, it may be an attempt to get out of the marriage by having the spouse file for divorce and, therefore, also carry the overt responsibility for the decision, thus minimizing the pain of guilt for the first party, who is now free to say that he or she wishes to continue the marriage, even to the point of ending the affair to save the marriage. The hooker is that the promise to end the affair in order to save the marriage is dependent upon the spouse continuing to pursue the divorce. If he or she backs off the divorce to see if the marriage can be restored, then the affair may have to come alive again in order to change the status quo.

An affair may be an expression of chronic anger or outrage on the part of a man or woman who feels abused or neglected or simply taken for granted in a chronic way within the marriage. The affair is then a piece of instrumental behavior, whether conscious or otherwise, the purpose of which is to punish and seek revenge.

An affair may be an attempt to sustain a faltering marriage by supplementing the intimacy or lack of intimacy by companionship from outside. It may be an attempt to heat up a cold, distant, and empty relationship by one party being aroused somewhere else and then coming back still hot to generate some spark in the marriage. (Whitaker 1973.) Or it may represent an attempt to cope with serious sexual incompatibility or dysfunction, whether for reasons of physical or psychological disability, by finding an alternative source of fulfillment, or at least a backup opportunity for release of sexual tension.

An affair may be an effort to seek reassurance as to a man's virility, continuing potency, and capacity to satisfy a woman, or as to a woman's femininity, continuing lovability, and capacity to arouse a man (Paul and Paul, 1975). It may be intended to quieten lurking fears about homosexual impulses. Or on the other hand, through a vicarious involvement with a same sex partner just one step removed, that is via the spouse's lover, an individual may bootleg some homosexual excitement and satisfaction but in an unconscious and socially acceptable way.

Chronic and multiple patterns of compulsive extramarital affairs by the same spouse or couple are likely to express fundamental structural defects in psychosexual development. At least to describe it like this facilitates an enormous sense of achievement in the marital therapist if change occurs or, alternatively, protects his self-esteem if change does not. Both of these are worthy goals.

The Fear of Growing Old and Death

An affair may be an attempt to deal with growing older with the accompanying loss of energy and both physical and mental prowess. Particularly will this be so where an individual experiences a diminishing capacity to initiate or sustain erotic sexual activity. Sexual conquest as a reassurance, sexual liaison as a distraction, and an orgasm as a cry of aliveness may well negate or at least neutralize the ever present universal fear of death (Becker, 1973) and nonbeing (Tillich, 1952).

The affair may bring a man or woman into intimate association with a much younger person, or at least a much more alive person, who then becomes a source of rejuvenation and from whom some new life and life force can be borrowed or even sucked.

The Yearning for Romance

An affair may express the universal human longing for romance and romanticism in personal life. Most courtships and marriages begin with a heightened sense of romance and for understandable reasons very few manage to sustain it with any consistency for any considerable period of time. So an affair may promise to do some redress for this deprived state of nonaffairs.

First, there is the excitement and unpredictability of the unknown, by contrast with the detailed and highly stylized scriptedness of the marriage. Each cannot anticipate every thought or word the other might utter in every circumstance, as perhaps is true in the marriage. There is an idealization of the new love object, by contrast with the tired disillusionment with the spouse. There is an opportunity for some new myths about marriage as well as about the new lover. This naturally is much less likely to occur during a second marriage or after a second divorce. (It is unnerving to the marital therapist to see how very similar the two persons in reality are, who appear so different to the eyes of love and maybe of hate.)

Second, in the interest of romanticism, the affair makes it possible for the marriage partner to have a sense of freely choosing and of being chosen on a day by day basis, by contrast with the trapped feelings he or she may have within the marital relationship. And, moreover, to have this sense of spontaneous choice, apparently without any commitment for the morrow, without any involuntary strings attached feeds the romanticism.

Third, there may be a richer erotic excitement in the affair, partly because of some fresh angles from the newcomer's repertoire and in part because the new relationship does not have a history of bad incidents to sour it. No memory traces of repeated failure and of lethal attacks upon the good faith and self-esteem of each are present to destroy the weave and tissue of the relationship. So the opportunity for spontaneous and intense erotic love is at hand again. The "transference" connection between the two has not yet been contaminated by any unpleasant aspects of the reality of the other. Extreme polarization may occur. The spouse is "all bad" and the lover is "all good."

Fourth, some romantic excitement may be stirred up in both parties, simply because they are doing something "naughty" and "bad" for which they may be punished if found out. Adam and Eve are at it again; and again the stakes are very high. Doing something forbidden, breaking the rules, and violating the family code—all of this writes the former parents into a role in the drama, which can add another spark, albeit at an unconscious level.

Finally, wit a well-developed sense of romance as the context, some healthy people have a burning desire to experience everything possible in life and to experience it intensely. This makes it difficult for some to accept the restriction of sexual encounter to what is available within the marriage relationship. Undoubtedly, men and women who are physically, sexually, and psychologically attractive will draw and be drawn to each other, like to like. Ironically, it is the narcissism in each which will encourage exploration of likeness in the other, even though the marriages in question may be rich. The chemistry of the situation will require thoughtful good judgment and a strong sense of personal boundaries.

Professional Therapy As an Affair

Earlier this chapter discusses "the affair as amateur psychotherapy." There is also the phenomenon of "professional therapy as an affair." A few years ago, a meeting of the American Academy of Psychotherapists discussed the pros and cons of sex between therapist and client and concluded tongue in cheek that sometimes it might be all right, but "never for the client's sake."

The therapist who offers sex as part of the treatment is likely to have such a big rationalizer that colleagues cannot but experience some initial envy. The therapist who has an affair with a client, apart from but contemporaneous with the therapy, may have unusual insight into the lonely position of the prostitute. The therapist who has an affair with a client after the therapy has "terminated," can never know for sure just with whom it is that his or her lover is in love.

In a significant but usually in a well-defined and controlled way then individual psychotherapy may have the character of "an affair." The spouse although knowing about it may be carefully excluded from the process in order not to "contaminate" it. Most often this is a benign if somewhat pretentious procedure. The biggest dangers are that the therapy will simply distract husband and wife from working on the marriage, or therapist and one partner may form a team "to take care of the patient partner", or one spouse may use the therapy and the practice it affords in healthy relationships to develop beyond the point where he or she is capable of renegotiation with the partner. (Learning to deal with complications like this helps to make the training for the practice of individual psychotherapy long and arduous.)

A Perspective

As complex a slice of human behavior as an extramarital affair is not yet fully predictable and is, therefore, not yet available to anything approaching complete psychological understanding. But any attempt at understanding should aim initially at complexity, in the interest of achieving at least a sense of appropriateness in the discussion.

First, each party to an affair brings his or her own unique individual psychology to the situation with whatever degree of health and whatever the character of the pathology (Lidz, 1968). The particular constellation of attitudes and traits, conditioned responses, parental introjects, developmental crises, level of self-esteem, destructive aggression, and so forth, present in each one, is like unto none other. If the fingerprint can do it, how much more impressively can a whole being in the world. Especially since there is something ultimately unpredictable, nonrational, and mysterious about each human personality.

Second, this unique self is the fruit of a unique and even more complex family of origin (Anonymous, 1972; Boszormenyi-Nagy and Spark, 1973; Bowen, 1971; Framo, 1975; Paul, 1967; and Paul and Paul, 1975). And the family of origin has a swelling flow of history from multiple tributaries, building up over several generations. This one affair in this moment in time may have been in the making for a long period with any number of craftsmen at work. Whoever knows fully just who is doing what for whom, and for whom else, at whose instigation, with whose encouragement, and to the benefit of whom? Who could get a bang out of a concept like that?

Third, the unique self with the unique family of origin, forsaking probably none of these, meets another unique self with a comparable entourage and together they unite two complex systems into a new giant conglomerate.

So when this new system, that is this fresh marriage, produces a hybrid event like an extramarital affair, who would claim fully to understand it? Fortunately, to make thoughtful therapeutic interventions, the marital therapist doesn't need to! In fact his "understanding" may more often be immobilizing than it is enabling. Many more clients are tuned off by too much "understanding" on the part of the therapist than are discouraged by too little. So even after the sophisticated psychodynamicist has developed the richest possible theory as to the "meaning" of the affair, using not just developmental psychology, but also group and family concepts, still in the last resort the most appropriate posture as far as understanding is concerned is one of considerable modesty. But if modesty should characterize understanding, imagination will enliven therapeutic intervention.

Therapeutic Intervention: A Brief Comment

In light of the scope and purpose of this chapter, only a brief comment is appropriate in conclusion, with regard to therapeutic intervention with a married couple "having an affair."

If the truth of the affair is unattainable without the benefit of transcendental wisdom, then the modest therapist might settle for a "useful way" of understanding the phenomena. A useful way has two characteristics. First, the therapist finds it relaxing and reassuring and, consequently, is likely to be more therapeutic to be around. Second, the clients find these new ways of thinking about their behavior intriguing and even disruptive of the marital script, in the direction of building some momentum for change. This kind of understanding has dynamic power. Its "truth" is defined in terms of its constructive issue. It is "true" if it works — and works in the best interest of the clients. The kind of technique intended here is, for example the "disruption" of the script so masterfully achieved by Jackson (Jackson, 1961), and the "confusion" induced by Erikson (Erikson, 1967; Haley, 1973), and the "reframing" of the Palo Alto group (Watzlawick et al., 1974).

Obviously the affair cannot be responded to in therapy as an isolated event or problem, but rather as expressive of a total family process which, presumably, since the couple has come to the consulting office is being experienced as very distressful. The writer has found the following strategies useful.

First, involve both husband and wife in "the happening." That is, to some extent scapegoat "the victim" that is the spouse busily "not having an affair." Among other things, this is likely to offer some relief to "the victim" who will feel less helpless and victimized if offered (and affirmed in) a major decision-making role in the drama.

Second, it is often appropriate to reframe the affair as a sign of (1) taking the marriage very seriously and (2) consequently taking extreme measures to save or recreate it by first bringing it to a point of crisis. So the one having the affair may be living dangerously for the sake of the marriage, but can do so only because he or she is confident of the encouragement and support of the spouse in taking these extreme measures.

Third, the therapist needs to clarify just what immediate purpose is being met best by the affair. As suggested above in this chapter, there are a number of possible causes to be served.

Fourth, it should be acknowledged that the couple may not yet be ready for change. If the affair is intended to benefit the marriage and has been carefully planned to that end, then it cannot be abandoned capriciously until that good purpose has been clearly realized. An abrupt giving up of the affair may indeed represent an insincere concern for the marriage from the beginning on the part of the spouse involved. Probably one of the most common causes of unsuccessful marital therapy is simply therapeutic interventions being made before people have decided to change. This is an occurrence which puts both therapist and clients in a very embarrassing position. A sensitive therapist will restrain clients from trying to change before they have decided to change.

Fifth, it can be helpful to bring out explicitly and openly the psychologically triangular character of the process where one spouse is emotionally and/or sexually involved with a third party. The therapist cannot get stuck with the secret himself, or he is trapped in triangles within triangles. The therapist needs to stay equidistant from all the moving parts—free to move in and out at will and constantly on the move in a way that combines the skills of a referee from both boxing and ice hockey. Conceptualizing the triangle will make the third party as present as possible, even to the point of physical presence, which would be highly desirable if this could be negotiated. In this way the spouse having the affair has to connect, compare, and integrate two polarized foci of intense emotions and expectations. The "good guy" won't look quite so good and the "bad guy" not quite so bad. The presence of each highlights the reality of the shape of the other. The spouse may find himself or herself suddenly equidistant from both, rather than being driven toward or away from one by the behavior of the other. This is good strategic ground to occupy with a view to resolution of the marital issues.

The goal of therapy with a couple actively involved with an affair is to help them resolve their intense, ambivalent feelings about each other and about spending their lives together. Whether the goal of the affair is individuation within the marriage (ironically through fusion with a third party), or is to leave the family of origin by leaving the recreation of it within the marriage, or is to change the structure and assigned roles within the marriage, or is simply an attempt to move out from a hopelessly diseased marriage, the final goal of therapy remains the same. For each, it is to resolve the ambivalence in one way and so find pleasure and peace with the partner. Or else where this is not possible, to resolve the ambivalence in another way and so end the marriage.

In light of this goal, the affair is at best a distraction from the pain of the marriage or the boredom of life and at worst a mask for the real issues. With livelier imagination the affair could be more frequently used to serve the constructive purpose that is often embedded in the turmoil.

REFERENCES

Anonymous: On the differentiation of self in one's own family. in *Family Interaction: A Dialogue between Family Researchers and Family Therapists* (Framo, James, ed) pp. 111–173, Springer, New York, 1972.

Becker, E.: *The Denial of Death*. Free Press, New York, 1973.

Boszormenyi-Nagy, I., and Spark, G. M.: *Invisible Loyalties*. Harper and Row, New York, 1973.

Bowen,: The use of family theory in clinical practice. in *Changing Families: A Family Therapy Reader* (Haley, Jay, ed) pp. 159–191, Grune & Stratton, New York, 1971.

Erickson, Milton: Confusion technique in hypnosis. in *Advanced Techniques of Hypnosis and Therapy*. Selected Papers of Milton Erikson (Haley, Jay, ed) pp. 130–157, Grune & Stratton, New York, 1967.

Framo, J. L: Family of origin., unpublished manuscript.

Haley, J.: *Uncommon Therapy*. W. W. Norton, New York, 1973.

Jackson, D.: Interactional psychotherapy. in *Contemporary Psychotherapies* (Stein, Morris, ed) pp. 256–271, Free Press, New York, 1961.

Laing, R. D.: *Knots*. Pantheon Books, New York, pp. 27–28, 1970.

Lidz, T.: *The Person*. Basic Books, 1968.

Paul, N. L.: The role of mourning and empathy in conjoint family therapy. in *Family Therapy and Disturbed Families* (Boszormenyi-Nagy, I., and Zuk, G., eds) Science and Behavior Books, Palo Alto, California, 1967.

Paul, N. L., and Paul, B. B.: *The Marital Puzzle*. p. 50, W. W. Norton, New York, 1975.

Peele, S., and Brodsky, A.: Stimulus/response: interpersonal heroin: love can be an addiction. Psychology Today, 8:22–26, August, 1974.

Tillich, P.: *The Courage to Be*. Yale University Press, 1952.

Warkentin, J., and Whitaker, C. A.: *Serial Impasses in Marriage*. Psychiatric Research Report 20, American Psychiatric Association, Feb., 1966.

Watzlawick, P., Weakland, J., and Fisch, R.: *Change: Principles of Problem Formation and Problem Resolution*. W. W. Norton, New York, 1974.

Whitaker, C. A.: *Family Psychotherapy*. Audiotape, Instructional Dynamics Institute, Chicago, 1973.

CARL A. WHITAKER, M.D., AND
DAVID V. KEITH, M.D.

5

Counseling the Dissolving Marriage

This chapter has three parts. The first segment describes a time line along which marriages come into contact with counselors. Clinical examples will give some flavor of our work with dissolving marriages. The second segment sketches our view of marriage and divorce, and the third is concerned with administration and treatment issues.

Presenting Problems

Marriage is first an existential metaphor for a complex, intimate interpersonal bond between two people. Divorce begins as a metaphorical way of dealing with a marriage problem and deteriorates into a legal process which attempts a just division of property and designation of custody for the children.

The three stages of marital dissolution are: (1) metaphorical; (2) metaphorolytic; and (3) postdivorce.

Metaphorical

We think of a metaphor as a vehicle which carries one across levels of meaning, separately and simultaneously. Divorce is a metaphor that evokes a whole gestalt of meaning and feeling. In this early stage of dissolution divorce is in the air as a way to increase the temperature in the marriage or as a way for one partner to increase his or her investment in himself or herself.

> Leo and Claudia had been married 8 years. They had two children. He had been working on his Ph.D. in microbiology for 6 years. She had been a promising violinist and had interrupted her career to follow him to the midwest and to rear their children. The marriage relationship had become increasingly divisive as her animosity had built up and his guilt had increased to the point where they were in a long-standing cold war

65

impasse. They had spent a year in couples' therapy and had made little progress except to slow the growth of marital divisiveness. They terminated and returned 6 months later because the pain was increasing. Two months after the therapy had restarted, Claudia discovered that Leo had spent $900 from their savings on camera equipment. She felt cheated. She was outraged and was planning to divorce him. One Sunday the war broke out in deadly earnest. Their 6-year-old daughter called and said that she needed help with her parents. A meeting was convened that afternoon. In the meeting Claudia worked Leo over verbally. He became first belligerent and then sheepish. It was clear that they were only re-enacting their usual, circular style. She said she was leaving. The therapist asked her where she was going. She said, "Back to New York." "Back to Mother?" the therapist questioned. "That would be worse." she said. "Why stop there" asked the therapist. "What do you mean?" she queried. "Why don't you go on to Newfoundland?" "What would I do there?" "You could play gypsy dances on your violin." All of a sudden Claudia brightened. "I could go to London." In the closing 20 min of the hour she decided to go on a trip to London—it happened to cost $875. She took a 2-week trip to London and returned quite excited. Two weeks later she reported that she'd had her first orgasm in 2 years. In this case the threat of divorce represented a push for more intimacy which developed into a contract for psychotherapy.

Roland and Barb, age 26, were referred by a gynecologist because she felt bored with their marriage. Barb felt as if her husband cared little for himself and less for her. She saw him becoming overweight and said that she did not want to grow old with him. In the initial interview it developed that they had both been very constricted, moralistic people who met and married because they were somewhat frightened of more active exciting people. In the months prior to their coming into therapy, Barb had had two brief affairs which she found very pleasing as diversion although she did not seem to be attached to either of the persons. She said she loved her husband and wanted the marriage to work. As the hour continued she also revealed that during the first years of marriage she had engaged in a lot of extramarital sex. They returned for a second interview. Things had become much worse since the first interview. They were further apart than they had been a week before. Roland stated that he had not known that she had been unfaithful to him in the early marriage. The revelation had been very upsetting to him. Instead of disintegrating, however, he had become even more withdrawn and affectively constricted. He seemed bent upon a kind of silent vindictiveness toward his wife. The therapist spent most of the hour trying to open up the secret that forced his isolation. He withdrew from the therapist as he had from his wife. He refused to get aroused. He happened to be a behavioral therapist and near the end of the hour asked, "What direction is this therapy supposed to take?" The therapist answered, "How about under your skin?" "Harrumph," he said. They did not return. It was later learned that they were separated and were soon to be divorced. Thus, they entered the second stage of marital dissolution.

Metaphorolytic

The marriage has deteriorated. There is a distance that is defended and does not seem flexible. Perhaps the lytic process begins when an attorney is consulted. Three of the ways in which a marriage in this stage presents itself are these.

1. "I'm getting a divorce. I feel depressed. I can't sleep. Can you do something for me, Doctor?"

2. The children have symptoms. This is a situation that people who work with children see frequently.

3. "We have tried all kinds of things but this marriage is intolerable. It just does not work. We would like to avoid making the same mistake again. The kids need some help in understanding what has happened."

> Kevin and Ann were both psychologically sophisticated and both worked in fields related to human behavior. Their marriage had gone dead. Both were disappointed and puzzled. They felt as though their professional training should somehow have protected them from marital failure. They sought therapy as a way to struggle with the parts of themselves which had caused the breakdown. A great distance had grown between the two of them. Kevin was living with another woman. Ann had the two kids. It seemed that in their marriage both were looking for someone who would talk like a child but act like a parent. Neither of the two boys had any overt symptoms but in the family therapy hours they were clearly tense and easily panicked. They were in therapy in the predivorce time, during the divorce proceedings, and beyond. Kevin's girl friend and Ann's boyfriend came to the therapy hours. Initially they were a playful, cozy foursome. The boyfriend stopped coming after several visits. His girlfriend stayed with the therapy for a long time. It seemed she was there to keep Kevin from going back into the marriage. The affect in the marital relationship gradually built up. They fought battles about time and money. They fought about the kids. They went through a period of profound enjoyment of one another. He almost proposed that they remarry. Ann was adamant that they not join again and thus they drifted further and further apart.

Postdivorce

These situations are less likely to be seen as part of counseling the dissolving marriage. However, it is one of the most frequent ways that dissolving marriages come to the attention of counselors. The symptoms emerge after the divorce is finalized. We think of it as working out secondary contracts. These situations are the most difficult and discouraging to work with. The healing processes are advanced. This kind of therapy involves reconstructive surgery which means new pains in old wounds and many people are simply not interested.

1. The most common clinical presentation is when the single parent comes in because of problems with the children.

> Sue, a divorcee, brought in her 13-year-old son Ken. Ken had wanted a boa constrictor for Christmas. Sue would not hear of it. An ongoing debate had developed. Ken went to talk with his father about it. The father said that he could have one; he thought that snakes were not a problem if properly fed. Ken went back to his mother and told her what Dad had said. In the argument that ensued, Sue and her son had a physical fight that scared her to death. She brought Ken to the clinic saying in effect that he was a naughty boy. It was also clear that he had taken on the role of spouse to his mother. At the end of the initial interview when the therapist suggested that the father come to the next interview in order to get the generational organization in the family straightened out, she became uncertain. She asked 13-year-old Ken if he thought that they should do that. He said "No." They did not return.

2. One of the divorced spouses presents with anxiety or depression. This situation is experientially similar to the one noted in the metaphorolytic stage when the *individual* comes for treatment. In the post-divorce period there is more rigidity.

3. The divorcee is involved in a new relationship and feels the need for help. These situations are difficult because of the covert contracts listed below.

    a. Personal demand: "I am scared. I find myself doing with him just about what I did with my husband. Sometimes when I make a demand on him he gets quiet just like Harry always did. I feel like something is wrong with me. Like there is a mystery related to loving that I do not understand. I feel lonely all over again."

    b. Psychotherapeutic demand: "Do something for us!"

       (1) They are each trying to do something for the other. They don't want therapy for themselves but supervision for their bilateral amateur psychotherapy.

       (2) The children, again, are the complaint. "No one can make them behave." Oftentimes mother is using them to keep the new daddy outside. Or, "Son John seems so dependent since Dale moved in with us. He is driving me crazy." This may be a form of amateur child therapy for which they want supervision.

    c. Cultural demand: This is a situation that has to do with a kind of transference to the group as a way out of the heat of marriage. "Hey, ain't divorce great. See Doc, I got divorced after I met Kim at this encounter group. I have been doing a lot of reading about group therapy and I thought I could make this a learning experience, too." This demand may also be represented by people who take on a politicized new life, e.g., the women's rights person who has wrenched herself out of marriage. Unless the counselor is politically aligned with such individuals, it is best to refer them on to someone who is.

Jill and Jeremiah, married for 3 years, were actively involved in the radical movement of the late '60's. They had developed a commune with a group of people with whom they were politically allied. Right across the street was another house in which a commune of the Students for a Democratic Society (SDS) movement lived. Jill had fallen in love with the leader of the SDS house. Jill and Jeremiah came in for counseling. The counseling and the marriage were fairly dead because of her transference to the excitement of the more radical group. The therapy went on for 8 months. Midway through she left her husband and went to live with the SDS leader.

A Perspective on Marriage and Divorce

The temper of the times causes us to wonder why anybody would want to get married. In our "do your own thing," "preserve your freedom" culture a person has to be crazy to get married. Some people are so ridiculous as to complicate marriage even more by having children. Children bring with them another set of problems that is dealt with in Chap. 6 and 7. For some persons marriage is merely a way of accomplishing a developmental milestone, especially if their own parents were divorced. Leaving the marriage can be a way to prove one's love for mother. Both marriage and chidren are unredeemable insults to one's individuality. Chekhov said somewhere, "If you can't stand loneliness, do not marry." If a person is single and lonely he can always hope, if he's married and lonely then what? The ridiculous thing is that not only are people seduced into burying their own potential in a marriage, but marriages end up driving some people mad, pushing others into homicidal and suicidal acts, producing hateful demons out of perfectly nice young people, and inducing alcoholism in others. Marriages that end in divorce oftentimes leave people suspicious of the opposite sex for the rest of their lives. Marriage is obviously more insane than taking flying lessons or collecting beer cans. Perhaps marriage could be thought of as a form of mental illness, a kind of *folie a deux* attempt to overturn the culture and the cure is divorce. If seen as a mental illness, we think that it makes it much easier to understand what is meant by creative divorce and the prodigal return to Mother Culture.

A 4-year-old friend explained how marriage works. "Once there was a penis and a vagina. They met at a party. They danced and played and had a lot of fun. Then they thought they would get married. The penis went and found a boy and got attached to him and the vagina went and found a girl and got attached to her and then they got married and they lived happily for a long time" (Meyer, 1975).

While we think of marriage as being absurd, we are also commited to it as being growthful. It is growthful to the extent that it is counter-cultural. The culture sponsors two kinds of marriages: (1) the stable, symbiotic dead model and (2) the individualistic ejection seat model.

In our way of thinking and working, marriage is the only way that one can get a Ph.D. in interpersonal relationships. But marriage, like getting a Ph.D., is not a process that leaves one's personhood untouched. Instead of getting a Ph.D. a person might be a lot happier if they sold real estate. They might make more money and they might have more fun. It is an experience which threatens one's being and wrenches one down to the roots. Like hypnosis, marriage is an altered state of consciousness. If one remains too skeptical and distracted by outside noise, one will get less into it and thus get less from it. The deeper that one goes the more possible it is for things to happen.

People who enter counseling situations do so as a way to grow. If they come about their marriage it is to make that relationship more growthful. We let crises arise our of our impulse for growth and out of our struggle with destiny or with loneliness in an attempt to become more intimate and more loving.

Marriages which have the most potential for growth occur between partners who have made it out of their families of origin, achieved individual adequacy, and lived on their own. Two I's combine to make a We. When children come along they increase the We-ness and provide an additional push toward intimacy. In terms of growth and interpersonal relationships, entering into a marriage is like a tennis player turning pro. He begins to play at a new level of intensity which brings in turn a higher level of skill. There is more at stake. He needs to be more committed and is allowed to be more committed. Once one plays at the professional level, it is hard to go back and play with amateurs. Playing with amateurs involves withholding a part of the self which can be boring and which reduces the possibility of shared excitement. Teaching beginners can be fun and brings the pleasure of showing off, but it lacks the intensity and thrill of using the whole self. Early on, it's the singles that bring the best enjoyment, the battle of the sexes. Later on as the marriage deepens, often with the advent of children, one learns the pleasure of teaming, in doubles. One learns how to invest the whole self and how to use restraint. There is a thrill in moving to the net together, it is a pleasure to back up the partner when he or she has the initiative and there are opportunities to take risks on your own, to let yourself get out of position knowing that you are backed up by a partner. Victory celebrations are fuller and losses better endured.

A form of delusional thinking which is seen in family or marital therapy is the statement, "I did not marry your family." Marriage is the union of two families and the two families help to make it work or help to facilitate the divorce. Divorce is a 3-generational problem until proven otherwise. When there are no children, their absence, for whatever reason, might have to do with the bilateral withdrawal of the marital pair. Usually the marital dyad is in the foreground but they are in fact embedded in a complex mix of intergenerational battles, traditional family-governed sex roles, and childrearing practices. Marrying the family white knight can cause the spouse to seem a failure if somehow he or she interrupts the family aspirations for their chosen one. Imagine how disappointed the Virgin Mary would have been if Jesus would have married someone who taught him how to compromise. Another example of the system-controlled marriage is the forbidden marriage which becomes committed to rigid pseudomutuality as a way to avoid the "I told you so" confrontation with the parents.

Marriage is a model of intimacy in our culture. A degree of intimacy is found in other relationships such as between patient and therapist, among co-workers, in a living together situation, and with one's seat mate on an airplane trip. Most other intimate relationships involve only parts of the person. Marriage is unique in its lifetime commitment, the physical sexuality, and the whole person to whole person quality of the relationship.

We feel depressed about divorces. We feel discouraged about the cavalier attitude that people take toward divorce. Our attitude is in part shaped by the anesthetizing effect that it has on personhood and by the impact that it has on children as they try to rationalize their parents' behavior, usually to protect the parents. It is very rare in our clinical practice to see a divorce that works. Divorces are too much like psychological amputations with all the sequelea of phantom limb pain, altered ways of functioning, changes in self-image, and the crazy sense of being a cultural object instead of a self. The reason for doing therapy with a dissolving marriage is simply to make it into an elective surgical procedure so that functioning is better postsurgically.

The craziest thing about marriages is that one cannot get divorced. We just do not seem to make it out of intimate relationships. It is obviously possible to divide up the property and to decide not to live together any more, but it is impossible to go back to being single. Marriage is like a stew that has irreversible and irrevocable characteristics that the parts cannot be rid of. Divorce is leaving part of the self behind, like the rabbit who escapes the trap by gnawing one leg off.

The reasons for therapy with dissolving marriages are (1) to help the partners get back as much of their original investment as possible by helping them to "decourt" and (2) to straighten out the issues of parenting when there are children involved. As Westman et al. put it so nicely " . . . Divorce is a process, not an event. Divorce alters the form of family relationships, rather than causing the comparatively abrupt loss of bereavement with its associated grief and guilt." (Westman et al., 1970.)

Divorce is a backlash against symbiosis (bilateral, nonautonomous, system-controlled living). The symbiosis is preset to prevent a change in the quantity of intimacy and to reduce the chance of separation anxiety. So many divorces come on the heels of a childbirth because children force an increase in intimacy.

In the symbiotic marriage, two incomplete persons combine to make an "I". Two 16 year olds combine to make a 32 year old. The marital fit is accomplished when the adequacies are complementary. The inadequacies are like holes which are filled by the spouses protuberant adequacies. He is afraid of rejection while she's mothering and tolerant. When the holes later start to get filled by children, by financial or professional success, or by psychotherapy, the partner gets pushed out and gets mad or panicky and then retaliates and the breakup begins.

> Dick and Mona had both been raised in attorneys' families. She was a middle child in a family that did not permit despair. Dick was the chosen one in his family, a very critical and controlling family that picked him out to follow in his father's footsteps. They married while in college. Their first child was born during Dick's 1st year in law school. After the child was born, Mona went cold and became critical both of herself and of Dick. Dick withdrew from her and became involved in a gay relationship. He found himself discouraged with law school. At that point they came into therapy. She came to help Dick get straightened out. Her depression and paranoia rose to the surface very quickly. After about three or four sessions, they came to an impasse in therapy related to their inability to move further apart or to move closer together. Dick had been pushing for a separation and Mona had been unwilling to notice it. It dawned on her one day in the therapy hour that they might get divorced. She said that it could not happen. She could not stand the idea of stopping. "I still feel close to him. I want to do things with him. I feel at times like there's a big hole in me and I cannot stand it." Acknowledging the hole was the beginning of her achievement of individual adequacy.

It is clear that a lot of divorces seem to work. That is due in great part to the cultural validation of the ejection seat marriage, alternate life styles, and the more stylized second marriage which is easier to leave and thus less necessary to leave. The whole self is not in and the level of intimacy is preset. The following example demonstrates the qualification which is placed on the lifetime commitment in subsequent marriages. It also shows the way that the qualified involvement in marriage may be introjected by the children and may become part of their interpersonal style.

> Lois, a woman in her late 30's, estranged from her third husband and going with another divorcee, brought her two children in because she was concerned about the impact of her marital failures on them. The therapist

asked her 12-year-old daughter if she thought her mother would ever find the right man. The daughter stammered and blushed, became confused, and said, "If my mother ever decides to get married again, she will think about it very carefully. I mean she will think about it carefully . . . you know she will think about it and she won't marry until she's certain she'll be divorced." She went on from there not even noticing her slip.

Another way that divorce works is when there has been no marriage. We think of this as happening in families where there are consecutive generations with divorces or in families where a first broken marriage is a developmental milestone or a stepping stone out of the family of origin. The other way that it works for people is that it reduces the need for dealing with ambivalence by injecting a lifetime inoculation of paranoia. We think that in that way divorce decreases vulnerability and the likelihood of involving one's self in future uncomfortable situations. It is like consecutive psychotherapies, the likelihood and the capacity for regressing and reintegrating are decreased.

To close this segment, we cite a case from the senior author's earlier work with marriages and families.

Matilda became pregnant after 4 months of marriage. Before her son was born, her husband beat her up and she divorced him. He moved to another state, remarried, and they lost contact with one another. She had been in individual psychotherapy for 5 years elsewhere. When her son was 15, she was referred to one of us because of their oedipal struggles. They remained in therapy for approximately 1 year. When her son was 18, he left for college and she became depressed. They returned for more therapy. At that point some of the author's thinking about the extended family was developing and he asked that she bring her parents in. He thought about asking the long gone husband but the situation seemed awfully dead. After some difficulty the grandparents finally came. They were divorced; it was easy to get the grandmother in but more difficult to get the grandfather. At the first interview with the 3 generations present, Matilda got into a loud paranoid clamor with her father. She accused him of all kinds of incest-tinted behavior and seductive fantasies. The blaming ended in a physical fight between the two of them with father finally restraining her on the couch. She screamed at him "You are just like that goddamned husband of mine"! She had never said anything with so much affect so the therapist said, "Can you get your husband to come here?" She said she'd try. She located him in California and he said, "I'd be glad to come, when do you meet?" He was divorced from his second wife, incidentally. The therapy session was scheduled for Wednesday. He arrived on Monday and she put him up in her apartment. He had not been there for 2 hours when *she* beat *him* up. The fight went on when they returned to the therapy session and abated during the therapy hour the next day. It was as if that part of her affect had been tied up for 17 years. And she was now getting a sense of her whole self.

Administrative and Treatment Issues

First, it is important to have some idea of one's own views of marriage. And it is important to define those for the divorcing couple. In our case we value marriage highly. Second, the marriage or relationship is a system. The whole is much greater than the sum of the individuals involved. When the individuals are getting no gratification but only bilateral suffering, it is because the system is in control.

Psychotherapy or counseling begins with the first phone call. At that point the structure is established. "Bring your spouse and the kids." Too often the counselor is covertly asked to take care of one spouse so that the other can leave more easily and with less guilt. The counselor becomes the rebound affair which we see as deadly both for therapists and patients. One to two visits alone with one of the spouses is all it takes to get the paranoia up high enough in the rest of the system so that they will not come in. The potential for a devastating result is increased if you stabilize only part of an unsteady system. If health increases in one-half of a dissolving marriage, it is not uncommon to see symptomatic behavior develop in the untreated spouse such as depression, psychosis, increase in psychosomatic problems, and increase in accident proneness and suicidal behavior.

Seeing a marriage that is coming apart can be difficult and anxiety provoking. It is hard to avoid getting hooked into supporting the adversarial framework. Teaming with another person helps. It is best if the co-therapist is a trained counselor; however, in case of emergency one can use a nurse, secretary, or business manager. If the counselor is an advocate for marriage it is useful to get a divorced person or someone who sees divorce as useful to be the co-therapist. When one is engaged in working with divorcing couples, it is important to have support from a group of colleagues. It can be personally devastating if one becomes the psychotherapeutic affair for one of the spouses or if one begins to feel inadequate as the divorce situation becomes more depressing and the therapist is given responsibility for the deterioration of the relationship.

Begin by taking a history of the marriage. Why are they doing this now? Why not 6 months ago? Why not wait 6 months more? How did they happen to get married? Oftentimes when married couples discuss the beginning of marriage it builds up the heat of attraction again. Ask how she helped him to escalate his drinking and how he arranged for her to have an affair with the office manager. Find out how the kids feel about the problem and invite them to the next interview, especially if the couple is confused about the kids' views. Find out about the in-laws, how they felt about the marriage and what their part in the marriage has been. Suggest that they bring the in-laws at some time in the future. If the in-laws accept the invitation, the counselor will learn a lot. If they resist at least the marital problem is redefined by implying the involvement of the in-laws and the conflict may spread into the whole system instead of being limited to the marital dyad. Changing the frame of the conflict is precisely the goal of early counseling; to change it from an individual's problem to a problem involving an affectively linked collective.

At this point it is worth thinking about where the marriage is along the time line that we developed in the first section. If they are in the metaphorical stage they are probably seeking psychotherapy and we seek to expand the metaphor. We might encourage divorce and inquire as to how much each expects to get of the property. "How long do you think it will be before she remarries?" "Will you try to find someone with more money?" "Do you think your parents will let you come back and live with them? Will you get your old room back?" Another method is to recommend separations; the fantasized trip to the Caribbean, the long repressed dream of joining the Peace Corps, or to suggest that one or the other take a motel room when things get too hot at home. The effect is usually to bring the divorce out of the shadows and to move the fight up to a different level. This may result in a resetting of the marital thermostat. It sometimes marks the end of the counselor's intervention and at other times the beginning of psychotherapy. The other possibility is that it may result in dissecting out the divorce and a decision to end the marriage. This latter decision moves them along to the metaphorolytic stage where lawyers are involved. The counselor is faced with involving himself in the always incomplete process of dissolution. This is crisis intervention, an attempt to minimize damage bilaterally in the marriage pair and also to assure the children's rights and to keep them out of the middle of the marital fight. This is a difficult therapeutic contract to negotiate. It requires a fair amount of initiative from the couple. There is a great need to resolve the ambivalence which comes up at this time and it often is resolved by assigning blame in order to get out. The therapist can interrupt a too quick resolution of the ambivalence by letting the couple know that it is impossible for anyone to be treated fairly. Everyone gets cheated and it is a question of how much they will be cheated.

When the child is the presenting problem both spouses need to be seen for the simple reason that while they may be sick of living and struggling with each other, they remain parents and they need to work out the ways in which they will deal with their children. It is important that the therapist make clear the reason for psychotherapy.

Lynn came to the clinic because her 3-year-old son Jon was too hyperactive for her to manage. She and Marshall were getting divorced. Lynn had the kids, a girl aged 6 and Jon aged 3. The marriage had gone sour; they had tried marriage counseling and found it not helpful. Lynn wanted out. Marshall and both families saw her as "crazy"; he was cool and reasonable about the divorce. "If she wants it, she can have it. I would like us to stay together." They planned to part amicably. Marshall said that he would like to have Lynn see the foolishness of her ways but he did not think that she ever would. He wanted a therapist to help Lynn and their son Jon work on their relationship. The intervention that resulted in rapid improvement of the mother-child relationship is described elsewhere. (Keith, 1974.) At the end when the father was invited back with the son, it was clear that the father had become increasingly anxious as the mother had become more adequate with the child. Marshall had become less responsible in picking up the kids and was disappointing them in his attempt to get even with Lynn. They declined the suggestion of further psychotherapy. In retrospect it seemed related to a failure to define the goals.

The intent of the early intervention with the marital pair and with their children is to get them to the existential place. "This is a mess, we are all in it. I still want out. I can see that it will be painful and we would like some help getting unstuck." Counseling the separating couple has three primary goals: (1) to help them make use of the ambivalence and despair to deepen their own personhood; (2) to help them with parenting; and (3) to help them regain as much of themselves as possible in the process of decourting.

Working with the divorcing pair is an attempt to keep the separation human so that it is not done pseudomutually with attendant individual emotional or somatic problems or problems in the kids, or so that extremes of vindictive, self-righteous anger do not emerge in the division of property. We suspect it is bilateral ambivalence and the attendant despair that brings the couple into psychotherapy. When we see grieving patients in psychotherapy, we tell them that the grief process is a psychophysiological one. They ought to expect to dream about the one who has died, to find themselves expecting to wake from a dream, or to open a door and find the dead one there, reborn. Anger and great love sweep over the grieving one. We encourage the same process in divorce counseling. Dr. Whitaker has referred to the process as decourting. It is the way that the divorcees regain as much of themselves, as much of their original investment, as possible. Decourting is done not only by expressing the rage and the disappointment, but also by sharing again the tenderness and the loving that first brought the pair together.

We discourage the common method of diverting the despair into a rebound affair, a rebound marriage, or into a substitute career. The divorcing pair needs every bit of the emerging despair to keep themselves alive. In most psychotherapy the struggle is to get the couple past the impasse where they are stuck. In divorce the impasse is not to be passed. It must be eaten piece by piece before any may leave.

The grandparents need to come in. Especially if they short circuit decourting. It is uncanny how much the husband's mother resembles his wife in her manner of speaking, how often the marital fight is a transplantation of an undone parent-child fight as demonstrated earlier. Decourting may also be interrupted by amateur therapists in the person's life. We always invite them in. The amateur may be a group, a roommate, or another affair. Usually they are more than willing to turn the treatment over to us. If they are not, we can resign and transfer care to them.

The main responsibility of the person counseling a dissolving intimate relationship is to provide a time and place for the separating process. It is often a depressing and discouraging business. Our affective experience tends to vary from very low with a sense of uselessness to occasional blips of gratification akin to that which a naturalist might experience as he watches natural processes unfold in expected ways.

It may be difficult, especially for the less experienced counselors, to think of themselves as simply a time and a place. The difficulty increases when hopeless or depressed feelings emerge in the counselor. While we usually encourage the use of one's own affect in psychotherapy, we feel that some caution may be needed in early contacts with the divorcing couple lest the counseling project be aborted prematurely. As we indicated in the beginning of this section, it is important to describe one's own views of marriage and divorce and of divorce counseling, as a surgeon describes a procedure before taking his patient to the operating room.

Two ways that counselors are apt to respond to their own depressive feelings should be mentioned. First, one spouse may be indecisive or the couple may continually project conflict onto the children, in-laws, or therapists. They may develop an immobile, rigidly defensive style. They are probably trying to avoid their own depression and the therapist might be most useful if he can be aware of and describe his own depressive feelings, rather than treating himself by mobilizing his own anger. Second, the decourting process often engenders moments of tenderness and closeness between the couple. Again, these are ways to soften the pain and anguish of separation. The counselor needs to let such moments happen rather than assuming that they are moving toward a reiteration of their marriage vows.

Finally, there are the postdivorce situations that one is brought into in several ways. These situations are usually fairly dead and frought with hopelessness. The systems are too complicated. Ghosts of marriages past whisper in the darkness and chains clank in the hallway.

In essence the first two divorce situations which we outlined, the lonely individual and the troubled child, are the same as those which we discussed in the metaphorolytic stage divorces and can be managed in very much the same way. It is these situations, occurring years after the divorce, that demonstrate the impossibility of divorcing. If the child is the problem the counselor has to sort out the problems of parenting from the marital fight.

Therapy or counseling with people in this group of conditions tends toward failure. Improving communication is less likely to increase intimacy as it does in another marriage. It is a knotty group of people with whom to work. Their suspiciousness of themselves is frequently projected onto the counselor. The whole self is not there and it is often difficult to get it there. As we noted above, secondary contracts are being negotiated. Our sense is that in most cases divorcing is not a move for individuation but is rather a matter of going AWOL from the marriage, and thus it is necessary to keep parts of one's identity secret later on.

Conclusion

Divorce has been increasing in great part because of support from the culture. The increasing prevalence has somehow diminished its tragic implications. Oftentimes the ambivalence does not emerge until years later in a seemingly very different context. Psychotherapists encounter divorce on many different surfaces. Therapists can make the situation even more complicated if (1) they see it as an individual problem and (2) if they cooperate in a too early resolution of the attendant ambivalence. Working with dissolving marriages because it is basically a crisis intervention can have a deadening effect on the counselor and be interrupting to his own growth if he does not have support from colleagues. We recommend making liberal use of consultants and co-therapists.

REFERENCES

Keith, D. V.: Use of self: a brief report. Family Process. **13:** 201–206, 1974.
Meyer, R.: Personal communication, 1975.
Westman, J. C., Cline, D. W., Swift, W. J., and Kramer, D. A.: Role of child psychiatry in divorce. Archives of General Psychiatry. **23:** 416–420, 1970.

Part II

Special Issues/ Dimensions in Marital Counseling

G. HUGH ALLRED, Ed. D.

6

Counseling in Parent-Child Relationships*

A critical dilemma confronting the counselor of parents and their young children is whether he should take the traditional approach and spend his time with the child identified by his parents as the problem child or whether he should spend his time on effecting changes in the social network of relationships in which the child is grounded.

Several decades ago, Alfred Adler (1958) postulated that all individuals are socially embedded and that people can be best understood and changed as this concept is understood and applied (Ansbacher and Ansbacher, 1956). He became the first psychotherapist to emphasize modifying the beliefs, attitudes, and behaviors of significant others in an effort to effect changes in the problem child. Communication and systems theorists, and some behaviorists, along with several others, appear to be operating from Adler's basic postulate. Even physicists are lending support to this position as they interpret the movement of particles of the atom as conforming to "purely social laws" (Cochran, 1966).

What Adlerians and many others are saying is that it appears that all actions are in the final analysis interactions. This suggests that the counselor in order to know and understand the importance and dynamics of any action of a child (or for that matter anyone else) must consider the whole network within which the action takes place (Dreikurs, 1955). This further suggests that the parent-child counselor is a family counselor who views all family members as in some way participating in the problem of the problem child.

---

* A substantive part of this chapter is derived from the author's book, *How to Strengthen Your Marriage and Family* (Provo, Utah, Brigham Young University Press), 1976. This information has been modified, however, to meet the needs of the counselor of the problem child and his family and social network.

If Adler's postulate is true, and I strongly believe it is, then the counselor of the problem child must accept the resulting complexity of counseling and the increased skill and courage that will be demanded of him as he attempts to deal effectively with the multiplicity of the variables that will result. Such challenges will provide opportunities for the counselor as he learns to view himself as the coordinator of a team of significant others whose strengths he musters in order to positively influence the problem child and the network of his relationships. I believe that the young child is an active agent in networks of ongoing interacting and interinfluencing sets of relationships and that the most efficient method of changing him is to modify the manner by which the significant people in his life influence him and are influenced by him.

The family counselor will be one of a team of individuals who are vitally concerned with the careful nurturing and training of the child and the social networks in which he is embedded. This team will include the young child's parents, his brothers and sisters, any other significant people living in the child's home or close by who have continuing contact with him, and, ideally, his teacher(s) if he is going to school. The counselor will meet with individuals in the network, with parts of the network, and with the whole network as appropriate to efficiently resolve the difficulties and maximize the strengths.

In this paper I present several concepts and principles that the counselor will need to be aware of in order to understand child and family dynamics well enough to work effectively with the other members of his team: (1) an important objective of child-family network counseling as it pertains to the problem child; (2) some basic assumptions regarding the child and his family; (3) principles for modifying the problem child's behavior; (4) some practices for living democratically with children that the counselor can teach the parents of the problem child; (5) the necessity for helping parents recognize and get rid of their faulty convictions about childrearing and the family; (6) the place of the marriage relationship in the problem child's network; and (7) how to help the family apply the concepts and principles previously outlined and discussed. Following these seven areas, and making up the last part of the paper, is a mental map of communication that counselors can use to improve their effectiveness and efficiency as it relates to the basic postulates of this paper.

An Important Objective of Counseling

One of the first tasks of the counselor is to help parents articulate the kind of character traits they want their children to acquire. This gives a more definite direction to counseling. We live in a democratic society and thus it seems that most parents want their family interaction to provide the kind of environment that will enable each child to acquire those traits that will help him become a happy and responsible citizen in a democratic society.

The democratic individual, the ideal, then, for which parents strive in their childrearing efforts, has a high level of self-esteem, a high degree of courage and spontaneity, and a strong desire to continually increase his repertoire of cooperative, democratic behaviors. His main interest and concern is the welfare of others as well as himself. He is sensitive to the workings of groups and responsibly contributes to making them work effectively. He bases his actions on what he believes to be right rather than on the capricious pressures of others. He sees with clear eyes the bad as well as the good and behaves responsibly to what he sees. He is honest and congruent; his verbal and nonverbal communication are consistent with each other. He tends to have much common sense, to be relaxed, and to be somewhat easygoing. He usually has a sense of humor that facilitates the effective functioning of people involved in group activities. His humor is not designed to elevate himself at the expense of others; however, it can be and is often used to dissipate tension so that others can work more effectively through their difficulties. The democratically oriented individual often has deep spiritual roots. His relationships with others and his attitudes toward them and himself are profoundly affected in positive ways by the spirit that emanates from him (Allred, 1976).

Some Assumptions Regarding the Child and the Family

Nine basic assumptions concerning the child and his family and social setting can help provide the counselor with a theoretical framework for understanding and working with the child and his family.

1. Each child has the *creative power* (Ansbacher and Ansbacher, 1956) to make choices that enable him to behave constructively rather than destructively in most if not every situation in which he finds himself. He has the potential to make the most of every situation by choosing to behave constructively, provided he has the courage to make such choices. He need not be at the mercy of past or ongoing poor experiences or the feeling that his behavior is but a result of his poor situation. Aristotle recognized this principle when he said that what lies in the individual's power to do lies in his power not to do (Hutchins, 1952).

The principle of creative power has far reaching implications for interpersonal relationships. It includes the concepts that each of us has the creative power to change himself, to influence those about him, and to be influenced by them. It is impossible for a person to exert no influence, nor is it possible for him to remain uninfluenced.

The concept of creative power suggests that there are times when the individual, whether a child or an adult, may be more influential in modifying other's behavior than they are in modifying his, due to his creative power. The concept also suggests that the child's behavior will be fluid and dynamic and not totally predictable. If we regard the individual as having creative power, the counselors, parents, teachers, and other influential figures will have to be continually on their toes if they are to help the child acquire those behaviors that will enable him to be a happy, productive human being.

2. Behavior, whether it be conscious or semiconscious, has *purpose* (Ansbacher and Ansbacher, 1956). The child behaves with the desire to achieve certain goals. In light of this, the important question that counselors, parents, teachers, and others must ask themselves in order to help the child to be responsible is not "Why?"—that has already been answered, but "What is the child getting out of behaving the way he does?" A follow-up question for parents or any others having continuing interaction with the child is "What am I doing when he behaves that way?" By using these two, or similar, questions, we can usually more clearly discover the purposes of the misbehaving child.

3. *Communication* is the vehicle by which the child achieves his purposes (Allred, 1976). The definition of communication here includes all of the verbal and nonverbal signs he makes to achieve his purposes: words, tone of voice, facial expressions, body stance, physical distance, and so on. Most emotional and most significant interpersonal communications seem to occur at the nonverbal level. For example, the child has the greatest impact on others and they on him through such things as a friendly or sarcastic tone of voice, a smile or a frown, and physical proximity.

4. All men are *socially linked.* Important questions surrounding the child's behavior appear to be in the final analysis social questions (Ansbacher and Ansbacher, 1956). In some way or other, they have to do with his relationship with others. There is a great implication in this principle that can help us relate constructively. We can increase our overall understanding of a child to the extent that we understand his movement, his purposes among his family members, and their purposes with him. In order to do so, we need to know something about the child's order of birth, the atmosphere of his family, what people significant to him may expect of him, and how he learned to achieve his goals with them.

5. The child's general, basic striving appears to be *to have a place to belong* with those who are significant to him (Dreikurs, 1971). One who feels he does not belong to those who are important to him may suffer great anxiety and pain and spend all of his energy and time attempting to gain a place. Many find their place with other people by being cooperative and by being helpful to them, but there are others

who, in their discouragement, feel they cannot find a satisfactory place in this manner and are content with such things as notoriety or infamy.

Too often parents respond to the discouraged child by taking more notice of his destructive, noncooperative efforts to belong than of his constructive, cooperative efforts, thus making his destructive efforts more worthwhile than his constructive efforts. Counselors, parents, and teachers who are in positions of influence have a particular responsibility to make the problem child's constructive, cooperative efforts worthwhile in helping him find a place. To the degree that they do not do this, they exhibit a lack of concern for the welfare of the child who needs help.

6. Closely related to the principle of belonging is the principle of *high self-esteem*, which is essential to a child if he is to have the self-confidence and courage necessary to approach life's problems with zest (Allred, 1976). It provides him with the greatest motivation for development and progression. He must take risks as he makes choices that he hopes will help him find a full life, and high self-esteem with its concomitants of self-confidence and courage enables him to take these risks and to progress at a healthy rate. He has little fear of making mistakes for he knows love from those significant to him will not be diminished if he should err for a time.

High self-esteem is also the essential ingredient for happiness and love. If a child does not have a high level of self-esteem, he will find it difficult to like himself and other people. Without love of self and love of others, he will not be able to experience real happiness.

7. At the very core of constructive, cooperative attitudes is *social interest* (Adler, 1958). Without this interest the child lacks the desire and ability to be concerned about the welfare of his loved ones and to behave cooperatively with them. Every child is born with the innate potential to work harmoniously and cooperatively with others, but his potential must be carefully nurtured. He must learn the skills of cooperation and effective living with others in order to develop fully.

It is possible that social interest is one of the critical elements lacking in the life of the delinquent, neurotic, psychotic, pervert, and criminal. The severely maladjusted person does not appear to be interested in the welfare of his fellows, nor does he appear to have developed interpersonal skills for cooperative living. It is true, then, that the child also has the potential to learn to be interested in his fellows in order to achieve his own selfish purposes and to move competitively against or away from them, the essence of destructive movement. It is, therefore, exceedingly important that those who would teach the child to interact constructively be very careful that they do not teach him to interact destructively.

It may be said that the child's concern for the welfare of others and his belonging to groups offer the ultimate meanings in life, those values and experiences that make his life worthwhile.

8. A child's *life style* is formed by the guidelines he creates for himself and by the patterns of responding he develops (Ansbacher and Ansbacher, 1956). The infant first seems to learn randomly by trial and error, but soon creates certain beliefs, attitudes, and principles for living that guide his future actions. Thus, the basic life style of an individual may be formed during infancy, probably before age 3.

The guidelines he creates may be quite logical or illogical depending on his own unique, subjective view of life. Whatever the case, he acts as if they are true and tends to make them come true, thus fulfilling his own prophecy. For example, the child who believes himself unable to play ball will consciously or semiconsciously manipulate his environment to avoid it. He will as a result not practice this skill, will say to himself, "I cannot play ball," and will make his belief come true. Conversely, the person who believes himself capable of playing ball will search for opportunities to do so. His skill will improve with practice and he will say to himself, "Yes, I can do it." As a result, it will come true.

Birth order (position in the family), age, sex differences or sex similarities among siblings, parental expectations, and the emotional climate in the family appear to influence the development of the child's life style. It is often found that the eldest in a family will tend to be rule-, authority-, and past-oriented, protective of and too responsible for others, conservative, bossy, nosy, a high achiever, and dependable. He may also be intolerant of himself and others. When parental expectations are perceived as too high to be attainable, the eldest may rebel by adopting values and behaviors completely contrary to those of his parents. The second or middle child tends to be quite different from the eldest, especially in a competitive family atmosphere where birth order takes on added significance. He will often be very active, rebellious, subtle, liberally oriented, a martyr, and creative. He is the one parents seem usually most concerned with when they come for family counseling. The youngest child is often spoiled as a result of excessive parental and sibling pampering. He may be considered cute and, therefore, be able to manipulate service from others through his charm.

The only child may be in an extremely disadvantageous position if his parents pamper, indulge, and overcaution him about life's problems and dangers. He may develop a life style of pessimism, timidity, low self-esteem, and low competence. However, when wise parents stimulate the only child to a high level of independence and courage, they may rear a child who becomes highly competent, experiences success, and thinks well of himself and others.

The only boy in a family of girls may become feminine as he models after his sisters or very masculine as he struggles hard to achieve a masculine identity. His chances of being masculine appear to be greater if he is the eldest, less if he has many older sisters. The only girl in a family of boys may have problems similar to the only boy in a family of girls as she becomes submerged in a world of masculinity, or she may struggle to achieve femininity and overcompensate, thereby becoming extremely feminine. A girl reared in an all girl family might view boys as strangers and may feel uncomfortable around them. Similarly, a boy from a family where all of his siblings are boys may grow up viewing girls as foreign objects to be avoided, and he may not develop the understanding and skills necessary to get along well with them.

Twins may respond extremely competitively in the competitive family. One may become highly aggressive and dominant while the other becomes passive and submissive, even to the point of giving up his identity to the other. Foster children may develop great manipulative skills in bossing others and getting service from them when parents, feeling sorrow and pity, pay off their disturbing, demanding behavior. The handicapped child often appears to develop a life style similar to that of the foster child.

The impact of birth order and special conditions (e.g., being handicapped) appear to be kaleidoscopic, depending in part on parental expectations, sex, ages, and number of siblings, and the emotional climate in the family. It is in the *highly competitive family that birth order appears to take on added significance* as children often enter the game of power politics in order to achieve the preferred place with their parents.

Effective counselors will help educate and train parents to consistently refuse to respond to the power plays of the child who attempts to appear better than others in the family, to consistently reward the child's constructive endeavors, and, thereby, help them rear an eldest child who is reasonably responsible and productive, a second child who is constructively creative, a youngest child who develops great skills in constructively working with groups of people, and a handicapped child who develops great courage and optimism and becomes effective in stimulating others to greater courage. In other words, effective counselors will stimulate parents to help the child take advantage of his unique family situation and to develop a positive and constructive life style. Stereotypes will not result, because of course no two eldest children who are raised in constructively oriented homes will be exactly the same.

The family situation in which the growing individual finds himself, with all of its vicissitudes and opportunities, is generally not nearly as important as how he learns to successfully overcome the vicissitudes and take advantage of the opportunities.

9. The child should be viewed with a *holistic* approach — as a whole person who functions within his total environment (Ansbacher and Ansbacher, 1956). All aspects of an individual and all significant aspects of his environment appear to be related and to interact in a continuing dynamic manner. Each of us functions within a system of self and within a system of interacting others — a cosmos of influencing interactions. It is by viewing the problem child in his entirety, functioning within a system of complex interbalancing relationships of people and things, that we come closest to a real understanding of him.

Principles for Modifying the Child

Now that we have in mind the nine assumptions regarding the child and his family, we can be concerned with several powerful principles for learning that are vital to the counselor who attempts to eliminate destructive character traits in children and increase those that are constructive. By using such principles, counselors and parents should find that the problem child's behavior can be efficiently modified in desirable directions.

Whenever two events occur simultaneously, there is a tendency for the individual involved in the events to connect the two, a process called *bonding* (Allred, 1976). For example, when a parent punishes a child at home by embarrassing him, speaking harshly to him, and/or spanking him, the child will generally feel angry, revengeful, sad, and/or humiliated. He will tend, to the extent these experiences recur, to get these same feelings whenever he is at home or thinks about it or anything associated with it. A punishing home environment is in fact one of the major causes of runaways.

In contrast, the child who experiences many loving touches and friendly words when he is home tends to feel joy and contentment. For him these feelings become bonded to home itself, his parents, and his siblings. His feelings for home and family tend to be warm and friendly.

The concept of *payoff* is of critical importance to the counselor and parent who attempt to diminish destructive behavior and increase constructive behavior in the child (Allred, 1976). Whenever the child achieves a particular goal, he achieves payoff, and this encourages him to repeat that same behavior when he again desires the same goal. This behavioral pattern is exemplified by the child who cries when he wants a piece of candy. When given candy at such times, he achieves payoff, and this increases his tendency to cry whenever he wants candy again. The purpose or goal of any particular behavior is to achieve payoff.

When the child's constructive and cooperative behavior leads to payoff, he tends to repeat that same behavior whenever he again desires the same goal. Conversely, when his destructive and competitive behavior leads to payoff, he tends to repeat that same behavior when he again desires the same goal.

The table (Allred, 1976) on the next page shows four goals — A, B, C, and D — of destructive behavior (Dreikurs, 1947, 1971) with suggestions for how the problem child can be encouraged to relate more constructively. It is necessary that the counselor understand the table so that he will be able to apply its concepts and hence help parents behave responsibly in their relationships with their child. Parents help the child achieve his goals when he behaves constructively by giving him positive payoff. On the other hand, they also help him by not giving him payoff when he behaves destructively. As parents work to pay off the constructive behavior of the child and to withdraw payoff when he misbehaves, they become responsible in their relationships with him.

Children tend to repeat those behaviors they see in other people, especially when these people are of significant value to them. For instance, if a child wants to acquire a particular skill, such as riding a bicycle, he will most likely select other people who possess this skill as appropriate models. *Modeling* (Bandura and Walters, 1963) has particular relevance to those working with young children, for it is the young who are generally most aware of their lack of knowledge and skills and are eagerly looking to those people they can imitate.

Most parents serve as the primary models for their children. Many have come to realize that words they speak to their children are not nearly as powerful a teaching device as their total behavior. Possibly the best single teaching device parents can present to their children is the example they set of self-respect, love for themselves, and love for their fellowmen. Parents who are good models of these behaviors and who effectively apply these principles of learning will tend to rear children who possess the same attitudes and behaviors and who will also rear respectful, responsible children. The principle of modeling also indicates that it is important for the counselor to be a good model of constructive behaviors for family members.

One of the most effective childrearing principles is the use of *natural consequences* (Dreikurs, 1971). When parents are taught not to intervene between the child and the consequences that naturally occur as a result of his behavior, they allow him to learn from his mistakes and, thereby, teach him to be responsible. Usually, parents need intervene only if a situation could be a dangerous one. An example of the wise use of natural consequences is the father who does not pay the installment payment on his young son's bicycle when the son has set a pattern of not budgeting wisely. The father even allows the bicycle to be repossessed so that his son will be able to suffer and thus learn the

TABLE 6.1

A guide for responding to the individual when he behaves destructively*

	Destructive goals			
	A	B	C	D
	To get attention	To be boss	To counterhurt	To appear disabled
Typical destructive behaviors	Individual may pull faces, talk long and loud, tattle, tell shocking stories, continually ask questions, not be able to hear others, leave things around for others to pick up, kick and poke others.	Individual may scream, yell, shout, throw self on floor, throw objects, criticize, whine, cry, display stubbornness, disobey, act superior.	Individual may destroy property, strike others, steal, say such things as, "You're stupid," "You're no good," or "I hate you."	Individual doesn't participate, doesn't answer questions, avoids looking at others, keeps eyes downcast, is alone most of the time.
Evidence for determining goals of destructively behaving person (tends to pay off destructive behavior)	Others give individual undue attention and/or service. Others are annoyed and irritated and often express this in words such as: "You take so much of our time."	Others fight individual for control, to be boss, and feel angry, often expressing themselves in words such as: "You can't get away with that." They may also feel sorry for him or even pity him.	Others feel hurt by individual and want to hurt him back; they may think, "I'll get even with you." Others may also feel guilty.	Others leave him alone, feel hopeless, don't expect anything of him, and often think, "I don't known what to do."

Behavior that will tend to stop or diminish destructive behavior	Ignore individual at this time, say nothing and do nothing. Control facial expression, tone of voice, and body movements that indicate he has achieved his goal. When he demands service, say, "You can do it yourself," and then focus on others.	Refuse to engage in power contest with him and say, "You could be right." Continue whatever you are doing, focus on others, keep cool, walk into another room. Refuse to feel pity for him.	Refuse to engage in battle of retaliation with him. Show no hurt or guilt in words, tone of voice, facial expression, body movement, or any other way. Calmly say something like, "It may be so," and focus on others.	Refuse to give up in the relationship and keep encouraging him.
Encouragement of constructive behavior	Have positive experiences with him when he is not demanding destructive involvement, not trying to defeat or hurt you. Relate to him in a warm, accepting manner (e.g., smile at him, put your hand on his shoulder, invite him to participate). Initiate positive relationships when he is behaving constructively.			Set your expectations so that the individual can have many success experiences and learn that effort is valuable in and of itself. Concentrate on having a warm, friendly, nonthreatening relationship with him.

* Based on a design developed by Rudolf Dreikurs, revised by G. Hugh Allred.

consequences of his irresponsible behavior. Such behavior on the part of the father demonstrates real concern for the development of character. Possibly one of the greatest errors of many affluent parents is their taking upon themselves the consequences of their children's irresponsible actions.

When parents structure the environment in such a way that their children experience the reasonable and logical impact of their irresponsible behavior, they are implementing *logical consequences* (Dreikurs, 1971). For example, the parent who excuses her child from the table after he has thrown food is using this principle. The parent acts on the logical assumption that when the child throws food he is disrespecting the rights of others and, therefore, loses his right to be at the table.

In order for logical consequences to work effectively, a good relationship must exist between parents and children. The children should have a say in determining the consequences of their behaviors; otherwise the use of logical consequences can stimulate competitive power struggles and thus result in destructive interaction between parents and children. There must be no hint of sarcasm, ridicule, humiliation, or revenge on the part of parents. The emotional content must be calm and matter of fact.

The use of natural and logical consequences is strongly suggested for parents' use as they work to prepare their families to relate democratically. There are, however, certain intangibles such as warmth and friendliness that are also vitally important and that have to do with the total personality that emanates from parents and is communicated to their children. It is from such emanations that children model their own behavior and either interact harmoniously or resist and rebel.

Certain *personality traits* of a parent appear to facilitate the teaching-learning processes (Allred, 1976). Since the counselor influences and teaches, these same traits are important to him or her also. Essential, time-tested traits of the effective teacher include sincerity, empathy, warmth and friendliness, a relaxed and easy-going attitude, flexibility, simplicity, confidence, consistency, being approachable, and being well-organized. Research indicates that friendliness is the most important attribute of those who attempt to help another person learn. This also includes friendliness toward one's self when self is the learner.

The effective teacher is also able to communicate well. He is direct, succinct, and congruent in his communication. He avoids being dogmatic, preachy, cold, abrupt, quick tempered, patronizing, or coercive. Criticism and discipline that are overly strict and coercive tend to produce rigid conformity, shyness or aggression, anxiety levels that impede learning, and deference to authority figures. As a result, the child bonds these negative feelings and attitudes to learning and feels it is threatening and, therefore, something to be avoided.

The traits of the effective teacher are consistent with those identified in counseling literature as being essential for the effective counselor (Bergin and Strupp, 1972).

Whether an individual is learning about things of a cognitive nature (e.g., ideas), developing certain body movements, or developing social skills, *practice* is a necessary prerequisite to his attainment of high levels of understanding and skill (Allred, 1976). A counselor rehearsing with a parent on how to respond effectively to a discouraged daughter is as important as a coach rehearsing with a student on how to follow through with a golf club. The old adage "practice makes perfect" tends to be valid in all areas where change to a new or different behavior is desired.

The following are additional principles of learning that the counselor can teach parents (Allred, 1976) as he counsels with them.

When a desirable new behavior occurs, it is important that it be paid off immediately and every time it occurs until it is well-established. This is known as giving *continuous payoff*. Once it is well-established, payoff should be given in a random fashion. *Random payoff* is given for the second, third, fourth, or fifth time the behavior occurs to keep the individual responding at a high rate.

The child needs to be *successful in learning* if he is to have the courage to continue. It may be that the typical child needs at least three success experiences to one failure if he is to keep trying. Counselors and parents should structure the experiences of the child in a manner that will enable him to experience much success. They should also structure their own lives so that they will be able to experience much success and thus provide healthy, constructive models for the child.

Shaping, another helpful principle, is based on the idea that it is beneficial in training to pay off any behavior that more closely approximates the desired behavior. For instance, as the child makes his bed and for the first time tucks in one corner, he is recognized for that behavior. And, if 2 days later he tucks in a second corner, this too is recognized. By applying this method, one can gradually shape his behavior until he becomes skilled at making the bed.

The most *rapid learning* tends to occur during *infancy and early childhood*. Because of this, parents, counselors, and teachers of children in the early primary grades are extremely important influences. If learning is to occur at a rapid but healthy rate, the idea or skill to be learned should generally *not be too easy or too hard*. It is generally best to *distribute* education and training over an appropriate period of time. Each child is somewhat different and will, therefore, *learn at his own unique rate*, depending in part on what he has already learned and his emotional experience with it.

For successful learning to take place, the child must have the *desire to learn,* for he will decide what is motivating — what is payoff and what is not. *Novel, fresh, and stimulating experiences* in which the child is an active participant tend to encourage and motivate him to learn.

Some Practices for Living Democratically with Children

What follows is just a sample of the many democratic practices for living with children that have been articulated by Rudolf Dreikurs (1966, 1971), the eminent Adlerian child and family psychiatrist. These practices have been very successful in the training of parents in democratic procedures and in helping them train their children in the acquisition of these democratic traits of character. Every counselor of the child and his family should also find these practices helpful.

It is important for parents to teach the child *self-reliance.* One of the effective ways of achieving this is for parents not to do for the child what he can do for himself. Parents who pick up a child who falls when he is learning to walk, when they know he can pick himself up, are undermining the child's feelings of self-reliance. Healthy feelings of self-reliance and competence are essential for the responsible democratic citizen.

Mutual respect, an idea based on the ethic of equality in human relationships, is the right of each child and parent. No parent should take advantage of his child and no child should take advantage of his parent. The family is no place for slavery or tyranny. The child is taught to respect the rights of others as parents are taught to respect the child's rights. Parents demonstrate respect for the child when they consider his ideas, opinions, and judgements and encourage him to become independent of them.

Parents should be encouraged to provide their children with *choices* at the earliest possible opportunities. They can do this by giving alternatives whenever they make requests, for example: "Johnnie, would you like to stop crying or would you like to take your crying to your bedroom?" Parents set the limits by requesting that the child either stops crying or takes his crying to his bedroom, but he can make the final choice as to which of these two he will do.

When parents allow and encourage the child to make choices from the alternatives they provide, they (1) help the child learn to make decisions and be responsible for them and (2) avoid imposing their will and thus sidestep much conflict.

It is important that parents *treat their children as a group* when they fight. Parents who try to be judge, jury, and executioner of their judgement when children fight put themselves in impossible situations. First, all children will not consider their judgement fair. Second, parents usually set a pattern of siding with the youngest, weakest, or smallest. Third, they take away from children the opportunity to practice resolving conflicts with others. Fourth, children are stimulated to fight even more to test their parents' love; each child believes his parents' love is evidenced by their siding with him. Fifth, many children learn very quickly to cooperate in their fighting in order to keep their parents busy with them.

Whenever children are fighting or quarreling, parents can be taught to disengage from their children's power plays to get their parents' alliance by learning to say such things as "Joan, that is between you and Jim. I know you two can work it out." These phrases are used, for example, when Joan comes crying to her parents that Jim is being mean to her.

Encouragement of the child is an essential ingredient of effective parenthood. Parents demonstrate encouragement when they accept and respect the child *as he is,* set reasonable standards for him that are neither too low nor too high, do not press him to fulfill their own unfulfilled dreams, provide him with opportunities to contribute to the welfare of the family, and recognize his contributions to the family, expressing appreciation for his efforts to contribute. A child needs continuous encouragement in order to grow, just as a rose needs continuous and large doses of sunshine.

The child must *feel secure* if he is to live a life of satisfactory experiences. The child, as has already been discussed, has creative power and thus his feelings of security are, in the final analysis, subjective and do not necessarily accurately reflect reality. This requires that counselors and parents need to be sensitive to the child's feelings of security. Feeling secure is an inner feeling of confidence and strength and is indicated when the child develops the stance of courage, confidence, and optimism toward life's situations. If he demonstrates courage, he is saying, "I am willing to risk"; if he demonstrates confidence, he is saying, "I will be able to work it through"; and if he demonstrates optimism, he is saying, "Things will work out."

Parents help their children acquire feelings of security by valuing their children, encouraging them, and by being models of courage, confidence, and optimism. Courage is as contagious as fear.

A *family council,* a place where family matters are discussed and decisions are made, can be an excellent school for children to learn to become responsible, democratic citizens. It provides each family member with the opportunity to express himself openly in all matters of both problems and pleasures relating to the family. The emphasis should be on "What is the issue?" and "What are the alternatives available to us?" The focus, therefore, is constructive. The family council can be destructive when parents allow family members to "wallow" in negative comments.

The family council should meet regularly each week with the parents presiding and each person taking his turn as chairman. Minutes should be kept and each member should have a vote in the decisions as much as age will permit. Poor decisions should stand until the next family council. In this way children can learn the consequences of their decisions. The book *Family Council* by Dreikurs *et al.* (1971) is recommended for those who desire to read more about the functioning of family councils. It can be acquired from the Alfred Adler Institute, 110 South Dearborn Street, Chicago, Illinois 60603.

Parents' Faulty Convictions

Most parents who come for counseling are eager to apply their new understandings and skills. Occasionally, however, a few are unable to take advantage of counseling until they become aware of their faulty convictions. This often requires individual therapy. The faulty convictions tend to have been formulated in the family of the parent's birth as he struggled for significance and worth in competition with his brothers and sisters.

Three of the more common faulty convictions developing out of competitive family relationships that tend to interfere in parents' childrearing efforts are: (1) "In order to have an important place in my family I must *dominate* my children"; (2) "In order to have a significant place in my family I must always be *right*"; and (3) "In order to have a significant place I must continually receive *service* and *comfort* from my children." The one who believes he or she must dominate will tend to boss, order, lecture, and condescend to his or her children. The one who believes he or she must always be right will tend to use criticism, faultfinding, and ridicule to make the children appear wrong, and the one who believes he or she must be served and comforted to have a significant place may appear helpless and dependent. All such behaviors tend to disrupt the effectiveness of parents.

The parent who seeks his significance in his family through these faulty ideas is usually only dimly aware of them. He becomes an unknowing reactor as he allows them to guide his behavior into destructive paths of unnecessary conflict with his children. Counselors can help parents become aware of their faulty beliefs and convictions and, thereby, gain greater control over their own behavior by helping them remember how they found a place in their family of birth. For example, if they remember that they always took care of their brothers and sisters and told them what to do, they may find that they believe they must dominate others to have a significant place with them and that this has carried over into their relationships with their children.

Here are some of the steps the counselor can take with parents to help them overcome their faulty convictions.

1. Help them *become clearly aware of such convictions.* This will tend to free parents to choose more constructive alternatives.

2. Help them *practice talking differently to themselves*. For example, if parents find that they are domineering parents who undermine the ability of their children to be self-reliant, they can be taught to say to themselves such things as, "I can be worthwhile and significant by allowing my children the right to make their own decisions rather than by making those decisions for them and thus undermining their self-reliance." If they are parents who have found their place by getting their children to wait on them and give them service, they can say to themselves, "I can be worthwhile and important by doing what I can to support my children in their school work rather than by demanding that they do special, unnecessary things for me."

3. Help them *practice behaving more cooperatively and respectfully* with their children. Parents can be taught effective communication skills and can be shown people who are good models whose more respectful words and phrases they can imitate and practice.

4. Help them realize that their fear of the unknown (the new behavior) is to be expected and that this *fear will leave* when the new behavior becomes the familiar and they find they can have a significant place through using the new behavior. Simply knowing that their fear of losing significance will diminish over time as they practice the new respectful behavior, and that they can achieve even greater significance and love by being more respectful with their children, can give them strength to persist until the unfamiliar becomes the familiar.

5. Help them have the *courage and self-discipline* to persist until the new behavior becomes firmly established. The counselor can enhance parents' courage and self-discipline by having them commit themselves to their children to change. And he can teach the children to give their parents supportive feedback regarding the progress they are making.

The Marriage Relationship

The marriage relationship provides the foundation for all other family relationships. A respectful and loving relationship between husband and wife sets up a model of respect and love for relationships that the children tend to imitate in their interaction with one another. The wise family counselor will be sensitively aware of the marriage relationship and will make this relationship part of counseling when it is appropriate. He must also be sensitively aware of the fact that just as a poor marriage can interfere with effective childrearing, a skillfully manipulative child can have a destructive influence on the marriage of parents who allow themselves to be so manipulated. Articles in this book of readings that focus on the marriage relationship should assist you to strengthen the marriage relationship when you discover this is needed to improve parent-child relationships.

Applying the Concepts and Principles Discussed

The following situation and accompanying discussion describes how I use many of the concepts and principles identified and described in the foregoing pages to effect changes in the child and his family (Allred, 1976).

The parents' eyes sparkled and their faces lit up as they described their eldest child, Gwen, a 5-year-old girl with a vocabulary beyond her years. The perceived her as being a good girl who tried to do what was right. She was obedient to her parents and a joy to them.

Three-year-old George was the reason they came in for counseling and their eyes were downcast and their faces tense as they described him. He flushed articles of his own and his parents' clothing down the toilet. He wrote on walls with crayons. He ran out in the street. It seemed that everyone was continually looking after and chasing after George.

The troubled parents had come to get help in an attempt to change George's behavior. A discussion of the situation revealed that Gwen watched his every move and told her mother when he was doing something he shouldn't do. Here typical phrases were, "Mother you'd better come quick. George is in the toilet again." "George has got one of your cuff links, Father." Gwen was continually tattling and George was continually misbehaving. Their mother especially was on the run throughout the day.

Further information about what was going on among family members showed that, in typical fashion, George's behavior had real meaning only as it was considered within the context of the total family. Gwen was an intelligent and good girl, but she was also good at George's expense. By continually tattling on him, she was able to demonstrate her goodness and George's badness. George, not believing he could compete with her goodness for the attention of his parents, chose instead to be good at being mischievous. And at this he became most skillful.

The parents were encouraged to change these patterns of misbehavior by telling Gwen that they were no longer going to pay attention to her tattling on George. Only when he was in real danger (i.e., going out in the street) was she to come to them. Otherwise they were going to ignore her tattling. They were also to be careful not to pay off George's misbehavior, but instead use the principle of logical consequences. George was to clean off his crayon marks when he scribbled on the wall. His mother or father could work with him to get the job done, but they were to function only mechanically in order to give no payoff to his misbehavior. He was to be denied crayons for a period of time after he used them improperly. His parents were to pay off George's attempts to be self-reliant and useful by recognizing such behaviors and encouraging him.

George's parents actually followed through on the recommendations and reported their progress. George was really coming out of it they said, and they were very happy with the progress they were making with him. Then the mother's face fell as she added "What is really worrying us now is that Gwen is becoming bad. She is getting hard to handle and is doing some of the very things that George used to do. It is as if George were becoming Gwen and Gwen were becoming George."

The parents were then taught to respond to Gwen's misbehavior in the same way they had responded to Georges'. They also attempted to understand Gwen better by walking in her shoes, by trying to understand how she felt and what goal she was achieving by behaving as she did.

It was also suggested that the parents redouble their efforts to help Gwen find a constructive place in the family by letting her help with tasks that interested her and that were helpful to the family without making another member look bad. Helping mother plan a grocery list, prepare a meal, and arrange flowers helped serve this purpose. Her parents were also taught to recognize her efforts to be helpful by saying such things as "Gwen, we surely do appreciate your helping plan the grocery list." "Gwen, your ideas for arranging the flowers in the vase were very helpful."

This case demonstrates the assumption that an individual's behavior is part of a network of interbalancing relationships; and when behavior is changed within one part of the network, it upsets the balance and results in changes elsewhere in the network. Therefore, anyone—counselor, parent, or teacher—desiring to effect changes with one individual, if he is to act responsibly and efficiently, must look to others with whom that individual relates.

Since Gwen had found her place by disgracing George, it was only natural that her secure feelings of belonging were threatened when she discovered that her mother and father were no longer responding to her tattling. This was most disconcerting to her. Because the mother and father no longer paid off George's bad behavior but paid off his good behavior, his relationship with them became better. This was not only disconcerting, but extremely threatening to Gwen's place of belonging. Things were changing and hence Gwen felt confused and insecure.

To the extent that her parents understood the above, they were able to walk in Gwen's shoes. Gwen gradually became secure within the new network of relationships as her parents paid off her constructive attempts to belong and refused to pay off her attempts to belong by reverting to George's old behavior.

As Gwen was helped by her parents in this manner, she learned while still very young that she could find a secure place of belonging

with those people who were important to her without making someone else appear less likeable than herself.

A Mental Map for the Counselor

In training marriage and family counselors at Brigham Young University, I have found that students need structured techniques in order to
accurately identify their recurring patterns of counseling behaviors. To
help with this need, I developed an instrument in 1973 that I have
called Allred's Interaction Analysis for Counselors, hereafter referred
to as the AIAC (Allred, 1973). I have patterned it after Ned. A. Flanders'
and Edmund J. Amidon's (1963) instrument for analyzing teacher-stu-
dent verbal interaction. The categories of the AIAC are identified and
described below and should be helpful to the counselor as a mental
map for helping him identify where he is at any given time in his
counseling, what he wants to do and where he wants to be, and where
he might need to go to improve his efficiency and effectiveness as a
counselor.

I have divided counseling behaviors into two broad areas, the "obstructive" and the "functional." To help counselors identify counseling behaviors that are usually obstructive to effectiveness in counseling, I have further divided the obstructive area into two categories of
behavior: (1) equivocates and (2) detaches/aggresses. For each category, I describe the specific behaviors.

The counselor who *equivocates* does so by making unclear statements, misunderstanding, appearing lost, wandering, and making in-
congruent statements. He may appear confused and not with his
clients intellectually. He may become silent when confused.

The counselor who *detaches/aggresses* responds in an aloof manner, withdraws, is not with his clients emotionally, uses a cool tone of
voice, appears insincere or not really caring, and/or responds in a
"professional" nonsensitive manner. As he aggresses against his
clients, he bosses, intrudes, fights to or for control, manages the
counseling session in an autocratic manner, and uses sarcasm, ridicule, blaming, and/or criticism.

These two categories can help the counselor identify relationship
behaviors that are the opposite of those that have been generally
found to be essential to effective counseling (Bergin and Strupp, 1972).
Counselors who find themselves functioning in recurring patterns in
either one of these two categories without a sound rationale are
probably undermining their effectiveness by interacting in these ways.

The personality traits of the counselor who is moving constructively
with his clients include sincerity, warmth, friendliness, appropriate
flexibility, and approachableness. He is also open and spontaneous,
confident, consistent, and well-organized. His communication is char-

acterized by nonpossessive warmth and respect, genuineness, and accurate empathy. His words, eyes, tone of voice, and body posture are congruent with one another. In this style of counselor communication, clients tend to experience feelings of acceptance, belonging, positive self-worth, and hope.

In the AIAC, I present a model I call functional communication that includes five categories that can aid counselors in determining the counseling behavior they may want to increase: (1) educates, (2) gathers information, (3) interprets and confronts, (4) seeks alternatives and recommends, and (5) supports. I recommend that you commit these categories to memory along with several of the facilitating phrases accompanying each category.

A counselor may *educate* his clients by structuring the interview, making observational statements regarding children and people in general, and giving facts or opinions. He must do this as with all functional counseling responses, in a context of respect, warmth, sincerity, and empathy; otherwise, the communication is classified in one of the obstructive categories (Bergin and Strupp, 1972). Facilitating functional educational phrases include:

● I would like to talk first with you and then observe your children.
● I find that children's crying usually increases when they find they can use it to get their own way.
● Children tend to repeat those behaviors that we pay off.
● Parents have to be on their toes not to pay off the attempts of the child to belong at the expense of his brothers and sisters.
● Parents tend to repeat the same mistakes with their children that their parents made with them.

A counselor who *gathers information* asks questions in order to obtain information, makes observational statements to his clients regarding their and their children's behavior, and summarizes his observations. Facilitating phrases include:

● What do you do when your child continues to whine and cry when you refuse to let him eat between meals?
● Then what you appear to be saying is that when you can stand his crying no longer you give in and let him eat.
● What you have told us then is that when you try not to let your child eat between meals, wear the clothes he wants, or eat from your plate and he then cries, you finally let him have his way?

A counselor who *interprets and confronts* is willing to guess about the meanings of the information he has obtained, clarify the meanings, and summarize the interpretations. He will respectfully confront his clients with their existing ways of thinking and behaving that are counterproductive. Facilitating phrases include:

● Could it be that your child continues to whine and cry when you refuse to let him eat between meals because he knows from past experience that he can get you emotionally involved with him and also undermine your resolve not to let him eat?

● Could it be that the goals of the child are the same whether his behavior is eating between meals, having his own way with his clothes, or eating off of your plate? Could it be that his goal is to show you who is boss and get your attention? What do you think?

● From what you have told me regarding your own childhood, could it be that you are laboring under faulty convictions and thus your desire to be a good parent is undermining your attempts to be firm and consistent with your child when he cries and whines?

The counselor who seeks *alternatives* and *recommends* will explore alternatives with his clients, suggest what they could or should do, and work to verbally commit them to carry out the assignment to which they agree. Facilitating phrases include:

● When your child cries and whines, how might you respond so that you will not pay him off?

● You believe that getting away from him by walking into another room will help you to be firm and consistent?

● Will you do it?

● No, not *try*. Will you *do* it? This means that each time your child whines and cries to get his own way you will walk into another room. You will also attend to him (give him payoff) at least twice each hour when he is being cooperative.

● We are agreed then. We will discuss your experiences with the assignment when you return next week.

The counselor *supports* his clients by working at securing a positive relationship with them, helping them to be at ease, making encouraging statements, accepting and clarifying feelings, and recalling and/or predicting feelings. The counselor's giving support to his clients is as necessary as the machinest's adding oil to his machinery. Support is facilitated by such phrases as the following:

● Please tell me more.

● And he made you angry.

You may feel like a terrible parent at first, for he may increase his crying to test your resolve, but stick with it. This feeling will leave.

● You showed much courage in only giving in to your child twice in 1 week.

● Keep up the good work.

The counselor can use the above five categories: (1) educates, (2) gathers information, (3) interprets/confronts, (4) seeks alternatives and recommends, and (5) supports to analyze the tapes of his counseling interviews and thus more clearly determine whether he is doing all he can do to be effective and helpful to his clients. I have observed that many counselors in training overuse certain categories and seldom use others. For example, my independently minded students tend to neglect support while those trained in nondirective techniques often acquire large numbers of responses in the categories of *gathers information* and *supports* but few in any of the others. Knowing the categories of the AIAC can help the counselor modify his patterns of counseling interaction as he attempts to acquire those he believes are more effective.

If the counselor finds that he wants to change his patterns but resists actually changing them, it may be that he has faulty beliefs concerning how he must behave in order to be worthwhile and significant and that these are getting in the way of his improving his effectiveness as a counselor. An example of this is the counselor who grew up in his family of origin creating for himself the conviction that to be worthwhile and significant he had to continually please others and, therefore, found it difficult to educate, interpret, confront, and hold his clients to their assignments. If the counselor finds that he has faulty convictions that are getting in this way, he will find that the suggestions for helping parents with faulty convictions can also be helpful to him.

Summary

In this chapter I suggest that the counselor can be much more effective in modifying the problem child's destructive behavior if he focuses on the network of the child's interactions rather than just on the child himself. I also suggest that counselors need to help parents articulate the kind of character traits they want their children to acquire. I have identified a few of the traits that I believe are consistent with democratic societies. I have discussed nine assumptions regarding the child and his family—creative power, purpose, communication, social linkage, belonging, high self-esteem, and social interest, life style, and holism. Some major principles for modifying the child's behavior and those people interacting with him that I have identified and discussed are bonding, payoff, modeling, natural consequences, logical consequences, personality traits of significant others, and practice. Self-reliance, mutual respect, choices, encouragement, security, group treatment for fighting, and family councils are also discussed as being important to the child if he is to learn to live democratically. The problem of parents with faulty convictions is presented and some specific suggestions were given. Last of all, I provide a mental map of counselor behaviors, obstructive and functional, that the counselor can use to better understand and improve his own communication and effectiveness in counseling.

REFERENCES

Adler, A.: *What Life Shoud Mean to You.* Capricorn Books, New York, 1958.
Allred, G. H.: *How to Strengthen Your Marriage and Family.* Brigham Young University Press, Provo, Utah, 1976.

Allred, G. H.: The Allred Interaction Analysis for Counselors. Paper presented at the Meeting of the American Society for Adlerian Psychology, Toronto, Ontario, 1973.

Amidon, E. J., and Flanders, N. A.: *The Role of the Teacher in the Classroom.* Paul S. Amidon and Associates, Inc., Minneapolis, 1963.

Ansbacher, H. L., and Ansbacher, R. R.: *The Individual Psychology of Alfred Adler.* Basic Books, New York, 1956.

Bandura, A., and Walters, R. H.: *Social Learning and Personality Development.* Holt, Rinehart, and Winston, New York, 1963.

Bergin, A. E., and Strupp, H. H.: *Changing Frontiers in the Science of Psychotherapy.* Aldine Publishing Co., Chicago, 1972.

Cochran, A. A.: Mind, matter, and quanta. in *Main Currents in Modern Thought.* March–April, pp. 79–88, 1966.

Dreikurs, R.: Adlerian analysis of interaction. *Group Psychotherapy,* 8 (4): 298–307, 1955.

Dreikurs, R.: *The ABC's of Guiding the Child.* Classroom handout at the University of Oregon, 1966.

Dreikurs, R., Grunwald, B. B., and Pepper, F. C.: *Maintaining Sanity in the Classroom.* Harper and Row, New York, 1971.

Dreikurs, R.: The four goals of the maladjusted child. *Nervous Child,* 6: 321–328, 1947.

Hutchins, R. M. (Ed. in Chief): *Great Books of the Western World,* Encyclopedia Britannica, Inc., Vol. 9, p. 359, Chicago, 1952.

A. LYNN SCORESBY, Ph.D.

7

Counseling in Parent-Adolescent Relationships

Introduction

Haley (1968) wrote that the manifestations of family problems reflect the particular forces acting on a family at a particular stage or time. Furthermore, he suggested that the outcome of counseling should be to help a family successfully move into a stage subsequent to the one it presently occupies. Because of its unique and complex nature, a family with adolescent children exhibits problems clearly related to the requirements placed on it. And, in a general way, the desired outcome of family counseling with adolescent children is their successful transition into responsible adulthood. The purpose of this chapter is to describe the nature of adolescent problems from a family perspective and to outline some appropriate counseling procedures.

In our culture, adolescence is typically viewed as the period of time when many social, physical, psychological, and emotional changes take place. The onset of these changes are often culturally recognized and ritualized as "rites of passage" into adulthood. It is likely true that many individuals experience change of greater variety and rapidity than any time since the first 2 years of life.

These changes place the individual in a position of having to accommodate and master several different elements which exert considerable influence. During the space of 4 to 5 years, an adolescent is typically expected to successfully learn dating skills, career habits and attitudes, friendship and peer associations, and heterosexual behavior. He or she in various ways is expected to move into society and demonstrate social competence in several settings. Beyond the social requirements of adolescence an individual experiences a rapid physical growth spurt where the body changes by adding secondary sexual characteristics, height, weight, and physical structure.

Coupled with social and physical development, adolescence is also a time of considerable emotionality where channels and controls are to be formed for feelings newly and intensely experienced. These emotions include a passion for some "cause" erotic experience, egocentrism, and self-consciousness. Showing the intensity of these emotions, Elkind (1967) wrote in regard to egocentrism, that adolescents believe others are preoccupied with their appearance and behavior. This keeps them in fairly continual examination of what is acceptable to others. Emotional behavior such as loudness, boarishness, faddish dress, or dramatic and exaggerated communication is an attempt to discover affectively what will be approved of by other people.

While the types of adolescent changes are only cursorily reviewed here, it still may be observed that the individual and his or her family face considerable newness and increased variation during this period of time. This, of course, may strain the family system requiring some adjustment to maintain satisfactory family relationships and simultaneously accommodate the needs of the adolescent. When families are able to do this adequately, adolescence is usually a positive time for the individual and the family. When the family system does not adequately adjust, adolescents tend to experience difficulty in progressing toward responsible adulthood.

The foregoing is corroborated by findings reported by Offer and Offer (1973). Their research showed that when family relationships are smooth with a history of stability, adolescents tend to progress toward adulthood in what they called a process of *continuous growth*. *Surgent growth*, another pathway to adulthood, is marked by less stable family relationships. When the family background of the adolescent is characterized by overt marital and family conflict, adolescent children experience *tumultuous growth* where considerable affect is present but uncontrolled.

How Adolescent Problems are Manifest

If we conclude that ineffective families are associated with adolescent difficulty, how are the problems manifest? Generally, the problems can be labeled as failure to successfully progress toward maturity. More specifically, the problems, disorders, and instabilities of youth are reflected in the very areas they are attempting to master. Consequently, an individual may enter therapeutic situations because of some form of social difficulty that may include drug abuse, alienation from others, or inadequate social skills. Heterosexual behavior, academic and career planning failure, delinquency, and/or cognitive disorders are also typical adolescent problems. Most commonly, family counselors will be confronted with families whose children have difficulty in one, usually more, of these areas.

There will, however, almost invariably be some family conflict associated with what is manifest by the individual adolescent. This generally stems from one of three sources: (1) chronic conflict within the family that has remained unresolved; (2) structural changes due to death, divorce, illness, or inability of a family member to fully participate; and (3) ineffective attempts to maintain the family and simultaneously accommodate the adjustments required by a particular adolescent's development.

Although the sources of family conflict may differ from family to family, some dynamics are associated with adolescent problems regardless of the particular source. These, as described by Lidz (1973), include (1) the lack of nurturance and an inability to maintain cohesive relationships; (2) a failure on the part of the family to adequately communicate with its environment so that the instrumental skills of language and role performance transmitted by parents to children do not match societal expectations; (3) rigid and restricted patterns of communication that are often vague and inaccurate; and (4) the impaired functioning of one or both parents due to marital conflict or incompetence.

We may conclude from how problems are manifest that a counselor is faced with two complex tasks. One is to learn about, understand, and improve the adolescent's ability to function in areas where he or she may be failing. Second, because of the close ties between family and the adolescent, the family dynamics associated with a problem are identified and successfully modified to better facilitate the adolescent's progress toward adulthood.

Therapeutic Assumptions

A counseling approach for adolescents and their families can be organized in one of two general perspectives. One gives focus to the individual adolescent with parents and siblings as resources. Most often the counselor sees the adolescent alone. The other procedure, described here, assumes the family itself must be modified and it, with its unique characteristics, is dealt with directly. For example, at least parents and the child are conjointly involved and when appropriate other siblings are included. The objectives of this approach are usually two-fold. (1) Emphasis is given to modifying and improving family dynamics. This means that patterns and sequences of communication among family members are identified and examined to determine how they may relate both to the adolescent problem and intrafamily conflict. (2) A correlating emphasis is given to the relationship between the adolescent and his or her environment of friends, school, work, and so forth. At the same time that the family system receives attention, efforts are made to help the individual succeed in his or her own world.

Prior to outlining some steps or phases of counseling, some underlying assumptions are described here to give logical foundation for subsequent treatment principles. One of these is the basic assumption of all conjoint family counseling. *It is that each person's behavior, desirable or undesirable, serves some needs of family members. Modification of one person's actions likely requires adjustment in the entire family system.* Otherwise, improvement may be slow in coming and short lived if achieved at all.

The second assumption underlying counseling with adolescent families relates to the first. *Since family members are tied together by tradition and communicational bonds, emphasis is given to modifying the total context in which the undesirable behavior occurs.* Instead of learning only about the actions of the individul adolescent, a counselor likely should identify a cluster of family events happening prior to, simultaneous with, or just after an episode when undesirable behavior is manifest. The actions of each family member as they occur in concert are examined in terms of: (1) the relationship to the performance of the adolescent and (2) the impact on the whole family system. As an illustration Sobel (1973) wrote about his work with the family of a youth who was expelled from school. In an attempt to learn about the total context, he found that in the previous 4 months the boy had experienced a sister's out of wedlock pregnancy, father's arrest for drunken driving, failing at math, breaking up with a girlfriend, mother taking a new job, failing at a try for the football team, and coming down with mono. It may reasonably be seen that focusing only on the school failure may have left out other important elements of this adolescent's problem. This implies that attending only to the presenting problem and not to the entire context may make efforts to help less effective.

The third assumption underlying counseling for families with adolescent children concerns the purpose or objectives. The family, by virtue of seeking counseling, defines itself as incapable of adequately responding to internal events or stressful conditions emanating from the environment. This probably indicates that the family system lacks alternatives of handling family member behavior. Consequent instability or rigidity makes it more difficult for the family unit to deal with the demands of society. At the time a child reaches the age of adolescence, the family has to accommodate children who have as wide a range of age as will ever happen, social expectations, and developmental needs. This along with the ordinary energy required to maintain the marriage makes for the greatest complexity and consequently stress the parents will experience. *This implies that counseling should be aimed at increasing the family's (parents) capacity to handle additional internal differentiation. Furthermore, the family system requires help to adjust its interaction with its environment so that smooth family relationships can be maintained.*

Families exist within a culture that has some influence in determining what is believed by and expected for adolescent children. In our American society, we typically view the adolescent years as the period of separation from the family and the establishment of independence. This coincides with the developmental notion that identity formation is the primary task of this period (Erickson, 1950). So deeply a part of our lives is this expectation that counselors working with families with adolescents almost invariably must confront this issue. Such questions as the following are often a part of counseling. How much freedom is desirable? How can parents exert control or influence and still foster independence? Will allowing freedom lead to more misbehavior or failure?

In a paradoxical way, the problem behavior of the adolescent and family conflict seems to further enmesh the individual with the family rather than promote a separation. Lidz (1973), for example, reports the difficulty of keeping parents away from schizophrenic children even though their encounters are often destructive. Or, consider one set of parents' reaction to a child suspected of smoking marijuana. To find out they began embracing the son in order to smell his breath and clothes. He interpreted their intent, became angry, and used their behavior as evidence he was not wanted by them. Shortly thereafter he engaged in some further deviant behavior resulting in additional parental controls. This pattern served to keep parents and son hooked together even though (but usually the case) the basis of their continuing relationship was undesirable behavior. Independence, freedom from restraint, and psychological individuation are prominent issues in counseling with adolescents and their families. Since this is so, one assumption suggests that *the paradox of influencing children while helping them to be independent can best be resolved by making parental control attempts implicit rather than explicit.*

This assumption is part of the basis for the approach described by Watzlawick *et al.* (1975). They suggest that rather than explicitly controlling a child through verbal means and application of rewards and punishments, parents implement behavior designed to place the adolescent in a position where he or she "discovers" what they think to be desirable. For example, instead of continually nagging and complaining to get a child to make his bed, they advise the parents to do it but put in cracker crumbs or short sheet it. In this way the adolescent "discovers" that mother is incompetent or perhaps not trustworthy and concludes that making the bed is the easier way out of the dilemma. In contrast to this implicit approach, many parents try to control children by means of exerting more power. Some try to revert to or maintain disciplinary strategies that worked previously when children were younger. Others use distancing-withdrawal mechanisms hoping that threat of rejection will influence the child. Still others resort to use of punishments and explicit rewards assuming that adding or removing something desired will be sufficient leverage to control behavior. Most often, as implied by this last assumption, parents must learn alternatives to either of these methods.

Counseling Procedure

Having stated some assumptions underlying an approach to counseling, this section describes some procedures that can be applied to a family with an adolescent child. Each counselor will of course apply any method in his or her own way and it is not intended here to prescribe what must take place. Some general procedures are explained instead along with a rationale for them.

Identifying and Defining the Problem

The purpose of this phase is to gather data regarding adolescent behavior and family dynamics associated with it. Then, translate the nature of this information in such a way that the family members view themselves as part of any problem or solution that may emerge. This step is successfully completed when family members can verbalize understanding of how they as individuals, the family unit, and the adolescent are tied together in interactional bonds. For the purpose here, it is assumed that the family unit is the parents and adolescent. Other family members may be included, however, when there is indication that they are directly tied to the problem.

Gathering Data—As the first counseling session begins, one initial and important step for the counselor is to create a procedure for the family to follow. The purpose of this is to legitimize the counselor's right to manage. Usually this is done implicitly by indicating that certain information is needed and then asking relevant questions, clarifying what is said, and stating what is observed. The counselor may say, "I want to spend some time becoming acquainted with you as a family." Some background or a family chronology may be taken similar to the process suggested by Satir (1967) or information may be obtained about each family member's birth order, age, whether this is a first or subsequent marriage for the parents, if all children are natural born, and how close or distant are ties between the family and other relatives. After identifying who belongs in the family and some of its history, the task is to focus on family behavior that is germane to the problem. This may include specific things like verbal or nonverbal communicative behavior that serves as elicitors or reinforcers for behavior. In addition, disciplinary procedures or people's role performances in the family may also be an object of inquiry. In some cases a structured activity may be given the family so that they can be observed during interactional situations. Many such activities may be created, each with a specific purpose. One tested method has been reported by Watzlawick (1966). He described a procedure of having family members mutually identify their main problems, plan something together, discuss how parents met, and resolve and communicate the meaning of a proverb. Then the family members are asked to sit in order and write the main fault of the person to the left of them. After collecting the cards, the counselor reads each at random and asks, "To whom do you think this applies." This author wrote this technique is useful because it, "reveals highly significant data on scapegoating, favoritism, and self-blame in a family."

While gathering information about the family system, the counselor also questions and learns about the adolescent. This may be done with parents present or, if advisable, the teenager can be seen alone. Often failure, inadequacy, or delinquent acts do not happen as isolated events. It is, therefore, useful to inquire about several areas where the teenager might be involved.

Linking Individual Behavior and Family Interaction—After learning about the nature of the individual behavior, an attempt is made to develop a link between circumstances within the family and the actions of the adolescent. This link may be in terms of a sequence of events which involves parents, siblings, and the adolescent. One frequently reported sequence can illustrate this. Suppose a child is spending time with friends whom the parents do not like. Some things are done which may be immoral or illegal. The parents respond by setting a curfew. When it is violated, an argument ensues and restrictions are made. These, in turn, are not obeyed resulting in another argument and additional attempts to control. In many cases, adolescent behavior will be linked in a sequence similar to this or others equally ineffective. Part of the task of gathering information is to identify those sequences that might relate in time and order to the behavior of the adolescent.

Family dynamics may be tied to the behavior of the adolescent and not be a part of a sequence in terms of the amount of stress exerted on the family. This may directly or indirectly have impact on the teenager. For instance, consider the example of the daughter, failing socially, disrupting her classrooms, and showing a rapid decline in quality of school work. She also began to exhibit signs of shyness and social isolation. An examination of her family yielded the following. (1) Her father recently experienced business failure and evidenced tension by yelling at and criticizing her and the other children. (2) He became temporarily impotent which contributed to depression and isolation from the family. (3) Simmering conflict in the marriage seemed to be aggravated during the last 3 to 4 months. A counselor uncovering these stresses on the family may, with good reason, hypothesize a link between them and the behavior of the adolescent. Associating family stresses with adolescent behavior and identify sequences helps the counselor and family members begin to view the total problem as a combined family-individual difficulty. This satisfies the criteria for the first phase of family counseling and provides a foundation for the intervention phase.

Intervening

The term intervening is used here to convey that the counselor is active in altering behavior. In this case, focus is on changing family communicative behavior and the adolescent's way of handling his or her environment. While there are differing views as to how the counselor should act to accomplish this, some common elements exist which run across the various theoretical positions. One of these elements is that the client family does not, by definition, have behavioral alternatives to what they are already doing. They may know that something is not successful, but they probably do not know what else to do. A second common element in successful approaches is the emphasis on pragmatics. Each has some mechanisms that bring results that encourage families to rely on and have confidence in what the counselor does. Failure to quickly address what families view the problem to be and bring about some family individual results often creates despair and increased frustration.

Operant Conditioning and Family Counseling—LeBow (1972) has applied principles of operant conditioning to family problems. This approach considers one person's behavior a reinforcing stimulus for another's. Chains of interaction are learned which are lawful and, therefore, subject to modification. Pinpointing certain observable and undesirable behaviors, he suggests that a frequency base rate first be obtained of each person's actions. One or more observers from among the family can be trained to tabulate behavior such as accusations, criticisms, tardiness, or sarcasm. Reinforcement contingencies are typically derived from things valued by family members and applied to modify behavior. Increased effectiveness is achieved by showing families models of desirable behavior which can be imitated. Patterson (1974) has been successful using this approach when parents modified the aggressive behavior of boys by using verbal reinforcers of praise and encouragement. This behavior was in this case both a model and a reinforcer. Alexander (1973) reported that operant methods successfully modified family communication and delinquent adolescent behavior by use of token reinforcers (poker chips) administered by one family member to another. In this approach, a positive alternative is identified and each person is given a number of chips to positively and/ or negatively reinforce the actions of one other person. At the end of a reasonable period of time (e.g., 3 days) each person's chips are counted. If the total equals or exceeds a predetermined number of positive reinforcements or is below the specified limits for negative reinforcers, some reward is available for each person. Often the rewards can be the type that further bring family members together in positive ways such as participating in fun activities.

Simultaneous to the application of these techniques to the family system, they may also be applied directly to the adolescent. He or she may be helped to set goals (e.g., improved grades or reducing delinquent acts) and work toward a reward for achieving them. The goal acts as an alternative to the undesirable behavior. The reward can be controlled by the parents, counselor, or self-administered by the teenager.

Application of operant principles can satisfy the therapeutic assumptions outlined previously. Focus is on modifying the family context of the adolescent behavior, and when all members participate in administering reinforcers, parental behavior can be changed from explicit control of the adolescent to a mutual control or reinforcing program.

Experiential Counseling — Kempler (1968) outlines what is called an experiential procedure. In this approach an alternative to what is happening among family members is supplied when a counselor "uses himself" as the means of altering events within the family. Emphasis is given to the counselor's ability to be spontaneous, to join in the family discussions, disclose his or her feelings, and invite family members to do the same. A primary objective is to help family members communicate accurately to understand each other and move toward increased openness and sharing of feedback with one another. Change mechanisms in this approach are the increased sharing of personal information and nurturant behavior, the sense of intimacy or cohesion found in the family, and reduction of distinction communicative behavior. To achieve these conditions the counselor is active by starting conversations, stopping them, and suggesting what could be said and how to say it. Simulated situations may be created or actual events recreated by family members with each person performing a role as he or she views it. These in turn are evaluated and each person is requested to share his or her observations and reactions.

This approach suggests that improvement for the family and the adolescent comes as a result of smoothing out troubled relationships and clarifying distorted communication. When attention is given to helping the adolescent improve in other situations, more effective communication skills are taught and feelings and values experienced by the adolescent are clarified.

Systems and Communication Theory — A third intervention approach is derived from systems and communication theory. These theories presume that family and adolescent problems are associated with communication, rigid or unstable, that forces a paradoxal bind in which parents and children are entangled. Dysfunctional interaction occurs when family members exchange a high frequency of either opposite (complementary) or identical (symmetrical) behavior (Watzlawick *et al.*, 1967). Dimensions of oppositeness may vary from family to family but some common ones include dominance-submission, quiet-talkative, or sloppy-clean. Symmetrical interaction exists when two people exchange identical behavior in juxtaposition to each other. This often manifests itself as a competitive status or power struggle. When several types of these exchanges exist they are said to be placed in cognitive categories or classes. Then when confronted with a problem, it often appears that acting just opposite or identical to what the other person is doing will solve the problem. Consider a wife, for example, who has quietly observed her husband's critical lectures until one day she decided to correct his behavior by doing the same thing to him. Instead of a complementary exchange, the shift in her actions, rather than solving the problem, paradoxically formed a symmetrical interaction which was equally dysfunctional. The person's attempt to solve the problem has kept their exchanges either in the complementary or symmetrical class.

Watzlawick *et al.* (1975) describe a four-step approach to resolving this paradox. Since anything logically opposite or identical to the problem behavior will compound it, they suggest a counselor (1) obtain a concrete definition of the problem (how all parties exchange behavior); (2) help a family define a specific goal; (3) identify what attempted solutions have already been tried; and (4) change the attempted solutions. Changing the attempted solutions means essentially to break interactional events that are complementary or symmetrical and create an exchange that is logically difficult or parallel. What is called an example of this would be a father and son who symmetrically accuse and blame each other. The counselor breaks this by giving beans and a cup to the father. Each time the son blames or accuses, instead of responding verbally, the father drops a bean into the cup. Exchanging a bean with a blame or accusation forces the interaction out of symmetrical and into a more functional type. The authors list several techniques designed to change opposite or identical interaction. One of these is to increase the flow of information between the family and its environment through more contact, more family discussions, and by relaxing of rigid interaction. This will create more alternative ways for family members to respond to each other. Another tool is to stimulate family members to metacommunicate or "talk about how they talk." This means that the counselor helps the family compare this nonverbal and verbal behavior and describes how each views himself or herself, how each sees the other, and how each perceives what occurs between them. Since rigid or other dysfunctional communication stems from a restricted language that each uses to communicate, a third technique implied by this approach is to help family members restore deletions they have made in the structure of their language. This according to Bandler and Grinder (1975) can be done when the counselor makes sure a person's statements are complete, not ambiguous, and refer to something or someone specific. They suggest that common detractors in interaction include cause and effect statements, mind reading which implies that a speaker knows the other's thoughts, and generalizations one makes about the nature of life and the world. This means that the counselor often asks, "How does this happen?" "To whom or what are you referring?" "What do you mean?" "Does this always happen?" In effect the counselor challenges the way parents and child explain events and requests that they give full, elaborate, and sufficient meaning to their comments. Such an approach is designed to alter the way a person construes family events. It is intended that making family members do so will result in alternative ways of responding to one another. This capacity for increased variation will, it is presumed, help the family more satisfactorily respond to the complexity it faces due to adolescent needs.

Conclusion

This has been an attempt to define the nature of the family in which adolescents with problems are involved. Then from the perspective of counseling the family conjointly, some assumptions were given and suggested approaches described. To this date, methods of counseling with adolescents and their families have not received much empirical attention. As a result, we can only assume that matching a specific technique to a specific family with a particular problem probably is the key to effective counseling. This implies that the counselor with the greatest flexibility and skill will have more alternatives and an increased likelihood of succeeding. Hopefully, what is included here will promote both of these.

REFERENCES

Alexander, J. F., and Parsons, B. V.: Short term behavioral intervention with delinquent families; impact on family process and recidivism. J. Abnormal Psych., 1973.

Bandler, R., and Grinder, J.: *The Structure of Magic.* Science and Behavior Books, Inc., Palo Alto, California, 1975.

Elkind, D.: Egocentrism in adolescence. Child Development, **38:** 1025–1034, 1976.

Erickson, E.: *Childhood and Society.* W. W. Norton, New York, 1950.

Haley, J.: *Uncommon Therapy.* Grune and Stratton, New York, 1968.

Kempler, W.: Experiential psychotherapy with families. Family Process, **7:** (1) 88–99, 1968.

LeBow, M. D.: Behavior modification for the family. in *Family Therapy An Introduction to Theory and Technique.* (Erickson, G. D., and Hogan, P., eds) Brooks/Cole Publishing Co., California, 1972.

Lidz, T.: *The Origin and Treatment of Schizophrenic Disorders.* Basic Books, Inc., New York, 1973.

Offer, D., and Offer, J.: Normal adolescence in perspective. in *Current Issues in Adolescent Psychiatry.* (Schoolar, J. C., ed) Brunner/Mazel, New York, 1973.

Patterson, G. R.: Retraining of aggressive boys by their parents: review of recent literature and follow-up evaluation. Paper prepared for the Jewish General Hospital and McGill University, Third Annual Symposium, Montreal, Quebec, Canada, November 1972. Also in F. Lowy (ed) symposium on the seriously disturbed preschool child, Can. Psych. Assoc. J., **19:** 142–161, 1974.

Satir, V.: *Conjoint Family Therapy*. Science and Behavior Books, Palo Alto, California, 1967.

Sobel, R.: Adolescence and family stress. in *Current Issues in Adolescent Psychiatry*. (Schoolar, J. C., ed), Brunner/Mazel, New York, 1973.

Watzlawick, P.: A structured family interview. Family Process, **5:** 256–271, 1966.

Watzlawick, P., Beavin, J. H., and Jackson, D. D.: *Pragmatics of Human Communication*. W. W. Norton, New York, 1967.

Watzlawick, P., Weakland, J. H., and Fische, R.: *Change: Principles of Problem Formation and Problem Resolution*. W. W. Norton Co., Inc., New York, 1975.

ALEXANDER B. TAYLOR, Ph.D.

8

Counseling Couples in the Middle Years

Definition of the Population

It is a difficult task to establish the parameters of the group referred to as middle-aged couples. It has become common practice to define middle age as the years from 45 to 64; however, there are some research projects which have used age 30 as the onset of middle age and several studies which consider age 70 as the end of middle age. If one were to ask individuals to classify themselves as being old or middle-aged, many individuals over the age of 80 still consider themselves middle-aged. For purposes of this chapter the population that will be focused on will be the group of 45 to 65 years of age.

It would be, of course, foolish to consider a 20-year segment of any individual's life as a homogeneous developmental cycle. When evaluating couples or individuals it is helpful to consider whether they are just entering the middle age period, they are in the middle of this part of their life, or they are reaching the end of middle age life. It is also necessary to make room for the fact that some couples who are well into their 60's are more like some couples who are just entering middle age, and that some couples who are just 45 behave and experience some of the difficulties typical of much older people. For example, a man who has a heart attack at age 45 may become both physiologically and psychologically more like a man much older than he is, depending on how he tends to handle such traumas. In addition, the couple will adopt a life style consistent with their response patterns to such traumas.

Defining the population under consideration must be done by several criteria. Generally, the author will be referring to couples that have been married for 10 years or more, however, will make reference to couples who are middle-aged chronologically but have remarried so that the age of their marriage will typically be much less than those individuals who are normally considered in this age group. It may also be necessary to use subjective measures when establishing the population under discussion. For example, when individuals begin to be aware of their physical decline (often followed by the familiar behaviors of attempting to recapture lost youth through sexual acting out, excessive make-up, etc.) this could be one definition of early middle age. Additionally, it is possible to define middle age as the time when one has reached stability in occupation with little likelihood of dramatic new achievement and just before the period of time an individual or couple is preparing for retirement. In any case, it is obvious that many definitions could be used to establish middle age both in terms of individual chronological age as well as age of the marriage of the couple, physical factors, etc., all of which are complicated by the subjective reactions and responses of the individuals under consideration. It is of value for the clinician to evaluate just where his patients fit in this total structure. The arbitrary ages of 45 to 65 considered in this chapter may not always apply to the clinician's population.

Conceptual Approach

Couples traversing the "middle years" must be viewed from a biological-psychological-sociological perspective to be understood and certainly prior to the establishment of any treatment plan.

The years between 45 and 65 normally result in significant physiological decline. As normal senses begin to decline with the loss in eyesight, hearing, and taste, individuals find that they no longer cope with their environment as they once did. Experimental evidence supports the conclusion that the capacity to coordinate physical motion decreases as we proceed across these years and that subtle changes in perception, memory, and motivation also begin to assert themselves. It must, however, be emphasized that these changes are generally subtle, they accumulate over time, and vary considerably from one individual to another. The differential rate of aging between husband and wife, the severity of physical decline, complications of serious illness or injury, and in some cases an improvement in health are all likely to affect family relationships. Some specifics of physiological change during the middle years will be considered in a separate section later in this chapter.

While physiological changes must be dealt with in their own right, it is equally important to evaluate these changes in terms of their impact on individuals and relationships. The impact will depend much more on individual life history, mechanisms available for handling change, as well as the total integration of that individual's personality. It can be argued that personality is established and fixed at an early age with only minor alterations occurring thereafter. On the other hand, it can also be argued that human beings are in a constant state of change, their personalities being dynamic with potential for growth, change, and capacity to adapt as well as the potential for negative processes caused by trauma, new conflicts, and the normal vicissitudes of life. The author of this article takes the latter position that the capacity for change is always present in the individual and that we are constantly responding *in significant ways* to environmental stimuli whether this stimuli be normal life experiences or the experience of counseling, and that the individual's personality affects how he experiences the stimuli and the stimuli will affect his future personality.

A great deal of change occurs in the lives of people who have lived 50 years. The rate of societal change increases significantly with each decade. Issues such as longer life-span, increasing economic freedom (especially for women), acceptance of divorce, the new humanism emphasizing the importance of individual worth, changing mores, as well as technological advances have produced a world which may for some be increasingly an anxiety-producing experience while for others the constantly changing world is a way to reach out for new excitement. However couples define these changes they must adapt to them. The quality of middle age marriage appears to be less than most of us would hope for. Family sociologists have noted that the divorce process is beginning to characterize not only young but middle age marriages. Pineo (1961) found in his longitudinal study of married couples that by the end of 15 or 20 years of marriage most couples report their feeling in marriage is that of disenchantment and growing emotional distance between them. Cuber and Harroff's (1965) study of upper middle class Americans classifies most middle age marriages as either "devitalized" or "habitually conflicted." In addition, many families appear to be going through significant stress as a result of the so-called generation gap wherein the breakdown in communication and understanding of the generations has produced extreme pain and disillusionment, typically among those parents who are entering their middle years. The interaction of physical change, psychological development, and sociological process in a dynamic system is the focus of evaluation and treatment.

Specific Issues

Financial

Several financial issues arise during the middle years of life. During the early middle years it is often the case that a couple's children are growing to maturity, they may be entering college, getting married, or they often require more expensive clothing and medical assistance. It is a time when financial resources may be severely taxed. As couples move more to the middle years they may be taking care of their children in college, as well as supporting parents who are no longer able to support themselves. During later middle years income may be reducing as the wage earner's energy level reduces and the couple begin considering the prospects of retirement. Kerckhoff (1976) states:

> "Economists and political scientists have described the financial pressures put upon the middle age, middle income categories of society by the young and the old; old people and young people cost a lot of money — money which to a large extent is being earned by middle aged people."

Peterson (1974) points out that 25% of the 21,000,000 aged population in the United States have income which is considered less than minimal level essential to bare existence.

In spite of the fact that middle-aged couples are often faced with important new expenditures, this period of time is usually one in which the wage earner has reached, or has approached, his highest level of income. As other problems arise such as declining health or technological changes many individuals find their potential for economic gain beginning to level out if not reduce. Financially some middle-aged couples are in excellent circumstances for the first time in their lives. However, many find that the pressures of providing for children who now have matured and whose demands are greater, as well as the beginning problems of assisting elderly parents, while at the same time trying to establish a retirement program overwhelming. Such pressures can result in severe anxiety, depression, and marital conflict as couples begin to fight over priorities. Great inner turmoil can occur as each individual attempts to resolve his or her inner needs and the needs of those around them.

Occupational

As has already been indicated, many middle-aged individuals must face the fact that they have reached the pinnacle of their careers, that many of their hopes of greater financial reward, higher status, and success are not likely to occur. For many, technological changes have begun to outstrip the individual's knowledge with many younger people coming along who have knowledge beyond that of the middle-aged person. For some, occupations have become routine, tiresome, and he finds himself with little motivation to go to work as he goes through this time in life. Kerckhoff (1976) points out that a middle-aged person may feel caught between his job responsibilties and family responsibilities. They have entered into an exciting time in their career where they are able to do many important and creative tasks. This conflicts with childrearing, marital, and other social responsibilities.

For many traditional American families the husband has been the primary wage earner. However, a higher percentage of married women between the ages of 35 and 60 are employed outside of the

home. While there was once a decrease in working for women between the ages of 40 and 60, that decrease no longer occurs. This
change may be connected to the role reversal process, which will be
discussed later. Conflicts between whose work will take priority as well
as the changing power structure in a family as couples move from early
middle age to late middle age can result in very significant conflict
between husband and wife.

Sexual Changes

A separate chapter covers the issue of sexual changes and counseling, therefore, this topic will be briefly discussed in this chapter.
Among the most significant fears of aging is the fear of loss of sexual
capacities and experiences. In spite of the work pioneered by Masters
and Johnson indicating older couples can have active and rewarding
sexual lives, many remain terrified and filled with myths about loss of
sexual potentials. It is not unusual for males during the middle years to
have episodes of impotence or retarded ejaculation. For some males
who at the same time are facing loss of physical strength, perhaps
retirement, and other reminders of aging, this sexual episode can have
dramatic effects resulting in more significant sexual problems such as
secondary impotence or the withdrawal from sexual activity altogether.
Some males who respond in such a negative manner may also attempt
to regain their youth by seeking sexual affairs (especially with younger
women) as one last ditch effort to prove their sexual worth. At the
same time their wives often feel a profound sense of rejection which is
aggravated by their own diminishing physical attributes. As breasts
begin to sag, hips begin to spread, and wrinkles begin to form this can
create panic in the female. Subtle hostility can often be observed
between husband and wife resulting from their sense of sexual frustration, rejection, and helplessness. This may precipitate impulsive separations and divorces in an effort to desperately regain ones sense of
sexual potency and beauty through the eyes of a new lover. When
these new alliances prove to be less rewarding than one had hoped, it
is not uncommon for the middle-aged individual to either react with
depression or abandonment of close interpersonal relationships. Depending on the individual's prior history, the reduction in sexual
capacities as well as the loss of physical beauty may not result in any
significant symptoms. If the individual has a well-integrated personality
and has learned to evaluate himself realistically and function in life
using a wide range of skills, such losses are taken in stride. However,
individuals who have learned to feel secure primarily via sexual and
physical reassurance often having a significant narcissistic process in
their personalities will frequently panic at any loss of these characteristics. While it is true that our society values youth and tends to over

emphasize beauty and sexual potency, most people manage to get through the middle years with relative grace and ease with only a minimal sense of loss.

Role Reversal

An important process that occurs during the middle years is role reversal. This role reversal occurs in two areas: first between the middle-aged person and their parents, and then later between the middle-aged person and their children. As the middle-aged couple's parents begin to age there is often a shift in dependency so that they become parents to their parents. This role reversal resulting from loss of confidence, failing health, loss of financial resources, etc., creates a significant shift in the relationship balance. The middle-aged couple are often caught between a sense of duty, resentment, and guilt. There may have been some distance between the parents and children for a time. If this has happened, their having to get reinvolved with their parents may release old hostilities which had long been buried. The resentment at having to give up financial resources is also quite significant. Furthermore, there is a sadness and difficulty in adapting as they are forced to view their parents who were once strong, powerful, and competent as now less so and very needy. This may result in either an overestimate of the degree of loss of the parents capacity or denial that they require any help at all. Most often there is a hope that if one takes enough action the parents can be restored to their old selves. Differences in values between parents and their middle-aged children often come to the front during these times when important decisions must be made and yet the two subsystems are unable to reach agreement on important priorities. Later in middle age the couple may become more aware that they have begun to have similar dependencies on their children. At first they fight this system being aware of what had previously occurred with their own parents, only to later find that they need to have some dependencies on their own children. It is of course not true that this occurs to all parents and their children.

Another major role reversal which frequently occurs is that beween husband and wife. During the childrearing years the husband's position of power is often at its peak with the wife's dependency being greatest. When the children are launched the wife's power in decision making and influence in the family begins to change. Often the male is older than the female and his decline occurs first. He is no longer as strong and he may become more retiring, quiet, and submissive. Peterson (1968) has suggested that part of the reason for the wife becoming more domineering during these later years may be connected to endocrinological changes. He points out that the wife loses more of her estrogen and produces more testosterone. The husband on the other hand is constantly producing less testosterone. In addition, sociological influences including the loss of status when a male leaves his work and is no longer the primary breadwinner resulting in a position whereby he gives very little to the family in roles that were once traditional for him may create important relationship changes. If a wife is earning more than her husband, his control, input, and influence tends to be considerably reduced. If a wife has been resentful of the way her husband previously handled his role she may use this time as a way to get even or at least to let out some of her hostilities. Once again it should be mentioned that not all middle-aged people go through this process of role reversal either with their parents, their children, or their spouses. However, if they do, it is extremely important that they be able to face the meaning of these changes, understand them well, and learn to handle them in nondestructive fashions.

Facing Death

At some time during the middle years each individual begins to add up certain inescapable facts. For one, the individual realizes that in all likelihood he has lived more than one-half of his life—that he is closer to the moment of his death than he is to the moment of his birth. The onset may be related to death of parents, aging of parents, death of friends, some traumatic event in the individual's health such as a heart attack, leaving home of the last child, or merely an awareness that one's life has clear limitations. It is a major fact in the developmental cycle in every individual that he must at some time come to the realization of his mortality. As each individual progresses through time and grows older his awareness of the possibility of his own death becomes more and more clear. Depending on individual history one may handle this circumstance with ease and a sense of peacefulness. On the other hand, this awareness can lead to despair or panic leading to inappropriate decision making or at attempts to deny this fact and recapture earlier vitality. The profound meaning of this existential moment may not be clearly recognized and is not discussed with his or her mate, so that those around are unable to understand the meaning of seemingly inappropriate behaviors and mood swings.

Retirement

Retirement as an issue for the middle years is a complex one. While some look forward to retirement as a period of relief and joy and the opportunity to travel, relax, or do other things in their lives they had not previously had the opportunity to do, others face retirement with a sense of despair, sorrow, and panic. If one has received great meaning, recognition, and involvement from his or her life's work the loss of this can indeed leave a major void. This added to the loss of financial resources which occurs to the overwhelming majority of Americans can create a whole series of problems. As work careers come to an end the individual faces a number of role shocks. As has been mentioned earlier, the husband and wife may find themselves in role reversals or, should they both be at home all day, they may be unable to tolerate the constant presence of the other. It should also be noted that by age 65 many individuals are no longer living with their spouses as a result of the death of a mate or divorce. Typically those who have remained with their spouses have begun to reduce their expectations and accommodate.

At this time in life some of those who have been alone attempt to find a companion for their remaining years. These "retirement marriages" also have potential for great difficulties. They are entered into at a time when individuals are not likely to want to make any significant changes in their life style. In addition, many of the new husbands and wives have a tendency to compare their new spouse with a previous spouse only being able to identify that which is missing in the new relationship. These retirement marriages also often face difficulty in relationship to the children of the couple who are having difficulty adapting to their parent's marriage. Although there has been very little study of these marriages the limited research which has been done suggests that marriages contracted during the retirement years have about the same degree of satisfaction as other marriages.

Marital Issues

It must be emphasized that the nature of marital adjustment in the middle years is likely to be very much like the adjustment of couples during other phases of their life. However, for the purposes of this chapter it is necessary to point out some difficulties that are typical, or at least more likely to arise during the middle years than at other times in the individual's life-span. Studies of marriage during the middle years have characteristically suggested there is an important disenchantment, disengagement, reduced communication, and often significant disillusionment (Pineo, 1961). Other authors, Blood and Wolfe (1960) and Cuber and Harroff (1965), have also indicated a general decline in marital satisfaction during the first 20 years of marriage with many unions, resulting in hostile interaction on the one hand or passive-congenial and apathetic interaction on the other. There were, of course, in all studies some marriages which remained vital, alive, and at the core of the couple's sense of aliveness. It is also during the middle years that children are launched from the home, leaving the empty nest. This can create a significant void, especially for those whose primary role has been that of parent or those who have failed to develop in other areas in their lives. A sense of despair and emptiness often follows. This experience with marriage along with the other factors previously discussed such as occupational awareness of limitations and physical decline, etc., may lead the individual to raise questions as to whether he or she should remain in the current marriage or try to find one last chance at happiness. Some decide to stay, but do so with a sense of resentment or cynical resignation. Kerckhoff (1976) states:

> "Marriage counselors have long noted when trouble arises in middle age marriages, it is often related to the boredom of the union, not to its traumatic qualities. Infidelity, alcoholism, hypochondria, and divorce and suicide must, in middle age, be as much related to the deadliness of the marital union as to any pain it can produce."

The extremely important decisions considered during this time of life produce self-examination characteristic of adolescent identity struggles. At this time many couples must begin to make important choices on how they want to live, do they want to change their life style, how do they want to allocate their resources, and how do they want to face the future together? In terms of marriage this is not an easy time, for husbands and wives may not reach conclusions about the same things at the same time and each has his or her own individual struggle along with that of their marital identity.

Self-examination

During the middle years many if not all individuals go through a period of self-examination, a re-examination of values. What one hopes to get out of life, what has happened thus far, and what is left in life. Questions such as: Who am I?, Where am I going?, Have I been true to my self?, What have I missed?, Have I been worshipping false gods?, etc., are very common. It is almost impossible for a middle-aged individual not to go through this thought process, for if he does not come to it spontaneously, certainly in discussions with his friends these issues will surely arise. This urge to re-examine oneself has been called middlescence and is in many ways similar to the identity crisis attributed to adolescence. There are probably many reasons why this identity crisis occurs at this time in life. For one, most individuals have now lived long enough to have experienced what their marriage is going to be, many have spent a life of accumulating things and establishing comforts which do not satisfy to the degree that they had hoped. The accumulation of these material items has not brought recognition, status, and a sense of well-being as one dreams. Second, in our society there has been an unrealistic view of marriage. With the disenchantment or loss of intimacy that occurs over the years for many people this begins to devleop pressure to do something about one's life. There is still a lingering feeling that one can somehow achieve that form of marital bliss that has been advertised. Third, the middle years are in a sense a time when one is truly at the middle of life. It is possible to look back at the past and see how one has developed and come to full maturity, and at the same time look to the future and what it holds for each individual and for the couple. This rethinking of life, reassessing of goals, and evaluation of one's contributions that have occurred up to now, along with what each of us wants to do with it in the future, is often done at this time in life. Other issues also contribute to this point in time when a person is likely to do this reassessing. For example, we have already mentioned that normally one has reached both financial and occupational limitations. In addition, there is the inevitable physical decline which can precipitate re-examination. All of these issues compounded by the fact that we live in a youth-oriented society which does not revere aging or wisdom and has only moderate respect for experience has potential for precipitating an enormous sense of loss. Once again, depending on the individual's typical way of handling crises in his or her life, the degree to which individuals and couples have been resourceful in establishing a wide range of experience and skills in large part determines how they will handle this crisis. For some it will become a depressing, self-defeating, complaining system with little action that will lead to any constructive solutions. For others there will be a sense of panic and attempts to deny the realities of life which they will act out by suddenly filing for divorce, having affairs with younger people, trying to cover up their age with youthful dress, make-up, and hair styles, by over exercising, or many of the other behavioral means of recapturing youth. For others there will be a graceful transition and maturing, for these people are at the height of their capacities in terms of their contribution to society and connection to people around them. For couples who are able to understand and who appreciate the normal flow of life, the middle life self-examination will be a smooth, pleasant, and maturing experience.

Physical Decline

Beginning at least in the early 40's physiological changes begin to become more noticeable and important. Perhaps a decrease in general energy levels is noticed first which then affects self-image and accordingly the adaptation process will begin for him or her. As energy is reduced it can affect occupational life, financial circumstances, social life, sex, as well as one's self-esteem. Around the same time some notice that there are also many sensory losses. There is usually the beginning of diminished eye sight, perhaps impaired hearing, and a general reduction in response time to the environment. There is some increased difficulty in reading, hearing, and fine coordination. At the same time, sexual capabilities are beginning to reduce with the individual noticing a slight loss of interest and sexual capacity. He may even experience episodes of impotence. In addition, physical health in general may start to decline. Beginning chronic conditions may assert themselves such as heart disease, arthritis, and diabetes, along with the most common complaint of chronic fatigue. Similarly most individuals find that their response and recovery from both illness and injury tend to be slower and in many conditions not complete.

Important endocrine system changes normally occur during this time in life. There are usually some alterations in the hormonal balances with women facing the loss of fertility, with many having menopausal symptoms. She faces an important physiological change that also has great psychological, personal, and marital meaning for her. While the same changes in the male are less clear there also appear to be changes connected with hormonal changes during the mid-years.

In addition to the vital physiological changes, cosmetic changes that occur also are obvious and can have profound meaning. Loss of hair, changes in the body weight, body size, reduced sexual attractiveness, along with noticeable signs of aging in the skin and muscles can create a most painful awareness for many individuals of their decline. It is generally at this time that the omnipotence of youth is lost and the all too real awareness of one's vulnerability is clearly perceived. Once again the actual occurrence of these physical characteristics may be much less important than individual and interpersonal reaction to such changes. It is also important to recognize the importance of each kind of change to a specific individual and couple. In any case, the awareness as well as the process of physiological decline is of basic importance in understanding any other processes involved in middle age interrelationship processes.

Broader Issues

Before establishing a treatment plan the clinician might find it helpful to consider some of the following broader issues which transcend the specific issues previously discussed.

In the treatment of any given population whether the couples are newly married, premarital, retired, middle age, or couples from various subcultures, the clinician must be careful not to take the couple out of their own history. That is, even though in this chapter we are dealing with couples in their middle years, these couples must be considered in light of their individual and marital histories. If an individual continues to have significant unresolved conflicts then these conflicts are likely to manifest themselves during the middle years. The typical way an individual has handled new experiences in life, or negative changes in life, is generally predictive on how he will handle situations of the middle years. If a couple has developed a history whereby they have not communicated well during the early years, they have grown apart to the point where they cannot be of assistance to each other, cannot exchange appropriate dependency, then when developmental issues of the middle years arise they will find them more difficult to deal with than had they been the type of couple who managed to stay alive and growing throughout their marital history. It would, therefore, seem wise that the clinician take a look at the individual and marital history of the couple. How have they handled new experiences, change, crises, decision making, etc.? How have they attacked their problems? What are their coping mechanisms? Have they attempted to prepare for each new stage in life? Have these experiences flowed for them easily? Do they maintain a mutual respect and intimacy throughout, or is this negative system brought to counseling characteristic of the way they have handled things? Many authors suggest that in addition to the developmental life cycle of individuals and couples in counseling, it is also wise to take a look at the developmental cycles of their parents in order to gain some understanding of the continuing life pattern for those people. In any case, the warning is not to take the issues of middle age and make those paramount and independent from the total being of a couple.

If an individual or couple were to be forced to face the loss of important fantasies or were to come to the realization that their expectations were not likely to be fulfilled, this would require them to do some reorganization or at least re-evaluation in their lives. If, for example, a young couple were counting on the husband going to medical school, but he was unable to do so as a result of a sudden financial loss or inability to gain admittance to a medical school, this couple would be forced to re-evaluate their lives, re-establish their goals, in short, this would be a significant crisis and a point of important change for them. This is just the circumstance that couples in the middle years are faced with. The hopes of our youth, the hopes of our parents, the expectations of our friends and loved ones must all be re-evaluated during this time. During the middle years most people are faced with the realization that that which they had expected of themselves in this life, that which was fantasied could be achieved or experienced is not likely to take place in some aspects of their lives. Many symptoms the clinician sees can be connected to this inability to cope well with loss of fantasy and unfulfilled expectations. Some will attempt to make old expectations come true. Others will attempt to change expectations dramatically. For many the realization that this is part of the normal process of life will flow easily and they will experience little or no difficulty with this problem. Some sudden personality changes or behaviors which seem inconsistent may be traced to the inability to reconcile life expectations and reality experiences.

It is difficult to live in Western society without being exposed to and perhaps seduced by myths of both aging and marriage. When a couple enters a counselor's office it is hoped that the counselor will be aware of these myths in order not to allow misinformation to distort his own point of view as well as helping the couple avoid traps inherent in such stereotypes. Although we have presented many of the potential problems in the process of aging for couples, these problems are not necessarily as extensive or damaging as many would anticipate. Some typical myths connected with aging are: (1) "As individuals reach middle age they clearly begin to lose their potency as human beings. They lose sexual potency, they lose memory, they lose their effectiveness around them, and by the time individuals reach age 65 they have very little left to do but to wait for their death." If someone age 30 forgets something, they are just very busy. If someone age 60 forgets something, they are bordering on senility. Neugarten (1964) studied mental health and adaptability of individuals ranging from age 40 through age 65. During these years she was not able to find a process of decreasing mental or emotional flexibility. (2) "With aging comes the loss of the opportunities of life and possibilities for gratification." This is an inappropriate evaluation since it is not a loss of opportunity that we are talking about, but a shift in opportunities to new or altered potentials. In many ways the older individual loses some of the constraints required during the early years of his or her life. (3) "Older people dislike both themselves and their age." Positive self-image is built throughout life and is not something that suddenly occurs during the middle years. Those who grow up with a positive self-image are likely to maintain this self-image during their middle and later years. In addition, many individuals also state that they enjoy the age they are and that this is a time of pleasure and enjoyment for them, not one necessarily to be viewed with terror. (4) "Older people are lonely people." Clearly there are some people who live alone as they age; those who have lost their spouses, who have not developed friendships over their lives, and lack personal resources tend to be lonely. These people often have tended to be lonely throughout their lives or at least have had difficulty in being active in maintaining relationships prior to this time in their lives. The overwhelming majority of individuals and couples (certainly up through the age of 65) have family, friends, and experiences which fill their lives. (5) "Retirement will lead to deterioration and depression." The overwhelming majority of people who have retired do not report this as their experience. There may be difficulties attached to it, but the inevitability of depression and deterioration is a myth. (6) "There is a precipitous loss of enjoyment of life with aging." There appears to be in many people's minds an attitude that old people do not enjoy food, or music, or experience, that they cannot take in new things, they cannot take up new habits, they cannot develop. This is one of the most devastating myths of a youth-oriented culture. Some hobbies that couples have had can be expanded and those that must be given up due to physical loss can be substituted with new and interesting experiences that the couple have wanted to do for years. In any case, questionnaires given to couples do not support the conclusion that they are not involved with and enjoying their lives. Generally speaking, studies have shown that flexibility in the ability to get involved in new activities and experiences, flexibility of mental processes in solving new problems, in growth in diverse areas of life, giving satisfaction to the self, the ability to use one's physical being and to enjoy life in spite of some difficulties, the freedom to give oneself to others, the satisfaction with one's own physical being, and a general satisfaction and sense of effectiveness in adapting to life's circumstances, appear to be not very different between those who are age 40 and those who are age 65 (Neugarten, 1964).

Another important set of concepts to keep in mind for the clinician are that individuals who are in their middle years are still after the same things and have the same needs as others do, even though they may be facing some specific problems associated with middle age, *i.e.*, we all have needs for recognition, productivity, involvement, response, security, etc. We have needs to interrelate well with those around us, to have an effective relationship with our mate and our community, and to be at peace with ourselves. The important issue is that individuals coming in as a result of not having these needs met may or may not have this issue brought to light as a result of middle age process. Furthermore, the clinician cannot attempt to work with individuals or couples in such a way that they would be required to give up any of these fundamental needs in their lives.

Finally it should be mentioned that we are all part of a larger network which includes our children, our parents, our friends, our community, and any important others that are connected to us in our lives. The clinician is at a significant disadvantage in that he is generally treating only a part of the social system. At the very least it is the clinician's and the couple's distinct advantage to find out as much as possible about the surrounding social system of which the couple is a part. What changes have occurred in that system and what impact has the change in that system had on the couple. What changes in the couple will then impact on the larger system. This systems models once again helps the clinician avoid the trap of concentrating too much on some specific event connected with middle age, whereas the larger system may be more important to what brings the couple for counseling.

Treatment

Essentially, treatment strategies employed by the clinician on the population under consideration would be the same as applied to most other populations, but included the specific issues connected with the process of personal and marital development during the middle years. Peterson (1968) outlines the pivotal tasks of middle age as the following: (1) "psychological adjustment to the loss of parental role; (2)

achievement of a new type of independent friendship with married children; (3) acceptance and cultivation of the essential role of grandparents; (4) extension of the network of friendships and organizational contacts to make up for the loss of intimacy with child launching; (5) successful coping with the fact of the male and female physical and psychological climacteric changes; (6) making sexual pleasure consonant with levels of energy and libido; (7) conservation of energy and cultivation of appropriate health habits in a well-balanced budget of exercise, hobbies, and interests; (8) expansion of intellectual interests with an upward reach to keep in touch with change; and (9) development of a life pattern that will form the foundation for successful retirement."

The clinician will need to approach these tasks, as well as any other problems brought to the office, using a wide perspective. First, the clinician may well have to offer direct advice or be a source of referral for his clients in several specific areas. Information in legal matters such as preparing wills, the disposition of property, and handling of legal matters for aged parents, etc., are common issues during the middle years. Financial matters also can become extremely important. Allocation of funds, depending on the demands of children or parents as well as the loss of financial income, requires planning. Medically, many couples need specific advice on health care, diet, and treatment of the process of aging. It is extremely important that the couple have a physician who understands, enjoys, and is in the practice of treating people who are in this process. It is incumbent on a clinician to be familiar with some aspects of the financial, legal, and medical concerns of his clients. Obviously, one of the best helps the clinician can be is as a referral source. He must know attorneys, physicians, and financial advisors who are competent, sympathetic, and within the financial resources of couples who seek his counsel. In addition, awareness of community resources including nursing homes, retirement assistance, housing, social security benefits, old age assistance, volunteer programs, and social outlets are necessary information for the counselor to have at his disposal. Should the counselor find this information is necessary, but not feel secure in offering such advice, once again to have proper referral resources available is a basic requirement. In order to obtain these referral sources it might be helpful to contact a local university or college, particularly the departments of sociology, social work, psychology, or psychiatry which may have a gerontology specialist or center available. In addition, the American Association of Retired Persons and the National Retired Teachers Association (jointly located at 1909 K Street NW, Washington, D.C. 20049) will provide useful information. This use of environmental manipulation or reality counseling is frequently necessary but rarely sufficient. Treatment plans centered around reality issues, but which exclude the dynamics of both the individual and the couple, rarely provide adequate assistance for couples.

It is helpful for couples to be aware of their reactions to the issues of middle age. It may be necessary to work on communication, old hostilities, old versus new roles, and systems of decision making and problem solving in general before the tasks of middle age and their impact can be fully explored. It is also rarely the best form of treatment to center counseling around one member of the dyad. Assuming that both mates are available it is generally wisest to include them both in the counseling process. Even though one member of the couple may be complaining of significant symptoms such as depression or anxiety, it must be remembered that they are both part of a system, and that whatever affects one can significantly affect the other. Furthermore, the other's behavior may be significantly involved in the production and maintenance of the problems brought to the counselor's attention. Some counselors may find it helpful to review each of the specific issues suggested earlier in this chapter in terms of the couple's awareness, reaction to, and solutions for them.

For some couples it may be necessary to do a much more in depth form of therapy. The counselor may wish to look into their individual and marital histories, to explore such matters as the nature in which they have developed their dependencies, whether they maintain a highly immature dependency system, or whether they have grown in such ways that they are able to handle dependencies in some areas but not others. Long-standing individual neurotic process, as well as long-standing inappropriate contracts between couples, may have functioned well enough up to this period in their lives, but with the onset of the crises of middle age these balances frequently break down. For example, some couples are able to tolerate a very poor relationship development so long as there are children in the home, but when these children leave the couple is left without an escape mechanism for their guilts, angers, or unresolved conflicts. Both mental illness and suicide increase with age. Whether this is due to increasing pressures on the individual or to their lessened capacity to deal with their conflicts is difficult to say. In any case, this may well be precipitated by the pressures and tasks of middle age.

Beyond the typical attempt to "cure" problems, there is an orientation which has at its theoretical core an optimism about human growth. A system which seeks to build on strengths rather than the continuous uncovering of pathology is strongly recommended. The marital enrichment movement could have a most important impact on middle-aged couples. Counseling oriented toward the expansion of self, the use of physical, mental, intellectual, and social expansion of self has value. Emotional expansion of self, new forms of communication, assisting in new ways of connecting with other people and other places, expressing feelings in new and more authentic ways, trying new solutions, developing new interests, and encouraging curiosity about self, others, and life in general are typical enrichment concepts. The use of couples groups, preretirement groups, consciousness raising groups, and marriage enrichment groups, which are initially centered around the issues of middle age, is an effective means to reduce depression, anomie, and anxiety connected with the problems of middle-aged couples. Such groups also offer opportunities to bring in specialists who can help group members who would not ordinarily be able to seek such advice individually. The enrichment model may also help some counselors avoid a constriction attitude toward his clients as opposed to one of expansion and greater life experience.

In summary, a recommended treatment plan would include assistance with the specific environmental and reality issues associated with the middle years, a review of the individual and couple reaction to each of these issues both in their history as a couple as well as their individual developmental styles, and assistance with the usual skills required in relationship and in dealing with life, along with some possible individual personality growth, all of this having as its goal both the relief of stress and a direction toward personal and relationship enrichment.

REFERENCES

Blood, R. O., Jr., and Wolfe, D. M.: *Husbands and Wives: The Dynamics of Married Living*. The Free Press of Glencoe, New York, 1960.

Cuber, J., and Harroff, P.: The more total view: relationships among men and women of the upper middle class. Marriage and Family Living, **25**: 140–145, 1963.

Cuber, J., and Harroff, P.: *The Significant Americans*. Appleton Century, New York, 1965.

Kerckhoff, R. K.: Marriage and middle age. In *The Family Coordinator*, Vol. 25, pp. 5–11, January, 1976.

Neugarten, B.: *Personality in Middle and Late Life*. Atherton Press, New York, 1964.

Neugarten, B.: A new look at menopause. Psychology Today, **1**: No. 7, p. 43, 1966.

Peterson, J. A.: *Married Love in the Middle Years*. Association Press, New York, 1968.

Peterson, J. A.: *Marital and Family Therapy Involving the Aged*, October, 1971. (Prepared for the symposium of the Gerontology Society, Houston, Texas).

Peterson, J. A.: Therapeutic intervention in marital and family problems of aging persons. in *Professional Obligations and Approaches to the Aged*. (Schwartz, A. N., and Mensh, I. N., eds), Charles C Thomas, Illinois, 1974.

Pineo, P. C.: Disenchantment in the later years of marriage. Marriage and Family Living, **23**: 3–11, 1961.

WILLIAM C. NICHOLS, JR., Ed. D.

9

Counseling the Childless Couple

The voluntarily childless couple, the husband and wife who decide for reasons of their own not to have children, undoubtedly have become more common in our society in recent years. Because statistics are not kept on motivations, it is impossible to know the percentage of childless couples in our society who are without children because they wish to remain childless. What is known, however, is that a greater proportion of the childlessness today is voluntary than in the past. Consequently, counselors and helping professionals from several fields are being called upon more often than previously to help the voluntarily childless couple live comfortably with their decision not to have children.

Noxious Social Attitudes

Counseling childless couples in the past tended to be a comparatively simple matter. Traditionally, couples received a very clear-cut message about childbearing, and that was that they were to have children. The majority did so in the past, and the majority do so today. Married couples who did not have children generally were assumed to be incapable of having them or were thought to have something wrong with them because they did not wish to have children. In brief, they often were regarded as being either incapable of having offspring or of being selfish. These attitudes of family and society toward the childless are repeated here because to a significant degree they still are found today.

Incapable: "They Would if They Could."

Pity frequently is a major social attitude toward the childless, toward those regarded as unfortunate because they do not have children.

Within families, it was not and is not uncommon to have the childless daughter-in-law regarded with less favor than the daughters and daughters-in-law who do produce them. The male, when family information or speculation places the responsibility on him for the infertile situation, often is regarded as something less than a real man. Childlessness in such settings is something to be explained. The assumption frequently prevails that, "It's too bad about John and Mary. They're such a nice couple. They would have children if they could."

For many in our society, including some counselors, it is unthinkable that a couple should desire not to have children, to remain child free as some have recently put it. Therefore, when a couple stay married for more than a few years without children, the tendency among some segments of the society is to assume that the situation is involuntary.

Selfish: "They Should Have Children."

Once people become convinced that a couple have no barriers to prevent them from having children except their own desire to remain childless, there is likely to be a switch from explaining in a pitying way why they are childless over to asking, "Why don't you?" Accompanying this question frequently is the attitude that they are selfish and think only of themselves. The assumption still runs deep, as it has traditionally, in much of the population that childlessness is a deviant state, that the couple who do not have children because they do not wish to have them are selfish, self-indulgent, materialistic, pleasure-seeking individuals who do not fulfill their responsibilities as married adults.

This is particularly true in view of the fact that we have become, as many have observed in almost cliche fashion, a "child-centered society." The parents of today's childbearing and childrearing young adults are the first generation in our society literally to be "caught in the middle" between being expected to obey and honor their own parents by being productive and reflecting credit upon them, while simultaneously being expected as the first child-centered generation to give their own children a prime place in their lives. The pressure to bow to both generations—the parental and the child—is unprecedented. Coming from a background in which children were expected to be "seen and not heard," we have reared children that the society has pressed us to "listen to and understand."

The counselor who fits into this situation—and that includes many of us who are in professional helping roles today—well may have to grapple with his or her own attitudes that would push the young marrieds toward having children or being regarded as either unfortunate or selfish. At best, the counselor may be ambivalent about the matter of voluntary childlessness.

The Counselor's Own Attitudes

The counselor who has reached middle age or older typically may have to recognize that he/she partakes of attitudes that place high value on childbearing and filial devotion and loyalty. The younger physician, psychologist, or counselor from another profession may have to recognize that he/she carries within conflicting attitudes concerning childbearing, being open to the possibility of voluntary childlessness on a cognitive level while being quite traditional on an emotional level. Admittedly, it is not this simple; some older professionals may be quite open and permissive on the childbearing question and some younger professionals may be more traditional than Methuselah, the Biblical oldest man.

Whatever the age of the counselor or helping professional, it is vitally important to understand and acknowledge that the counselor's own attitudes play a significant role in his/her work with young couples who have decided to remain childless. Similarly, it is important to understand that the prerogative of deciding whether or not children shall be borne rests with the married couple and not with the counselor.

As one professional person put it, "I have recognized that when it comes to human behavior, I have three different attitudes or codes within myself. One is the code for myself. A second is the code for others. A third is for my children, who are both others and a part of myself; they fit into a unique third category." Such recognition is vitally important for all counselors. To require of others the same things one requires of oneself is not especially fair or sensible. To recognize what we personally consider important, desirable, and so on is essential if we are to work with others in an effective way. Sorting out our own values and attitudes from the things that others value and do is not only desirable but also vital if we are to be open to working with young couples concerning their childbearing decisions and behaviors as capable professionals. It is equitable and truly professional to become aware of our own values and to segregate them from our work with others so that we serve as helpers and not as apologists and adherents of our own particular points of view.

Questions for Childless Couples

Once the counselor has been able to put aside his/her own attitudes and values and enters into working constructively with a married couple about their childbearing situation, it is important to know what questions to ask and what motivations to probe into with the couple.

Part of putting aside one's own attitudes and values involves recognizing that a childless couple may not have any problems regarding their childlessness that they either wish or need to take up with a counselor. The counselor should not make assumptions, in other words, about childless couples needing help. For some couples childlessness is not a problem, whatever concerns about it that they may have had already being resolved.

Those who do need some help may approach the professional in one of two ways with their concerns, either directly or indirectly. The first task of a counselor or other helping professional always is to ascertain what those who have come to him/her are seeking. "Why are you here?" is always the pertinent first question, whether asked that explicitly or phrased in another way. For those who do not state explicitly their problems and require some assistance from the counselor in order to elucidate the concerns that they have about childlessness, the counselor will need to listen sensitively to what they are saying, make his/her inferences, and ask the direct questions that lead the couple into uncovering and talking about their problems and reasons for seeking help.

As it emerges that the partners are struggling with some problems and questions about their own voluntarily childless state, it is important to probe into such matters as the following:

"What Are the Feelings of Each of You about Having Children?"

Are they in agreement about remaining childless? Or does one wish to remain childless and the other to change their game plan and situation and have children? It is important for each of the partners to speak for themselves and for themselves alone, not for their spouse. As they talk, one can watch for discrepancies between their verbal and nonverbal actions and for other indications that there is some conflict between them or within one of them individually with regard to the professed desire and agreement not to have children. Noting that such conflict is present does not mean necessarily that they will change their minds and decide to have children. On the contrary, it may indicate that they simply have some residual pockets of feelings that need to be worked through in order for them to live comfortably with their decision and situation.

Individuals typically have some ambivalence about many things and do not ever come to the point of completely resolving all of their feelings about them. The most that can be expected, if one is realistic, is for the ambivalence to be tipped primarily in one direction so that the decision stays slanted in that direction. Any person or couple who decides to remain childless may well retain some questions about the decision and some wishes that they could have it both ways. Working out such residual feelings may mean essentially helping them to recognize and to live with the fact that some ambivalence will always be present.

"Who Decided That You Would Not Have Children?"

Typically, the counselor may expect to find a variety of patterns prevailing concerning decision making about childbearing if we are to trust what little research we have on this matter. This often is a sensitive question for the female, who may have become resentful at continually being asked to explain why she does not want children. It is important to convey to both partners that the question is not intended as a criticism, direct or implied, but as a request for information in order to assist the counselor's understanding of them and their wishes and needs.

The question of who makes or made the decision may not be separable from the next two questions given below.

"How Was the Decision Made Not to Have Children?"

The decision may have been made by one of the partners and concurred in by the other. It may have been made by the female, for example, when she was in her teen-age years, even before marriage had been seriously considered (Veevers, 1973). She eventually married a male who accepted her decision against childbearing as a part of her. On the other hand, the decision may have been made by the couple in concert, being arrived at during their courtship or subsequent to marriage. Whatever the timing of the decision, the more it was a bilateral matter rather than a unilateral one, the more likelihood it would seem that there would remain no feeling that one of the partners had been coerced or seduced into accepting a previously made decision.

Another important aspect of this question is that of whether it was consciously made or came about as a result of drifting and the acceptance of tacit assumptions on the part of the spouses. It is not unusual to find that couples have drifted into a situation without ever examining openly and directly how each of them feels about it. "Did you talk about it? Have you talked about it enough so that both of you are satisfied that you know how the other feels and that he/she understands how you feel?" If not, exploration of such feelings may need to be conducted with the counselor. It may turn out that a considerable amount of energy has been tied up unnecessarily in refraining from dealing with the childlessness matter because of anxiety over how the partner may have felt about the decision.

"When Was the Decision Made Not to Have Children?"

If this question has not been answered earlier in the interview with the couple as they dealt with other questions, the counselor may wish to pose it at some point along the way. As implied above, there are some differences between a pattern in which the female decided in her adolescence not to have children and a pattern in which the couple decided together sometime after marriage to remain childless. Research by Veevers (1973) has disclosed that there is with some couples a postponement pattern in which they temporarily postpone childbearing and eventually find that they have moved to a stage in which they are never going to have children. Such a couple may be unable to pinpoint the time when the transition came from postponement to permanent childlessness, but be in agreement on their implicit decision and be content with it (Veevers, 1973).

"If there is disagreement . . . " If the partners are in disagreement about whether to continue with their childless pattern, what are the feelings that each has about the disagreement? What effects do they think the disagreement is having on their relationship? How have they attempted to deal with the disagreement? How are they handling it?

What the Counselor is Looking for

The counselor is interested in determining the depth of the feelings of the marital partners. Specifically, he/she is concerned with ascertaining the degree of healthy, mature choice in the decision of the couple to remain childless (or to have children, in another case), as opposed to reactions of rebellion, anger, and alienation with regard to their own parents, how much mutuality there is in the decision, the amount of stress that may or may not be present as a result of family or other social attitudes and pressures that run counter to the couple's decision, and how well the couple is coping with external pressures and attitudes such as those that view them as inadequate or selfish.

Couples today frequently get a double message: it's valuable not to have children (because of population resources problems), but such childlessness is for somebody else, not you. If the partners with whom the counselor is working are receiving such a double-edged message, what are they doing in response? The most important source of such messages probably is the family of origin of each of the young persons.

That Older Generation

When counselors deal with a couple about their childlessness, it is always wise to consider their relationship with their parents, the ties that they have with their mother and father. Particularly significant is the recognition that the young adults cannot be understood apart from their relationship to the older generation and perhaps even apart from their relationship with their grandparents. The interlocking of generations plays a role that must be deciphered as best we can in order for us to work out the pieces that play a part in the couple's decision to forego having children.

In exploring the relationship with the parents, one would do well to look for indications that there is estrangement or rejection of the parents, or rejection of their way of life, resentment about the manner and conditions in which the young wife and husband were reared. Similarly, one looks for attitudes of negation and resentment toward the siblings. Do Mary or John give indications that they feel that the parent/s neglected them in contrast to a brother or sister? Many such feelings may be present and should be looked for in searching out the meaning of the family relationships with the couple. Such attitudes and feelings may affect childbearing motivations in significant ways.

Bitterness, pain, or simply a firm resolve born out of such experiences may be enough to make the decision irreversible and the dealing with the parents or siblings problem ridden. The counselor's task is not that of persuading a couple either to have children or to refrain from having children (except in certain circumstances in which childbearing may be contraindicated for the sake of either wife or husband), but that of determining the nature of the couple's feelings and the relationship to the older generation and family of origin. A key issue here is that of determining whether the young married partners have obtained freedom from ties to parents and perhaps to siblings and grandparents to a sufficient degree to make their own decisions and to live with them as comparatively independent adult persons.

Parents and grandparents sometimes tend to assume that the decision of young adults concerning childbearing is a province in which they have some liberty and license to assert their opinions and wishes. Many, perhaps most, parents and parents-in-law at least tacitly, and sometimes explicitly, expect their child and his/her spouse to produce offspring. When such offspring are not forthcoming after a period of a few months or years, the parental generation may begin to bring various kinds of pressure upon the couple to produce children.

Not the least of the results that the pressure of older generations may produce is the feeling among the young married that they have failed their parents. Feelings of guilt and of disloyalty frequently are found in such situations.

The Other Side of Social Concern

A society has a deep and abiding interest in the replacement of its population and in the production of useful citizens. As a consequence of these and other factors, we have tended to focus our attention on the impact of the parent on the child and on the "duty" of married persons to produce children. Much less have we focused our attention on the impact of the child on the parents.

Only recently have we come to recognize that children are a mixed blessing. Research is beginning to accumulate that supports the idea that children bring stress to a marriage and may result in lessened satisfaction for married persons. Stated most simply, the research that is piling up shows that couples experience the highest degree of marital satisfaction before they have children and after the children leave home. In contrast to some of the earlier notions that the "empty nest" stage which occurs after children leave home is a period of stress, we are beginning to learn that marital satisfaction may increase following the children's departure and that at least some of the dissatisfaction that occurs with married persons in middle age may be related to other factors (Zemon-Gass and Nichols, 1975).

All of this, along with other things, should help the counselor to recognize that pressures placed on a young married couple to have children may be quite damaging to the couple, whether such pressures come from family, friends, society, or the counselor himself.

When a marital couple have decided that they do not wish to have children and desire to remain voluntarily childless the counselor has the task in my judgment of helping them to understand what they have chosen for themselves and how they can implement their decision in the most responsible way possible. (The same principle would apply if they had chosen to have children and sought help with matters attendant to that decision.) Although the counselor's own values may be involved here, it is impossible to avoid making value judgments and decisions in working with couples around such problems. Having helped John and Mary to examine the relevant facets of their decision, the counselor may be called on to assist them in differentiating themselves from the expectations and coercions of their parents, family, and other social groups.

There is such a thing as "healthy selfishness" in that persons need to learn how to differentiate themselves from others who would push them into taking or continuing roles that restrict their growth and development. The counselor frequently faces the difficult task of helping individuals to recognize that there is no solution to a given situation that would result in happiness for all parties who attach themselves to it; e.g., that doing what is best for themselves may result in making parents, siblings, or other close individuals unhappy.

Similarly, the counselor needs to recognize that many ideas that have been considered true and socially desirable may not be all that desirable. For example, it has been assumed by many that adult personalities are not fulfilled unless the adults become parents. While the primary socialization of children and the stabilization of adult personalities generally are found to occur together, it is more likely to be marriage rather than parenthood that tends to bring greater stability and satisfaction to chronologically adult males and females.

What the emphasis on having children often boils down to is not so much a question of benefitting the young married persons as it may be of trying to get them to do something that would fulfill the wishes and desires of others.

Childlessness and Sterilization

Some married couples are not in disagreement or in conflict over whether or not they will have children. They have no intention of having children, regardless of how others may feel about it and are perfectly content with the decision that they have made. They still face the question of how they will implement their choice to remain child-less. Inevitably, the matter of permanent contraception surfaces.

The recent popularity of vasectomy as a form of birth control has given rise to a new specialty or subspecialty, vasectomy counseling. Vasectomy counselors may be concerned with the psychological aspects of this procedure, with such things as the psychological health and motivation of the candidate which may serve as indicators of his reaction following the surgery. The vasectomy counselor also may be concerned with dealing with such questions as whether vasectomy works, whether it hurts, whether the man will be the same afterward, whether the physicians know what they are doing, whether the man can change his mind afterward, and others (Wright, 1972).

Counseling with marital partners on the issue of whether one of the partners is to be sterilized—and this is a two-way street now that female sterilization has become more feasible—carries the responsibility of helping them to recognize the ramifications of making a decision that involves both of them. Sterilization made solely on the basis of individual choice may lead to future difficulties.

As obvious as it may seem, for example, Robert may need to explore individually with the counselor his feelings about the fact that in deciding to undergo a vasectomy he is not merely cutting himself off from the opportunity to procreate, but also that he is deciding to do something that may affect his future relationship with his wife Lucy. Lucy also may need some sessions to explore her feelings about the matter. If Robert is able to recognize that he does not wish to pro-create, completely apart from his relationship with Lucy, he is in a much better position to proceed than if he is not able to do so. What if Lucy subsequently decides that she wishes to have a child? How will this affect her relationship with Robert and his with her? There is a possibility that she could divorce Robert and have a child by another male, or that she could conceive as a result of coitus with another male or by artificial insemination by donor. What does all of this do to Robert and Lucy? Exploration of the possibility of sterilization of one of the partners without involvement of the other partner is a risky business insofar as the relationship of the married couple is concerned. It well may be that some couples will decide to have both partners sterilized. Such a decision would not be the most unusual marital contract on record.

Robert and Lucy, in the foregoing example, had no children and no intention of having any at any point in the future. Their motivations were basically individualistic and selfish, and they felt no guilt about not having children or about desiring to use their time and talents in order to fulfill their materialistic wishes. Equally important, they had decided individually before meeting the other that they did not wish to have children. Robert had a vasectomy and both were satisfied with that mode of birth control because Lucy's decision not to have children was as strong as his intention not to procreate. Their decision was a sound one for them.

Not all situations that the counselor encounters are as simple as that of Robert and Lucy. What are the reactions of the counselor who finds that in the couple before him a considerable amount of disagreement exists or that there had been a change of mind on the part of one or both partners following sterilization? For example, a couple now 30 years of age decided early in their marriage that they wished to have no children and the wife had a tubal ligation. How is the counselor to deal with the situation, including his own feelings about a physician's actions in tying off the tubes of a 24-year-old female some 6 years earlier, now that the husband has decided he wishes to have children? Such a situation probably will call for referral to an experienced marital or individual psychotherapist who can work with one or both of the young persons over an extended period of time.

Living Without Children

What do couples do who decide to remain childless. This question should not be construed as implying that the childless couple must find something to fill a void in their lives and relationship. On the contrary, many childless couples do not give any evidence of missing anything significant from their lives as a result of having no children. There are childless couples for whom the designation "child free" is a very accurate description of how they feel about their situation. Some couples, however, who do not have children find that they do have a void and set about consciously or unconsciously to fill that spot. Those couples are the ones who may need the help of a counselor. Some will feel the void out of their own personal dynamics and others will be feeling the pressure of being regarded by friends and relatives as deviant because they are childless.

Active participation in organizations whose aims are opposed to childbearing or to extensive childbearing provides an outlet for some couples. For a few, joining such organizations as Zero Population Growth (ZPG) or organizing their life around not having children and thus rendering a social service is helpful. The number of couples for whom this proves therapeutic appears to be small. The same thing holds for the National Organization for Nonparents (NON). The counselor cannot assume that the childless couple he is working with will find satisfaction and meaning in such organizational activities and endeavors. Rather, he/she must seek to ascertain the motivation of a couple for remaining childless and work from that point to help them find the meaning that they desire. Referring all childless couples to ZPG or NON is no more appropriate than suggesting that every individual who has problems with alcohol should go to Alcoholics Anonymous or sending every person who is using drugs to Synanon. Some will be helped by such organizations and some will not. It may be that engaging in the activities of such organizations is a phase in the lives of some childless couples that loses its meaning with the passage of time and is replaced with the wish and need to do something else.

Some who remain childless may feel the need to have some contact with children. Adoption may be a viable option and solution for a few couples. Again, it is less than wise to assume that a given couple may have any need or desire to adopt children. Those who do—and this refers to the husband and wife who express a preference for such a course and whose wish appears to hold up under careful examination and to be separate from their desire to escape family or social pressure—may be referred to a reputable adoption agency for assistance. At the same time, they may need continuing help in probing their own motives and reactions to taking children into their home and life.

Other childless couples who manifest a desire to have contact with children may do so for shorter periods. Not all marital partners wish to take on the task of rearing children, their own or adopted children, or of having contact with youngsters for the majority of the 168 h in a week. Some find that they can fulfill their quota of desire and quotient of tolerance in a matter of an hour or so a week. Volunteer activities fill the bill quite neatly for such persons.

Others may work with children in their occupational pursuits, e.g., teaching school, and be completely fulfilled. Professionals should think twice before speaking disparagingly about the motives or contributions of such individuals. There are persons engaged in teaching and working closely with children in primary and secondary schools or in preschool and day care centers who derive vicarious enjoyment from the behaviors and achievements of children and who do so in a quite healthy fashion.

Similarly, there are individuals who can spend a few hours each week sharing with a youngster as a Big Brother or Big Sister in a relationship that is healthy and helpful for both the otherwise deprived child and the adult who is content with limited amounts of contact and responsibility involving children. This is not to imply that all adults who serve in such roles can tolerate children or adolescents only for limited periods, but it is to say that such structured relationships can be exceedingly helpful for some adults and children. Primarily, the task here is one of fitting the needs of children and adults as closely as possible.

Other adults do not desire or need contact with children. Some can either "take them or leave them" insofar as children are concerned. Still others would prefer to leave them. Everything that is known about good mental health principles and sound personality development would indicate that such persons should not be coerced into having children or having contact with them. Both generations are benefitted by being left apart in such situations. While the matter is far more complex than one in which the observation can be made that some persons like spinach and others are allergic to it, there is a similarity in that there is no particular rational reason why all persons should like or enjoy children.

The married couples who do not care to have children or desire to be around them can, in many instances, simply set up a life style and pattern which does not include children. They can pour the interest and energy which otherwise would go into children into other things. This channeling of emotional and physical interest and activity into things other than children need not be a matter of second choice and poor substitution or anything of that nature. On the contrary, it may be a matter of healthy choice for some couples, their focus and goal being different than that of couples who choose to have children. As difficult as it may be for some professionals to recognize, this may be a rational and mature choice for some partners to make.

A Concluding Observation

There are no good reasons why a voluntarily childless couple should not be able to obtain help from those of us in the helping professions in implementing their decision. The role of the counselor is not that of judge or advocate but that of helper. The voluntarily childless situation of marital partners is one that calls upon the counselor to examine his/her values in depth and to help persons who have charted their course to sail on it as best they can in a pattern that we recognize as variant and not as deviant.

REFERENCES

Veevers, J. E.: Voluntary childless wives: an exploratory study. Sociology and Social Research, 157: 356–365, 1973.

Wright, M. R.: Psychological aspects of vasectomy counseling. The Family Coordinator, 21: 259–265, 1972.

Zemon-Gass, G., and Nichols, W. C.: Take me along—a marital syndrome. Journal of Marriage and Family Counseling, 1: 209–217, 1975.

VINCENT D. FOLEY, Ph.D.

10

Alcoholism and Couple Counseling

Epistemology is the area in philosophy which deals with knowledge. It is critical for philosophy; it is also critical for counseling. This is a bold statement to make. Nevertheless, how the human mind organizes its experience is the prime determinant in how one does counseling. Just as a counselor expresses a value system by what he emphasizes and/or neglects, so also the counselor organizes the material presented to him according to a model which highlights either what goes on inside an individual, what goes on between two individuals, or what goes on among a group of individuals who are closely related into a system.

In the light of the above, it follows that the locus of pathology will be found either inside a person, between two people, or in the manner in which a system operates, according to the model adopted. In this chapter we are going to examine the "alcoholic spouse" from all three points of view with particular emphasis on the system concept.

Paradigms in Therapy

Intrapsychic Model

Sigmund Freud began his long and fruitful career as a therapist by examining the role of the unconscious in an individual. Freud looked at the various processes going on inside a person from a model which stressed this aspect. This first model is known as the *intrapsychic*. As a result the locus of pathology, the problem, is seen as something residing inside a person. This is not to deny the influence or the importance of others but it is to stress the individual. A problem, any problem, therefore, is seen as residing in a given individual. An alcoholic, then, is viewed as a person who uses alcohol as a coping mechanism, as a way of handling mounting anxiety. More specifically such a person is seen as orally dependent, as one who is fixated at a particular point in terms of psychosexual development. Counseling with such a person, using a Freudian model, will focus on the unconscious determinants of the alcoholism and strive to resolve these conflicts by bringing them to the surface. Presumably when the unconscious has been made conscious, through a process leading to insight, the alcoholic wll be cured. The goal of therapy is insight, a complex phenomenon involving several distinct operations: namely, confrontation, clarification, interpretation, and working through. (Greenson, 1967.)

Interpersonal Model

Harry Stack Sullivan (1953) accepted the basic concepts of Freud but added a critical dimension: the other. This other is not peripheral to a given situation but central. Sullivan began with the idea that a person is the way he is because of another. It is a response to the other. The shift, seemingly simple, in fact was revolutionary. The other in Sullivan's model is no longer peripheral but essential. The alcoholic, for example, is now regarded as one who is responding to his environment by his drinking. Drinking is no longer regarded as a property of the person but is viewed as a response to a given situation. It is a communication; it is a cry for help. Counseling, using such a model, focuses on the interaction between the client and the counselor. The goal of therapy is not insight as in the Freudian model but understanding, i.e., the client's becoming aware of the interaction between himself and the counselor. Cure in this model is not a going back as much as it is a working with the here and now. In this model the locus of pathology is not viewed as something inside the person but as something between the client and the counselor. This second model is known as the *interpersonal* model.

If the other is viewed as part of the problem it follows that cure must involve both parties. The counselor in this model is no longer a blank screen upon which projections are made but a part of the process, a participant observer. Whether the issue is anxiety or alcohol, the other is part of the process.

Anxiety for Freud was the response of an individual to a conflict going on inside himself. When the demands of the *Id* came into conflict with the needs of society, the *Ego* experienced anxiety. The conflict was within. Anxiety for Sullivan, however, was not the result of such conflict but due to something between two people such as a mother and a child. Sullivan writes: "Anxiety relates to the whole field of interpersonal interaction; that is, anxiety about *anything* in the mother induces anxiety in the infant." (Sullivan, 1953.) The issue is that of communication, i.e., what transpires between mother and child.

The communicational process between mother and child becomes for Sullivan a model or paradigm of all communication. Uncovering the communicational network, both the verbal and the nonverbal, is emphasized.

Alcohol in this model is viewed as a vehicle for communication, a nonverbal way of making a statement. Treatment then will focus on helping the person to verbalize the pain which causes one to retreat into alcohol. Theoretically if the alcoholic can express his pain, specifically his anger and hostility in words, the need for alcohol will diminish. Cure in this model is improved communication due to an increase in self-awareness and understanding.

We have seen how one can use a model which focuses on the individual and see pathology as residing within. We have also seen how one can conceptualize the process as a communication between two people and how the pathology is seen as the result of poor communication. There is, in addition, another model which looks at interaction as the result of underlying patterns of structures. This third model has been called by various names but is most often known as the *organismic* because it examines the underlying structures of an organism.

Organismic Model

The model is based largely on the work of Ludwig Von Bertalanffy (1968). Although a biologist, Von Bertalanffy was interested in how a general system theory might be applied to human interactional systems such as a couple or a family. Even though a system is a system is a system yet there are differences between one system and another. For example, whether a given system is alive (a family) or not (a heating system) is critical. The former is characterized by continuous input, whereas the latter is not. Nevertheless, the basic concept of a system, namely, that the various parts are interdependent and interrelated holds true for any system.

An alcoholic in this model is seen not just as an orally dependent person as in model one, nor as one who uses alcohol as a way of communicating as in the second model, but as a person who is in a system which both influences and is influenced by his drinking. Therefore, it is not enough to examine his communication, both verbally and nonverbally, but it is necessary to look at the underlying structure of the system which both creates his need to drink and supports its continuation.

Consequences of an Organismic Model — Each of the models mentioned has certain properties which have consequences for the counselor. What one does is the result of what one sees. The consequences of a system approach are: wholeness, relationship, and equifinality.

Wholeness — In geometry we learned the axiom "The whole is greater than the sum of its parts." This most aptly expresses wholeness in a system concept. A couple is not the sum of the personality of husband and wife alone but the result of the dynamic interaction that occurs between them. One plus one does not give two but three in a system concept. Wholeness is the uniqueness that is the result of what happens between two people.

Therapeutically wholeness means that to look at one person in the system apart from the other is to get a distorted picture. To label an individual as depressed, anxious, or alcoholic is to disregard the concept of wholeness. It is true to say that a person is an alcoholic but it is not the whole truth. Drinking is the result of a context and cannot be looked at apart from the context without leading to a distortion. More simply stated: the alcoholic spouse must be considered but the nonalcoholic one as well. In a system concept one is not the sadist and the other the masochist or vice versa, but each is involved in the behavior of the other. One drinks but the other supports that drinking by his behavior. Therefore, change if it is to be permanent must deal with their ongoing patterns of behavior, with the organization of their system, and not just one aspect of it.

Relationship — In an organismic model *relationship* becomes the focus of concern. This follows naturally from what has been said about wholeness. If husband and wife together constitute an entity, a system, then one must be concerned with the links by which they are joined rather than with what is happening inside them. The issue then is to see what it is they do to each other rather than why. The emphasis in this model is on *what* more than *why*.

The shift from what to why is a quantum leap therapeutically. No longer is there a concern with the psychodynamics of the system but the interest is centered on their mutual involvement with and responsibility for the system. Their dance of life is examined. The movements between husband and wife in this model are viewed not as cause and effect but as synchronous. One cannot say in an organismic model that Mr. Jones did such and such to Mrs. Jones, *i.e.*, was the cause of her behavior. Rather more accurately one would say that Mr. and Mrs. Jones did such and such together, *i.e.*, each contributed to the final product. The movements between them are not like those of tennis players but more like those of dancers. In tennis I move toward the net as a response to my opponent's hitting the ball just over the net but in a dance my partner and I move at the same time. My partner and I dance the tango together. I move forward as she moves back. The organismic model sees the alcoholic spouse and the nonalcoholic one in the same manner. Alcohol is part of the system, the context within which each one moves.

Equifinality — The last consequence of the organismic model is what has been labeled the self-perpetuation of a system or by Von Berta-lanffy (1974) *equifinality.* This means that a system is constituted by its here and now parameters. The initial conditions of a system are not the only means by which the system operates. In an open system (a family) in contrast to a closed system (a heating system) the parameters are time independent of the initial conditions. This third property of the organismic model has important therapeutic ramifications.

Silvano Arieti (1969) has noted that the major contribution of Von Bertalanffy (1968) to therapy has been to point out the importance of equifinality. To forget equifinality is to be guilty of what Arieti calls the "genetic fallacy," namely, a going back to the initial parameters of the system. This means getting caught into finding out why a system has gone wrong rather than what is wrong with it in the here and now.

Therefore, a system can be changed by new inputs made by the therapist currently without becoming involved in the past. In an orga-nismic model the emphasis is on the process of the system more than the content. The underlying structure of the system, its organization, is the focus of therapy and not a concern with this or that aspect of it. Alcoholism then is seen as a *content issue* in the relationship and not the only issue or problem of the system. The *real problem* of the system in this model is the *process issue, i.e.,* how the couple relates or interacts regardless of the issue presented. Alcohol, sexual dysfunc-tion, and communicational problems, etc. may be cited by the couple as the problem, but the counselor using an organismic model will see the problem as a process result of a dysfunctional patterning of the system. The goal of counseling in the organismic model is awareness, *i.e.,* helping the couple become aware of their interaction, of their dance, so that it may be changed from a dance of death into one of life.

The theoretical differences among the three models can be seen in the following:

Model	Locus of Pathology	Goal of Counsel-ing
I. Intrapsychic	Individual	Insight
II. Interpersonal	Communicational Network	Understanding
III. Organismic	Structure of the System	Awareness

The practical differences in the three models can be seen in an analysis of Edward Albee's (1964) play *Who's Afraid of Virginia Woolf?*

Three Approaches to Counseling

The play is a convenient vehicle for seeing how one might do counseling with George and Martha according to the three models presented. One could treat them as individuals, seen separately, and work on their intrapsychic problems. One could also see them conjointly and focus on their communicational patterns. Or finally one could observe their ongoing interactional patterns, their structure, and help to make them aware of what it is they do to each other. By far the most effective approach would be the use of an organismic model.

The play opens with Martha asking George the name of the movie in which Bette Davis delivers her famous line "What a dump!" George retorts by saying he doesn't know. Martha persists and George finally says he thinks it was from the movie *Chicago*. Martha, shocked by George's limited grasp of movie trivia, tells him that *Chicago* starred Alice Faye. She adds as a final comment, "Don't you know *anything?*" George responds "Well, that was probably before my *time*, but . . . " (Albee, p. 5). Martha has won round one, movies; George has won round two, age. The conflict will escalate, the issues will change, but the patterns will tend to endure. At times one or the other will attempt to bring the conflict to an end, to have closure, but it will not happen.

For example, in Act I, Martha will ask George for a kiss but do so in such a way that he perceives the invitation not as a gesture of closeness but as a threat. He will respond to the invitation by telling Martha that she is so attractive that to kiss her would excite him passionately and he would have to take her by force. Martha laughs and George, trying to keep his distance, will attack her drinking. This provokes Martha and she becomes angry.

In Act II the stakes have been raised. Now Martha and George are no longer fighting over games of trivia or who can outdrink the other but are involved in the issue of whether or not Martha will go to bed with Nick, one of their guests. Clearly Martha is using this as a ploy in their marital game, as a way of getting George's attention. His response is to ignore Martha and pick up a book. This inflames Martha even more, and driven by her frustrated anger, she tells George, "You come off this kick you're on, or I swear to God, I'll do it. I swear to God I'll follow that guy into the kitchen, and then I'll take him upstairs, and . . . " (Albee, p. 173).

Martha marches off to bed with Nick and George equally angered and frustrated takes the book he has been reading and hurls it with fury against the chimes on the wall.

This in essence is the marriage of George and Martha. It is a series of conflicts, of fights, of struggles, which go on endlessly. Better educated than most couples, certainly more articulate, nevertheless, George and Martha are not atypical of the kind one meets in marriage counseling. How might they be treated?

If they are seen according to model one counseling will proceed along intrapsychic lines. Martha's over involvement with her father will be examined in depth and how this relates to her distorted perception of George. His guilt over the loss of his parents, seemingly due to his carelessness, will be investigated. In addition, the need George has to use his acerbic wit as a means of keeping Martha at a distance also will be examined.

If one opts for a communication model, their verbal pyrotechnics will be looked into. In addition, the overuse of alcohol as a symbolic means of communicating will become an issue. One of the goals in this approach will be getting George to deal openly with Martha's aggressiveness and she with his distancing. Understanding how they communicate will be the ultimate goal. Unfortunately learning how to communicate may not be sufficient. Edgar Levenson (1972) has labeled a communicational approach as one which he calls the fallacy of understanding. It is a fallacy because underlying it is the concept that understanding in and of itself is curative and will lead to change. It may of course but then again it may not.

Some years ago a cartoon appeared in *The New Yorker* magazine showing a husband reading his paper totally unaware of his wife. She was pointing a revolver at him and the caption read "Dear there is going to be an interesting story in tomorrow's paper." Perhaps the woman in question had gone to a communication expert and he pointed out that her husband was saying something to her by reading his paper. She had finally gotten the message that he would rather look at the paper than at her. In their case would communication alone help? Similarly, could one suggest that George and Martha had communication problems? Hardly! George and Martha are experts at communication. In fact, George tells Nick that he and Martha are aware of their games and merely exercising. As George puts it " . . . walking off what's left of our wits." (Albee, p. 33.)

An organismic model would look at George and Martha and observe their interactional patterns, seeing how *they created their system*. In a system viewpoint, you will recall, the members of the system are interdependent, both creating and being created by the other. George is George because of Martha and vice versa. Their system is created by the here and now parameters. Therefore, perceiving these and making new inputs into the system (the role of the counselor) is the way in which George and Martha can change. It is a question of changing the process and not the content of the relationship.

Alcohol plays a role in their system. But what must be observed is that it plays a *positive* role in their interaction in the sense that it helps the system stabilize itself and continue. In the language of system theory it has a *homeostatic* function. This means that alcohol acts in the George-Martha system as a balance mechanism preserving the system intact. Alcohol, therefore, has a system function apart from its personal (intrapsychic) meaning and its interpersonal (communicational) meaning. It is a property of the system fulfilling an important role in maintaining its balance. Therefore, any kind of counseling with George and Martha would have to take careful account of the role of alcohol. If the counselor were to neglect its positive function in the system he would destroy their relationship by removing one of the balance mechanisms in it.

We can conclude this analysis by saying that symptoms can be viewed in a variety of ways. They can be properties of an individual, or a means of communication, or a balance mechanism of the system. Each of these is important and cannot be neglected. Nevertheless, in practice, the traditional approach to counseling has been to focus on the individual, only in passing on the couple, and very rarely is the system interaction, the underlying patterns, examined. This accounts for the frequently observed phenomenon of how symptoms seem to bounce around in a family system. This is most often noted in alcoholic families as we shall now see in a case study.

The Problem of Problem

How does one go about defining a problem? Again it is a question of perception. In a family, for example, one can hypothesize that each member has a problem, the marital couple has a problem, and the system itself, the family, has a problem in its interaction. This means that Mr. Jones has internal problems, problems with his wife and children, and the Jones family may also have problems with forces outside itself, inimical to its survival. In the light of this what gets labeled as the problem depends on what is perceived by one or more individuals as the problem.

Usually when a couple comes for counseling or a family seeks help there is a presenting problem. The wife, for example, complains that "My husband drinks." In this instance the problem is defined as the husband's. In another case the wife might say "My son has a school phobia." Both of these analyses are true insofar as they go but they don't go far enough. Mrs. Jones is correct when she complains about her husband's drinking but she fails to see either her role in the drinking or how alcohol may keep the system functioning, albeit poorly. This occurs because she is not aware of alcohol as a property of the system and probably not even aware of the family as a system.

The unwary counselor wades in and starts making inputs. If he is fortunate some changes may occur. The husband perhaps stops drinking and all is well. But is it? Within a short time, frequently, symptomatic behavior begins occurring elsewhere. The wife gets depressed or a child begins acting out. Why? Because the system has not been changed. The role of alcohol as a family stabilizer has been forgotten and new homeostatic means of balance must be found. To produce lasting change in a system requires a change in all parts of the system. Recall that the first property of a system is wholeness—the whole is greater than the sum of its parts. Therapeutically this means that Mr. Jones cannot be considered apart from Mrs. Jones and John and Mary, his children. If he is going to change then each one of them must make an adjustment. Until a new system balance has been found, symptomatic behavior will continue to occur. All too often, after a period of time, the original symptom will reappear. After Mrs. Jones has been depressed and son, John, has acted out, Mr. Jones will start to drink again and the original balance will be found. And none of the family members will understand why.

A Case Study

The client had been drinking for 19 years. He began a short time after the birth of his only child, a boy. During all that time the family survived—painfully—but it survived. Finally, after a prolonged drinking bout, the client went to his minister for help and was referred to a counselor who proceeded vigorously getting his client to join AA, become active socially, and in general restructure his life. In addition, he called in the wife and interpreted the husband's drinking as a symbolic way of communicating. He suggested that if the client could verbalize his anger he would not have to drink. The wife agreed and the couple proceeded to work on their communication.

Three months later, the wife went into a serious depression and the son was arrested for stealing. What had happened? How did the counselor fail? What went wrong?

The counselor looked at the alcohol as a property of the client and also as a vehicle of nonverbal communication between husband and wife but he failed to see it as a property of the family system. His failure to do so led to further symptomatic behavior. Another way of saying this is that he did not grasp the significance of alcohol as a homeostatic balance but saw it merely as a content issue, as something negative, as a problem in the system. It was all these things to be sure but it was something more.

An analysis of the case can be revealing. Two errors were made by the counselor. The first was a neglect of the positive role of alcohol in the functioning of the system. The second was the counselor's failure to understand how he helped the dysfunctional system continue by his behavior toward the client.

Man is a being who cannot exist without meaning or purpose. It is not enough for a person to live from day to day but it is necessary to find in the life process some kind of continuity which makes life a meaningful whole. Mr. Smith was a man who had a weak ego. He did not cope well with stress and handling pressure caused him to become anxious. He needed to rely on others.

Given such a character structure, Mr. Smith would seek a wife who might give him support and lend him some of the attributes he needed but didn't have. Mrs. Smith, on the other hand, was a woman who found meaning in taking care of people. She felt this to be her Christian duty, an expression of her charity. Mr. and Mrs. Smith would complement each other. Their choice of each other as a marriage partner might be called "exquisite."

The 1st year of marriage was a good one. He worked and she took care of his needs, cooking and cleaning for him. They related very much as a child to a mother. The relationship changed, however, with the birth of their son which occurred in the 2nd year. Mrs. Smith no longer had time for her husband since the child was demanding. He brooded about this and then retreated into drinking. The more he drank, the closer the wife moved toward the child. As the horizontal line between husband and wife grew further distant, the vertical line between wife and child grew closer. Mrs. Smith, nevertheless, regarded herself as Christian woman and this meant taking care of her husband. As time passed, Mr. Smith began to miss days at work and this necessitated Mrs. Smith's going to work. She assumed more and more responsibility for the family.

Mr. Smith was a man of considerable talent. He had intelligence and personality, despite his immaturity in regard to alcohol. One of his employers promised him a good future with the company if he would become sober. After the "lost weekend" mentioned above Mr. Smith decided to go to his minister for help.

The counselor to whom he was referred did not understand the positive role of alcohol in the family system. He did not see that Mrs. Smith found meaning in taking care of her husband. Consequently, getting him to become sober and getting him to be more responsible required, at the same time, the necessity of his wife relinquishing some power in the family. To do this, however, meant to lose meaning in her life. In addition, the son had to give up his substitute husband role and become a son. He too lost meaning for he no longer had a mother to give special meaning to his life. If the family system were to change all the members would have to adjust and not just Mr. Smith. The counselor unfortunately did not see this and so ignored the needs of the wife and son.

Getting Mr. Smith to express his anger in words toward his wife relieved his need to express it through alcohol but it did nothing for the wife. She had lost power in the system and also meaning. She responded by becoming depressed, expressing her anger in symptomatic form. Mr. Smith had displaced his son as husband; Mrs. Smith had gotten wrapped up in her own needs; there was no room for son John. He still did not have a father and he had lost a mother. John began expressing his anger by becoming antisocial. The homeostatic balance in the family, father's drinking, had been taken away and so the family system began drifting in search of something which would again give it balance. The function of scapegoating in a family is positive as well as negative. It supplies the system with a homeostatic mechanism. When the scapegoat stops taking that role it causes a crisis in the system. If it can't blame this or that person anymore then how will it find a way of coping with stress and how will it find meaning? If I stop tormenting you then how will you continue being a martyr? My change in behavior has created a crisis for you and for us as a system. In brief, this is what happened in the Smith family. The first error of the counselor was to ignore the positive role of alcohol in the Smith family.

There was, however, a second problem which the counselor ignored as well. It concerned the way in which Mr. Smith patterned his relationships with others. Mr. Smith was a passive, dependent man. He did not initiate action, preferring others to take responsibility for him. He came into counseling at the urging of his minister, not by his own choice. The subsequent joining of AA and the various other changes that were made were done so on the suggestion of the therapist. Throughout the counseling process Mr. Smith remained passive. He still did not assume responsibility for his behavior. Whereas his wife once took responsibility for him that role now became the function of the therapist. The underlying pattern of dependency, the ongoing structure of his personality, was not dealt with and so unwittingly the counselor was prolonging the problem instead of curing it. By failing to understand the interaction between himself and Mr. Smith, by failing to take into account their relationship as an extension of a life long pattern, the counselor was merely dealing with the surface and not patterns of behavior which had to be changed.

Therapy with the client would have involved two essential questions. First, "What role did alcohol play in the family system?" Second, "How did Mr. Smith structure his relationship with others?" Ignoring the first issue meant that the counselor would not see in what way his wife and son were involved in his drinking. Ignoring the second question meant that counseling would not involve character changes, new patterns of behavior for Mr. Smith. It would mean simply that the changes made would only be ephemeral, of a passing nature. An introduction of stress into his life would probably result in a return to drinking since Mr. Smith did not know or see his passivity and dependency on others. Being unaware of this meant that the real problem of passivity would remain while the content or issue might change. Before counseling Mr. Smith was a passive, dependent man who drank. After counseling Mr. Smith was still a passive dependent man but one who now did not drink. He was still passive but unaware of this and, therefore, essentially unchanged.

The case of the Smith family illustrates the value of an organismic approach. Seeing Mr. Smith in relationship to his environment is important because it allows the therapist to see what role others play in the maintenance of symptoms. Looking at patterning also allows the therapist a chance to see what the client is doing to others by examining the relationship between them. A counselor must always say to himself, "What is it the client is doing to me?" How is he patterning the relationship? What feelings does he evoke in me? What kind of a response does he want?"

Again the reader should notice that our emphasis is not on why but on what. This is critical for an understanding of what we are suggesting as a viable means of counseling. Mr. and Mrs. Smith form a subsystem; Mr. Smith forms a subsystem with the therapist. Both systems are constituted by the here and now parameters. If these are changed the subsystems will change. It is not necessary, therefore, to go into why Mr. Smith is passive or why Mrs. Smith needs to be needed as a mother in order to function. What is necessary for change is to see what it is that he/she is doing, getting them aware of the patterning of the relationship.

Stages of Treatment

It should be clear from the above that stages of treatment with the problem of alcohol using an organismic model will involve three phases: observation, intervention, and consolidation.

Observation

The first stage is one in which the interaction between the couple or the family is noted or observed. What are the ongoing patterns of interaction? What is it they do to each other? What role or part does each one play in the system? This means paying more attention to the process than to the content. It means a careful observation of what occurs between the couple. In particular, attention must be given to the nonverbal interchanges. The discrepancies between what is said (verbal) and what is done (nonverbal) are to be noted since frequently these will be in conflict. Is Mrs. Smith, for instance, saying she doesn't want her husband to drink, yet, at the same time, making it easy for him to do so by taking responsibility for him? Does Mr. Smith play into this role by his passivity? One cannot function without the other.

Intervention

Stage two is one in which interventions are made. This might mean several possibilities. For example, in the Smith family eliminating John physically would force the couple into dealing with each other. Their detouring mechanism would be removed. Another intervention might be to suggest a relationship between father and son as a way of getting some distance between mother and son. A third possibility is to ignore the existing pathways in the family and to create new ones. For example, telling husband and wife they have to go to their room each night at 9 p.m., lock the door, and talk about their relationship for 5 min, forbidding them to talk about the child they have triangled. Another possibility is making them begin each sentence with "I feel such and such and I take responsibility for it."

The use of video tape, where available, has proven invaluable in this phase. Mr. and Mrs. Smith may not see themselves in their interaction but will be most astute in observing how others interact. They can watch a video tape of a similar couple, Mr. and Mrs. Jones, and quickly perceive the "real problem." Also the use of a marital couples group of three or four couples lends itself to the possibility of role playing as well as identification. Such groups can lessen the amount of time needed to foster change. Again the focus is on what is happening and not why it is happening. The practical consequence of equifinality is the bypassing of why and when issues and a focusing on what and how ones. Therapeutic pay dirt is to be found in what is happening in the couple system and how it keeps occurring. Change is the setting up of new parameters and not the examination of old ones.

Consolidation

Stage three involves the consolidation of changes made. The counselor is part of the system in which he is involved. He is also a most powerful member of the system. His presence creates a new system; likewise his absence changes the interaction of the system, creating either a new effective system or allowing the old system to be recreated. Lifelong patterns are difficult to break or change. There is a need to reinforce changes in a system, making sure that when the counselor is no longer involved, the new system will function in his absence. This means that the questions raised in stage one regarding the patterns of interaction, the role each plays in maintaining the dysfunctional system etc. must be examined again. Can the counselor honestly answer that these are different. If so then the counseling process can move toward termination. Appointments can be spaced out as a way of diminishing the powerful bonds that exist between the couple and the counselor. The transition from dependency on the counselor to self-reliance can be made with a minimum of difficulty and the task of the counseling process will be ended.

Summary

This chapter has attempted to outline the current approaches to marital counseling following three paradigms: the intrapsychic, the interpersonal, and the organismic. Each paradigm presents a different locus of pathology. The intrapsychic sees the problem residing in a given individual. The interpersonal sees it as a breakdown in communication. The organismic sees it as the structuring or patterning of the system.

The organismic model has three consequences for counseling: wholeness, relationship, and equifinality. Wholeness means that one spouse cannot be viewed apart from the other. Relationship means that the therapeutic focus is not on what goes on inside a person but on the interactions that take place between the person and others. Equifinality means that the interaction of the system is determined by its current structure (parameters) and not by its initial conditions. This means that a change in the here and now can produce a change in the system and not just give symptom relief. The goal of counseling, using an organismic model, is awareness of the structure, whereas it is insight in the intrapsychic model and understanding in the interpersonal.

Edward Albee's play *Who's Afraid of Virginia Woolf?* was presented as an illustration of couple counseling using all three models. The organismic model was suggested as the most effective approach because it perceived the positive, homeostatic role alcohol played in their relationship.

Finally, a case study was presented and the interventions of the counselor analyzed. Because he did not use an organismic model, the counselor failed to see how alcohol lent stability to the family system. In addition, he failed to see how he played a role in maintaining the system by his taking responsibility for his client, thereby perpetuating his lifelong pattern. Suggestions regarding effective interventions, *e.g.*, couples group and video tape were also made.

Perhaps the simplest way of summarizing our approach to marriage counseling is to say that the relationship of the intrapsychic to the interpersonal to the organismic is that of good to better to best. The organismic model is not the only model but years of experience has found it to be the most effective one.

REFERENCES

Albee, E.: *Who's Afraid of Virginia Woolf?* Pocket Books, New York, 1964.
Arieti, S.: *General Systems Theory and Psychiatry* (Gray, W., Duhl, F., and Rizzo, N., eds), p. 49, Little, Brown & Co., Boston, 1969.
Greenson, R.: *The Technique and Practice of Psychoanalysis*. pp. 37–45, International Universities Press, New York, 1967.
Levenson, E.: *The Fallacy of Understanding*. Basic Books, New York, 1972.
Sullivan, H.: *The Interpersonal Theory of Psychiatry*. p. 74, W. W. Norton, New York, 1953.
Von Bertalanffy, L.: *General System Theory*. George Braziller, New York, 1968.
Von Bertalanffy, L.: General system theory and psychiatry. *American Handbook of Psychiatry*. (Arieti, S., ed), Vol. I, p. 1100, Basic Books, New York, 1974.

MORRIS TAGGART, Ph.D.

11

Medical Aspects of Marital Conflict

Any contribution to understanding the interaction between marital conflict and the broad aspect of human life we know as physical health and illness is clearly part of psychosomatic medicine. It may be useful, at the outset, to indicate how the term "psychosomatic" is used in this chapter. The modern study of psychosomatics received much of its early impetus from the work of Freud who, although he parted company with official medicine, provided the important theoretical ideas as to how the leap from mind to body may be understood. As Rifkin (1974) has indicated, the fact that the early workers in psychosomatics placed the "psycho" first indicates that the psychological state is primary or causal or both. For example, psychoanalytic usage during the first one-half of this century has generally restricted the term "psychosomatic" to those "organic changes consequent on affective changes, the organic manifestations of dammed up instinct and physical consequences of unconsciously determined behavior patterns." (Glover, 1949.) The emphasis in such usage is indeed on the unidirectionality of the traffic between psychogenic antecedent and organic consequent. In this chapter, however, "psychosomatic" is used in a much more general and perhaps looser manner, i.e., to refer to any situation in which the emotional components intrinsic to marital conflict and physical function come together in a process of dysfunction called "illness."

This course is taken for several reasons. First, it is becoming increasingly difficult to assign cause and effect roles in interactions between psyche and soma. If, for example, one talks about a physiological predisposition which then interacts with an emotional state of affairs to produce, say, a gastric ulcer or adolescent diabetes, which is cause and which is effect? Perhaps all that one can talk about in such situations are conditions which together are necessary and sufficient for illness to result, but which considered separately are necessary but not sufficient.

Second, taking a broader view of psychosomatics enables one to deal with emotional factors in illness in ways that go far beyond etiology. Such ways include, for example, the way in which marital conflict may exacerbate the course of a physical illness, the way in which marital factors may interfere with the successful treatment of a physical Ilness, and the way in which a physical illness may affect the course of a marital relationship or a marital therapeutic process.

Readers who are physicians may wonder at this point what advantage is to be gained by taking a point of view which asserts that the relationship between emotional factors and physical illness is more complex than was thought by earlier researchers. It has been difficult enough in the practice of medicine to integrate traditional psychosomatics. Hyams *et al.* (1971) report data which support the view that primary physicians do not consider their medical role to include the management of emotional disorders. They suggest that the proliferation of medical information has made it difficult, if not impossible, for the physician on the front line to keep up with the psychiatric implications of his practice.

Marital therapists may be even less sure about the usefulness of the viewpoint urged here. The proliferation of medical knowledge may indeed be a problem for the physician, but it is an almost unthinkably added burden to those whose medical knowledge is skimpy in the beginning. Added to this is the fact that an issue of major importance to marital therapists—the impact of illness upon marital dynamics—has almost been totally neglected by researchers (Vincent, 1973). Theories within the field of marital therapy itself have burgeoned in recent years. Marital therapists have their own overload problems. Why complicate further an already complicated field of professional activity?

There is no easy answer to the questions raised by both marital therapists and physicians. Part of the resolution, as always happens when new ground is broken, will be seen in the emergence of specialists in both professional groups who will translate the new insights into the pragmatics of everyday practice. For the most part, however, the hope is that both physicians and marital therapists will become more sensitized to the overlap between their respective areas of activity. Thus sensitized, they presumably will appropriate the insights as they are able but, more importantly, will recognize the need for and implement the setting up of mutual referral networks in which the traffic will go both ways.

The breakthrough which promises to vitalize an interest in the overlap areas between medicine and marital therapy, and which helps articulate in a formal way the more general way of looking at psychosomatics, is the application of General Systems Theory to both psychosomatic medicine and marital therapy.

The development of General Systems Theory (GST) and its application are so well-known that most are familiar with it. Stated very simply, GST represents a radical shift away from the older concept of objects as individual entities to a new focus on their function and relationships. One of the first results of this new way of looking at things has to do with causation. The linear notion of cause and effect, e.g., emotional problems cause illness OR disturbed individuals cause a conflicted marriage gave way to that of circularity of cause and effect. This may sound like a terribly naive and simple shift to make. In fact, GST revolutionized the physical sciences with the introduction of relativity theory and quantum mechanics, and it bids fair to do something similar for the social and biological sciences as well.

Durkin (1972) has provided an historical and conceptual framework which helps one understand the application of GST to various forms of psychotherapy, especially group psychotherapy. No longer is the focus on the individual person as such but "scientists soon discovered that goal-directed behavior, growth, and creativity could be accounted for scientifically by the dynamic interaction among the component parts of any living system." Framo (1972) makes a contribution in the area of family therapy which deals with the implications of a systems approach for all traditional concepts of etiology, diagnosis, and treatment. He argues that symptoms "can be looked upon as disordered relationship events," and that "psychiatric illness, craziness, or odd disordered behavior is a socially intelligible response orchestrated to an odd, crazy, or disordered system." Knapp (1971) illustrates the impact of a systems approach on how one views the relationship between psychological state and physical illness. Knapp, in his presidential address to the American Psychosomatic Society, says that, "psychosomatic medicine deals transactionally with relations between three broad fields — the biologic, the psychologic or symbolic, and the social."

The thread which runs through the views just expressed is that which captures the essence of a systems approach — that an analysis of and intervention into the functional relationships among components of a system of human events may be more fruitful than a "Newtonian" concern with the components separately. That a systems approach is already in process of being established in both the fields of psychosomatic medicine and psychotherapy is an encouraging sign for it makes all the more possible for cooperation to take place between the two fields. In the article cited earlier, Durkin (1972) notes that one of the properties of systems theory is that the laws of organization can be generalized across the boundaries of scientific disciplines. Psychosomatics is itself a product of this phenomenon in that it, stated crudely, attempts to understand some human events in terms of not biological medicine alone or psychology alone but some combination of the two. Similarly, marital therapy represents a moving beyond the traditional viewpoint of psychotherapy which attempts to understand what is happening to an individual in terms of intrapersonal events. To be sure Freud was not uninterested in relationships—his use of the Oedipal conflict is an eloquent testimony to the contrary—but marital therapy was a beginning attempt to intervene directly into the functional network. Thus, what is being contended for in this chapter is not really anything new. It calls rather for the further implementation of processes which are quite explicit in the two fields of psychosomatic medicine and marital therapy.

Interactions between Marital Conflict And Illness

Etiology

Much of the earlier work in psychosomatic medicine has proceeded according to the so-called *hypothesis of specificity*. This states that there is a definite correlation between a physical condition and a particular emotional conflict, e.g., the role of repressed hostility in hypertension. In attempting to move beyond mere description of the role played by the emotional conflict, researchers have tried to postulate a connection between certain personality types and specific disease syndromes. Meissner (1974) considers that this attempt to relate specific personality types to specific diseases has been, on the whole, disappointing. He notes the current revival of interest in relating personality types to certain kinds of heart disease (Friedman, 1974) but concludes that "the impact of such studies, even when the data look reasonably good, has not been very profound." In Meissner's own search for the stressors which may make for illness, he argues that exacerbations at least tend to coincide with periods of marital tension.

An example of the point just made is given in the now classic study of Duncan and Taylor (1952) who showed that patients with pelvic pain reported high rates of marital dissatisfaction, meager sex drive, resentment of their children, and even onset of pelvic pain in conjunction with marital or family distress. Stein and Charles (1971) were interested in the early life experiences of adolescent diabetics. They discovered that the families of their patients were characterized by severe family disturbance and marital discord to an extent not seen in the control families of adolescents who had equally serious illnesses but not diabetes. An interesting finding in the same study was that, while loss of a parent through death did not distinguish between diabetic and control families, loss of a parent through divorce did. When one puts this finding alongside the well-known study of Hinkle et al. (1951)

which demonstrated that family distress exacerbated diabetes in family members whereas insulin requirements tended to drop as family and marital distress were removed, the implications are fairly clear.

The fact that marital distress may be related to illness in another family member is underlined by Herzberg and Wolff (1972) in an article in which they tried to tease out the etiological pattern in factitious fever among adolescents. Family factors, especially those having to do with the quality of the marital relationship, seemed most powerful in the etiological puzzle. Interestingly enough, Herzberg and Wolff take the crucial step in translating their picture of the etiology into therapeutic intervention. It was treatment of the marital dyad which seemed to have the most beneficial effect on the cases they present.

A particularly dramatic example of the ways in which events within the marriage may affect the "illness behavior" of other family members is reported by Tuch (1975). He found that paramenstrual women (in the period between 5 days before and 6 days after menstruation) were much more apt to bring their children in to see the doctor even though the children did not appear in all that much need of medical attention. It is perhaps speculative, but not unreasonable, to assume that these women's feelings about their own bodily processes, affected by and affecting the marital relationship, somehow got displaced onto the children. Thus, illness in a spouse or another family member can serve the function of diverting attention away from the vicissitudes of a marriage. Indeed, Hollender and Abram (1974) point up the danger of medical personnel colluding in such a process by reserving all of their attention for the person showing the physical symptoms. This may have the effect of supporting and encouraging the "scapegoating" pattern rather than challenging it. As Meissner (1974) has shown, somatic symptoms in a spouse or other family member may take on the role of a control mechanism, serving a stabilizing function in an other wise relatively brittle and conflicted marital relationship. An example well-known to practitioners of family medicine and family therapy is the one where an adolescent develops symptoms designed to block an impending divorce between his parents. Often the symptoms are behavioral. At other times, the acting out may take the form of physical symptoms such as eating disorders, mysterious infections, etc. It is as if the adolescent "knows" that his parents have only the parenting function as their reason for staying together. By manifesting symptoms of one kind or another, he provides them with a reason to close ranks and either postpone or abandon altogether the plans for divorce.

An important question in all of this is to ask which illnesses, etiologically speaking, are prime candidates for the kind of inquiry which attempts to tease out the significance of marital factors. Perhaps the question can be stated more succinctly in the context of some statement of the hypothesis underlying a general approach to the whole psychosomatic issue. Meissner (1974) gives his version as follows: "the hypothesis underlying the intensive study of the relationships between patterns of physical illness and varieties of emotional traumata has postulated that the connecting link is stress, specifically that the emotional disruption from traumatic events causes a disorganization of autonomic and hormonal regulatory systems, possibly mediated by the limbic system." If we were to accept that the use of the word "causes" in the above statement actually refers to a series of feedback interactions between emotional traumata and physical events, the statement is a useful one. The question then becomes—which emotional traumata are such that marital stress plays an important role?

The radical systems therapist would undoubtedly answer that all significant relationships in which an individual is engaged play an important role in any distress he may be experiencing. Thus, relationships with children, former parents, extended family, significant others who are not family members, etc., are all taken into account in a thoroughgoing systems approach. Emphasis on the marital relationship, however, can be derived from at least two important considerations. First of all, it is as important as any other aspect of the total system. Second and perhaps more important from a tactical point of view, the marital relationship is *seen* to be important by most people in the culture. While a few patients may request help to deal with their family of origin, most would have to be convinced that such relationships, whether good, bad, or indifferent, are central components in their distress. A well-functioning marriage, on the other hand, is seen as a good by most people. This makes the marital relationship accessible to both study and intervention, and it may represent the best chance for the professional, whether physician or psychotherapist, to penetrate the systems aspects of the patient's life. Thus, the liabilities and assets of the marital relationship can become a vantage point from which to view stress in either or both partners or indeed other family members.

The consequence of the line of argument adopted here is then that the marital aspects of any physical illness thought to have an emotional component ought to be considered. Since the role of marital factors can range all the way from being very obvious to very subtle, inquiry into the functional and qualitative meanings of the relationship perhaps ought to be part of routine evaluative procedures.

While the marital relationship is at risk of being involved in any link between emotional disturbance and physical illness, the involvement is more obvious at some points than others. Diseases which affect marital roles directly are cases in point. Flapan and Schoenfeld (1972), while tending to pay more attention to the female half of marital dyads, consider the whole area of reproduction, infertility, adoptive parenthood, contraception, artificial insemination, motivation for childbearing, etc., as one which ought to be understood and dealt with in the context of the marital system. There are, however, other problems with which physicians have to deal where the connecting links may have less face validity but nonetheless are there. For example, Bess *et al.* (1972) were interested in the factors related to successful narcotics renunciation. Of the 17 patients they examined, 13 reported poor relationships with the father and 9 reported good relationships with the mother, whom they experienced as warm, concerned, and protective. The vast majority of the sample saw mother as the dominant parent in the family. The study also revealed that in every case, more than one-half of the sample, where a parent aided and abetted the narcotics habit through economic support, etc., that parent was the mother. Granted that the sample of patients here is quite small and perhaps biassed, it is findings such as these which prompt more and more physicians and others engaged in drug abuse treatment to view the family, and therefore the marriage of the parents, as the unit of intervention.

Another area of special interest where the role of marital factors in physical illness is concerned is the connection between depressive tendencies and psychosomatic illness (Hollender and Abram, 1974). The fused marital relationship, the enmeshed family, the affective suppression in favor of cohesion at all costs, especially the avoidance of anger expression, the not dealing well with issues of separation, in short, all of the signs and symptoms one sees in relationship to depression in patients may contribute mightily to the development and maintenance of physical symptoms. Because of the area's period of economic growth when most parts of the country were experiencing a recession, physicians in Houston have seen the rise of what might be called the "Houston syndrome." This constellation of symptoms appears to be related to the stress which occurs when families relocate here from the rest of the United States. In its classic form, the move has not really been negotiated between husband and wife and she resents it as something which has been imposed upon her by an unfeeling spouse. The husband, as a result of job transfer, moves into a ready-made community of peers, whereas the wife and the children may have a somewhat rougher row to hoe. Wives get depressed and fall heir to whatever physical vulnerabilities they posses already. Children may also get depressed and confused, showing increased school difficulties, worsened allergy conditions, and the like.

If a physician is convinced of the need to include some study of marital factors in his overall evaluation of the physical symptoms presented to him, a practical question arises as to how best to get at the kind of marital and family data most helpful. The growth in the use of the problem-oriented record in the practice of medicine may provide a solution. Smilkstein (1975) has described the nature and use of a Family Problem-Oriented Record which helps gather such data routinely. Using such information-gathering devices, the physician can see at a glance how the marital relationship has survived past crises, what strains and stresses were operating in the family when it last consulted him, what the current developmental tasks of the family and the marriage might be, what the ages of the children are, etc., etc. Having this kind of information at hand makes the physician's task much easier as he sets about the work of assessing the significance of marital factors in the current symptomatology. How he translates a discovery of important marital involvement into appropriate professional activity will be dealt with later in the chapter.

Therapeutics

If it is not always obvious how marital factors may effect the etiology of physical illness, the picture is often much clearer when it comes to appraising their effects in the treatment of disease. Since, in any case, we are adopting a systems approach with its emphasis on a series of feedback interactions between physical conditions and marital factors, *antecedent* and *consequence* no longer carry the logical distinctions from one another which they did in the earlier view. Thus, the ways in which the quality of a marital relationship affect the course of a disease, or interfere with its successful treatment, are just as important as those ways in which marital factors seem to be implicated in etiology. If there is stress related to illness, that stress will have to be coped with by the marital dyad to some degree. The premorbid state of the marriage will affect that coping process which, in turn, may affect the course and treatment of the illness *and so on*.

The most striking effects of marital factors on course and treatment of illness are seen, as one might expect, in situations where the stress is most acute. Life-threatening events such as a diagnosis of cancer, a cardiac arrest, open heart surgery, etc., can cause severe stress on a marriage no matter how solid the relationship. Coping reactions are set in motion immediately when the stress aspects are felt. Faced with such crises, people and marriages tend to fall back on patterns of adaptation already part of their repertoire and which may have served them well in the past. Unfortunately, such patterns may not always be adaptive in the current struggle.

Intervention into the family and into the marriage while the acute stress is being felt is underlined as important by Salk *et al.* (1972). Reporting on the psychosocial impact of a diagnosis of hemophilia on both primary patients and families, they point to the period immediately after the diagnosis has been made as the most important crisis to be addressed. The long-term well-being of the family may be seriously hampered unless it is helped through this initial emotional upset. Indeed, the kind of educational work so important in coping with the vicissitudes of a long rehabilitative process or other aspects of chronic illness may simply not get done if the acute stress is not dealt with when it happens.

Acute stress, however, is not only defined in terms of the discovery of some exotic disease or the occurrence of spectacular surgery. What might appear to be inconsequential to an outside observer may turn out to be a very traumatic experience. Even those events which are part of normal development such as the first experience of impotence in a male or the earliest signs of menopause in a woman may be the occasion for severe distress in a marriage. It is doubtful if the mere passing on information in such cases will do much good. It is the stress which has to be dealt with, particularly in terms of how the marital dyad is able to cope with it.

Dealing with acute stress immediately after the traumatic event is, however, only one aspect of the problem. Illnesses which require a long rehabilitative process affect and are affected by the marital relationship. Helping couples handle acute stress at onset simply makes it easier for the long-term rehabilitative regimen to proceed usefully (Huberty, 1974). Again, one can see this most readily in cases where the spouse's involvement in the recuperative period is most crucial. Few situations approach the poignancy, in this regard, of chronic home dialysis. Abram (1970) notes that few studies deal directly with the spouse of the dialysis patient even though that spouse is intimately involved in and may be actually responsible for the patient's treatment. In a later publication (Abram, 1972) he focusses specifically on the role of the marriage in home dialysis. Unfortunately, much of the comment is speculative. How will the wife react? Is she really the way he says she is, or is what the husband says simply his projection onto her? Such speculations can be cut through very nicely if the marital dyad is evaluated as a dyad. It is the functional quality of the *relationship* which becomes crucial to the treatment, and it is focussed intervention into the *relationship* which will pay off later.

The work of De-Nour and Czaczkes (1970) with families involved with home dialysis points to an almost universal response of marriages and families to long-term illness in a spouse or family member. They noted that the predialysis patterns of handling aggression within patient families tend to go underground in response to dialysis as a treatment modality. This same "protection" of the primary patient is seen in the families of labile diabetics (Baker and Barcai, 1970), in cases of ischemic stroke (Adler *et al.*, 1971), and in coronary artery surgery

(Hollender and Abram, 1974), and anyone who has experienced serious illness in a family member is no stranger to the phenomenon. Dobson *et al.* (1971) found it useful to include wives of patients who had suffered cardiac arrest in discussions during the recuperative period. Once again, however, wives were interviewed separately from their husband patients. Given the delicate and often affectively loaded nature of the negotiations called for in such situations, one wonders if these can be achieved fully unless the couples are interviewed conjointly. White and Liddon (1972) appear well aware of this point in that they tried, wherever possible, to include spouses in interviews with patients who had survived cardiac arrest. The conjoint interviews allowed the typical pattern, *i.e.,* overprotectiveness on the part of the spouse and a corresponding anger reaction by the primary patient, to surface in such a way that the marital system became aware of it and could perhaps deal with it.

Even elective procedures such as plastic surgery, artificial insemination, the use of fertility drugs, and voluntary sterilization, etc., appear to be fruitful fields in the matter of considering the marital dyad as the unit for both evaluation and intervention. It is, after all, the marital relationship which has to live and cope with the consequences of such procedures. Everyday problems met by the family physician, such as duodenal ulcers (Schmidt and Messner, 1975), underachievers (Frank and Frank, 1970), and learning problems in children (Taichert, 1973), are responsive to the kind of inquiry which sees marital dysfunction as a possible factor to consider.

The Impact Of Illness On Marital Health

If the foregoing appears to be directed mainly to physicians, this is not to suggest that marital therapists can afford to be sanguine about their role in this whole area. That illness may have an impact on marital health is a truism, to be sure, but the implications of that truth have not played a powerful role in either the training for or the practice of marital therapy. The explosion of medical knowledge in the last 15 years may sometimes depress competent doctors who try to keep up with the new information, but it leaves the lay public, including most nonmedical psychotherapists, more ignorant about medicine than their fathers. In addition, the earlier practitioners of marriage counseling were service rather than research oriented. In the decades during which marriage counselors alone preserved interest in both marriage and family relationships, not a great deal of research of any kind was done. Marriage counselors, like other nonmedical psychotherapists, have been engaged in a struggle for independence from medicine as represented by psychiatry. Small wonder, then, that little research has been done on the impact of physical illness on marital health (Vincent, 1973).

Just as it is important for physicians to become aware of the marital factors inextricably embedded in patients' presenting symptoms, so it seems equally important for marital therapists to be more aware of the physical illness profile of the marriage which comes in for help. Greene (1970) has described extensively the use of his Biographical Marital Questionnaire which, among a lot of other things, provides data on the couples' physical illnesses and complaints. There are some diseases which produce quite definite emotional responses in people, like the depression often associated with hepatitis or mononucleosis (Vincent, 1973) or the irritability which sometimes affects users of thyroid extract. Such conditions do no obviate the need for marital therapy but the therapy will be much more informed if the therapist gathers the data and then is able to appreciate its possible significance. Illness behavior is, after all, another important aspect of the ecological context in which marital conflict is expressed. The marital therapist's becoming more familiar with how a marriage may be affected by illness of one kind or another represents a further way to fill out the systems approach to which he/she is already committed.

No doubt, someone will someday write a definitive text on psycho-somatics expressly for the nonmedical therapist. Before that happens, research will most likely have to be done in order that the territory be more adequately mapped. Until then, marital therapists are faced with the same challenge as are their medical colleagues, that of becoming as familiar with the twilight zone between the two areas of professional activity as one can with the tools at hand.

Some useful tools do exist. Precisely because of the systems approach adopted more and more in psychosomatic medicine, material which informs the physician informs the marital therapist as well. The rise of the new specialty of family medicine, with its distinctive journals and professional associations, has done much to encourage the kind of research useful to both groups. Joint conferences and workshops between marital therapists and the family practice physicians bear promise of providing opportunities for each group to learn from and with the other. Training programs for marital therapists, although hard pressed to incorporate new emphases like sex therapy, will hopefully move to provide more training in the new psychosomatics.

Translating Point Of View into Professional Activity

The question remains as to how the physician and the marital therapist can respond to cases where there does indeed appear to be significant interaction between physical illness and marital factors. For the physician, a lot depends on the nature of his practice and his own sense of competence in working directly with couples to resolve conflict. Obstetricians and gynecologists can and often do see marital pairs routinely as part of their normal practice. Some family practitioners are setting aside specific time periods when they see families and marital dyads, such as Friday afternoons. Fees can be adjusted to reflect longer interview sessions if necessary. Surgeons and other hospital-based specialists may do some conjoint interviewing themselves but perhaps are more likely to utilize a team approach in which a specialist in family or marital therapy is intimately involved in the whole enterprise.

For most physicians and marital therapists, however, the increased sensitivity to the interaction between marital conflict and physical symptoms will lead to collaboration of various types. Even given the vicissitudes of having to make a living, busy schedules and the like, there are many forms the collaboration may take. Some marital therapists practice in close conjunction with family physicians, sometimes located in adjacent offices. For others, collaboration means the setting up of mutual referral networks with free flow of information in both directions. Health Maintenance Organizations may contract with marital therapists to provide the necessary services. Whatever the form of collaboration, its institution is likely to follow efforts on the part of both professional groups to break out of the mutual isolation in which they find themselves. This is sometimes done at joint professional meetings but probably happens more often between individuals. No doubt there are difficulties in getting such collaboration in motion. Territorial squabbles frequently need resolution and proprietorship of patients negotiated. The fruits of genuine collaboration are not insubstantial either—professional practice which goes beyond mere lip service to the proposition that physical illness and marital conflict, like any other areas of human experience, are multifaceted and complex.

REFERENCES

Abram, H. S.: The psychological stress of chronic hemodialysis. Psych. Med., **1:** 37–51, 1970.

Abram, H. S.: Death or dialysis. Psych. Med. **3:** 151–161, 1972.

Adler, R., MacRitchie, K., and Engel, G. L.: Psychologic processes and ischemic stroke (occlusive cerebrovascular disease). I. Observations on 32 men with 35 strokes. Psychosomatic Medicine, **33:** 1–29, 1971.

Baker, L., and Barcai, A.: Psychosomatic aspects of diabetes mellitus. *Modern Trends in Psychosomatic Medicine.* (Hill, O. W., ed) Vol. 2, Appleton-Century-Crofts, New York, 1970.

Bess, B., Janus, S., and Rifkin, A.: Factors in successful narcotics renunciation. Am. J. Psychiatr. **128:** 861–865, 1972.

De-Nour, A. K., and Czaczkes, J. W.: Resistance to home dialysis. Psych. Med., **1:** 207–221, 1970.

Dobson, M., Tattersfield, A. E., Adler, M. W., and McNicol, M. W.: Attitudes and long-term adjustment of patients surviving cardiac arrest. Brit. Med. J. 3(5768): 207–212, 1971.

Duncan, C. H., and Taylor, H. C.: Psychosomatic study of pelvic congestion. Am. J. Obstet. Gynecol., 64: 1–12, 1951.

Durkin, H. E.: Analytic group therapy and general systems theory. *Progress in Group and Family Therapy.* (Sager, C. J., and Kaplan, H. S., eds) Brunner/Mazel, New York, 1972.

Flapan, M., and Schoenfeld, H.: Procedures for exploring women's childbearing motivations, alleviating childbearing conflicts and enhancing maternal role development. Am. J. Orthopsychiatry. 42: 389–397, 1972.

Framo, J.: Symptoms from a family transactional point of view. in *Progress in Group and Family Therapy.* (Sager, C. J., and Kaplan, H. S., eds), Brunner/Mazel, New York, 1972.

Frank, I., and Frank, R. K.: The management of the academic underachiever in a family practice. *Psychosomatics,* 11: 183–187, 1970.

Friedman, M., and Rosenman, K. H.: *Type A Behavior and Your Heart.* Knopf, New York, 1974.

Glover, E.: *Psycho-analysis.* Staples Press, London, 1949.

Greene, B. L.: *A Clinical Approach to Marital Problems.* Charles C Thomas, Springfield, Illinois, 1970.

Herzberg, J. H., and Wolff, S. M.: Chronic factitious fever in puberty and adolescence: a diagnostic challenge to the family physician. Psych. Med., 3: 205–212, 1972.

Hinkle, L. E., Evans, F. M., and Wolf, S.: Studies in diabetes mellitus, III and IV. Psychosomatic Med., 13: 160–183, 1951.

Hollender, M. H., and Abram, H. S.: Coronary artery operation: psychological and medical problems. International J. Psych. Med., 5: 67–80, 1974.

Huberty, D. J.: Adapting to illness through family groups. International J. Psych. Med., 5: 231–242, 1974.

Hyams, L., Green, M. R., Haar, E., Philpot, J., and Maier, K.: Varied needs of primary physicians for psychiatric resources. Psychosomatics, 12: 36–45, 1971.

Knapp, P.: Revolution, relevance and psychosomatic medicine: where the light is not. Psychosomatic Med., 33: 363–374, 1971.

Meissner, S. J.: Family process and psychosomatic disease. International J. Psych. Med., 5: 411–430, 1974.

Rifkin, A. H.: A general assessment of psychiatry. in *American Handbook of Psychiatry.* (Arieti, S., ed), 2nd Ed, Vol I, Basic Books, New York, 1974.

Salk, L., Hilgartner, M., and Granich, B.: The psychosocial impact of hemophilia on the patient and his family. Social Science and Medicine, 6: 491–505, 1972.

Schmidt, D. D., and Messner, E.: The role of the family physician in the crisis of impending divorce. J. Family Practice, 2: 99–102, 1975.

Smilkstein, G.: The family in trouble—how to tell. J. Family Practice, 2: 19–24, 1975.

Stein, S. P., and Charles, E.: Emotional factors in juvenile diabetes mellitus: a study of early life experiences of adolescent diabetics. Am. J. Psych., 128: 700–704, 1971.

Taichert, L. C.: *Childhood Learning, Behavior, and the Family.* Behavioral Publications, New York, 1973.

Tuch, R. H.: The relationship between a mother's menstrual status and her response to illness in her child. Psychosomatic Med., 37: 388–394, 1975.

Vincent, C.: *Sexual and Marital Health: The Physician as Consultant.* McGraw-Hill, New York, 1973.

White, R. L., and Liddon, S. C.: Ten survivors of cardiac arrest. Psych. Med., 3: 219–225, 1972.

12

Resources for Couple Growth and Enrichment

"We thought we had a good marriage, but now we realize that we were settling for much less than our potential."

"We were married 32 years ago, but our *real* marriage began 6 weeks ago."

"It's hard to believe that we have lived together as husband and wife for 9 years, and only in the last 6 months have we really come to know each other."

"We had given up our dreams of married happiness as idle fantasies. Now we are discovering that we can really make them come true."

These are testimonies from couples who have participated in group experiences which we call "marriage enrichment." They represent tens of thousands of other couples all over North America, and a growing number in other parts of the world who are making an exciting discovery—that stale, superficial, dull marriages can, under the right conditions, be sparked into new vitality in a matter of 15 h, and that this can open the way to ongoing growth and enrichment of the total relationship.

To a veteran marriage counselor of some 40 years, this has been an exciting revelation. It offers new and promising possibilities. Although we are still at the stage in which we are testing out these new programs and experimenting to discover what works best, there is already enough evidence to indicate conclusively that we are on the threshold of significant new developments.

What Is Marriage Enrichment?

The concept is simple and obvious—that marriages which are already quite acceptable can, in most instances, be made decidedly better. This can take place in two ways—from within, by reorientation of the relational component; and from outside, by creating a more

173

favorable environment. Marriage enrichment is concerned with both of these, but we will confine our discussion here to the first—improvement of the husband-wife relationship as such.

Although marriage counseling is equally concerned with this objective, the marriage enrichment approach differs from the traditional counseling approach in at least three ways. In enrichment programs the focus is on couples who are not in serious trouble; the objective is to stimulate growth rather than to provide therapy; and the process used is couple-group interaction rather than interview (individual or conjoint) with a particular couple. These differences are not basic; and there are evidences that marriage counseling itself is in transition from one approach to the other. The distinction between the two is, however, clear enough to warrant treating them as different operations requiring somewhat different skills.

Since the basic supposition of marriage enrichment is that most couple relationships have potential for considerable growth, this must first be examined.

Our culture has tended to see marriage in *static* terms, as a "state" or "estate" into which two people entered through a legal and religious contract which was sealed by the wedding ceremony. Once married, the couple "settled down" to the performance of several clearly defined tasks, such as establishing a home, raising children, and functioning as a recognized social unit. These duties were fulfilled by appropriate role performance, and the roles of husband, father, and breadwinner and of wife, mother, and homemaker were clearly defined, although they made allowance for some degree of individual variation. The culture also gave a formal nod of approval to the idea that the couple should be "happy" in their life together. Tradition has not, however, been much concerned about how that goal might be achieved. If happiness did not come their way, the couple were expected to continue the marriage out of a sense of duty.

As the sense of duty became less and less effective in keeping couples together, marriage counseling was developed as a rescue operation. The title of a well-known series of magazine articles, "Can This Marriage Be Saved?" exactly expresses the concept. A similar idea lay behind the description of marriage counseling as "reconciliation." A good deal of our early thinking about counseling with couples was also based in the "medical model"—the counselor discovered what was "wrong" with the marriage and applied his knowledge and skill in putting it "right." The couple's relationship was then either restored to the *status quo ante* or was made to approximate to some rather vague norm that was taken to represent the state of affairs in the average marriage. The counselor's goal, whether this was expressed or not, was to maneuver the marriage into a condition of *stability* that would make it possible at least for the couple to tolerate their life together and at best to enjoy their relationship.

Stability was, in fact, society's norm for a successful marriage. This is reflected in such terms as "adjustment," "getting along together," "solving problems," correcting "dysfunction," and "getting back together." In all this language there is no hint of the idea of growth or the achievement of potential. Stability was the goal, and stability was all that was generally expected or hoped for.

The marriage enrichment movement challenges this whole way of thinking about marriage; and in doing so it immediately meets vigorous resistance. When you speak to the average couple about "marital growth," their minds at first go completely blank. They have no frame of reference into which to fit such a concept. Their next reaction is to feel threatened. "Here is someone telling me that my marriage could be *improved*. That can only mean that there's something *wrong* with my marriage, which is of course just another way of saying that there's something wrong with *me*." So the suggestion is interpreted as a personal insult and treated accordingly.

Our culture has thus created a situation for the average married couple which represents an absurd contradiction. In effect, we are saying—"We hope you'll be very happy together—but be sure to resist vigorously the advances of anyone who offers to *help* you to achieve this goal"! This has the result of keeping couples away from marriage counseling until they are in an advanced state of alienation and dysfunction and of keeping most of them away from marriage enrichment altogether.

Despite this formidable barrier, the marriage enrichment movement makes steady progress. But it does so only by the slow process of couple-to-couple testimony of the kind quoted at the beginning of this chapter. Any couple willing to share with other couples in specific terms how they themselves have achieved significant marital growth provide the sort of incontestable evidence that shatters the conventional illusion. And it is in this way, and in no other, that the marriage enrichment movement steadily grows.

The Marriage Enrichment Movement

It is generally agreed that marriage enrichment developed out of the human potential movement. It is a short and logical step, when one begins to think about *individual* potential, to extend the investigation to *relational* potential.

The sequence of historical development began, interestingly enough, in Spain and with a Catholic priest. Father Gabriel Calvo, following his ordination, went to a slum parish in Barcelona to work with youth. After a time he saw clearly that the problems of most young people stem directly from deficiencies in the families in which they were raised. So he switched his attention to working with families, as the best way to serve youth. But again, after a time, his probing mind was forced to the conclusion that the effective functioning of the family depended on the quality of the marriage. In his own words, "I began to realize that. . .I would have to go to the heart of the family— the couple. . .In many families I could see a characteristic, something special they had which was lacking in other families. I tried to discover what these special qualities were, and I concluded in time that the unique quality was the confidence and trust these couples had in each other."

In order to increase the essential "confidence and trust," Father Calvo began in 1958 to organize retreats for married couples. These were so successful that the Marriage Encounter, as it is called, has now spread extensively across the world. It came to the U.S.A. in 1967. By this time, however, a similar movement had already begun among Protestant groups.

So far as we have been able to ascertain, my wife and I developed the earliest continuing program in North America. Our first retreat was in October 1962, in a center called Kirkridge, in the mountains of Northern Pennsylvania. We had, of course, never heard of Father Calvo; and being Quakers, we developed our own type of weekend, later training other couples as leaders through the Friends General Conference. By 1966, Leon and Antoinette Smith, of the United Methodist Church, had developed another program which they called the Marriage Communication Lab and which was later adopted by several other Protestant denominations.

Since these first beginnings the movement has proliferated, and at this writing there are some 14 national organizations which offer marriage enrichment programs, as well as a host of local organizations and agencies. In 1973, my wife and I established the Association of Couples for Marriage Enrichment (ACME, P.O. Box 10596, Winston-Salem, North Carolina 27108) in an attempt to coordinate the movement as a whole and give it purposeful direction. ACME, which has now become international, has recently estalished standards for the selection, training, and certification of leader couples and has united the various North American groups in the Council of Affiliated Marriage Enrichment Organizations (CAMEO).

Although the various programs that have developed differ from each other in detail, the basic principles and procedures are closely similar. They all work with groups of married couples, not through counseling and not through instruction, but through experiential learning designed to stimulate a commitment to relational growth. Most of these experiences take place during residential weekends; but they can also be spaced out over 6 or more weeks in a series of evening sessions.

The three original patterns, despite some borrowing from each other, have preserved in general the procedures which they separately evolved. Marriage Encounter includes no couple-to-couple group interaction — the focus is on providing the most favorable setting and support for an ongoing and private couple dialogue. All the couples are first assembled together, and talks are given about various aspects of marriage by the leadership team, which consists of a priest and several experienced couples. After each talk, the participants write down their thoughts separately and then go to their rooms for individual couple sharing. This process is repeated a number of times throughout the weekend, concluding with a group celebration.

The other two patterns focus on couple group interaction, although private couple dialogue is also incouraged. The main difference in their approaches is that the Marriage Communication Lab follows a prepared structure, taking up different aspects of marital interaction in turn and encouraging couple and group interaction by the use of experiential "exercises." The Quaker Retreat uses a minimum of structure and no prepared program — the group of couples take responsibility for making their own agenda and pursuing their own goals, the leader couple acting as "participating facilitators."

Apart from the priest in Marriage Encounter, all leadership teams consist of married couples who are already committed to marital growth and who have undergone selection and training. The modeling role of the leaders seems to be of high siginificance, and there is general agreement that this can be most effectively undertaken by a married couple who can demonstrate, by their own honest and open sharing, the growth process on which the participating couples are being invited to embark.

What Happens in Couple Growth Groups?

By common consent, it is very difficult to describe adequately what happens at a marriage enrichment event. Since it is essentially experiential, only through participation can all its dimensions be comprehended. Although couples generally approach it with some degree of apprehension, they invariably find it a pleasant and fruitful experience. It has no precise counterpart in the entire range of events in which couples normally take part and is, therefore, always experienced as something new and different.

Several studies have been made of marriage enrichment weekends with pretest, post-test, and later follow-up (Nadeau, 1971; Brudes, 1972; Wittrup, 1973; Swicegood, 1974). All have demonstrated convincingly that significant positive change takes place in the couples concerned. This is borne out by the testimonies of the couples themselves. We have no evidence that one ot the three patterns is superior to the other — all prove to be very effective.

Careful observation shows that for the average couple a marriage enrichment experience has three results. First, they come to know just where their marriage now stands. It might be supposed that they knew this already, but that proves not to be the case. Almost invariably, they find that they have never before openly confronted the realities of their relationship.

Second, on the basis of this evaluation, the couple reach some agreement on the desired directions of their future growth together. They see their present shortcomings in positive terms, not a demeaning as "problems," but as "obstacles" which they can overcome together. Often they make a growth plan and a commitment to the group that they will continue to work to achieve their goals.

Third, the couple learn new skills which will enable them to achieve their new objectives. Good resolutions are not enough in themselves—you not only have to decide *where* you're going, but find out *how* to get there. The couples learn from each other's experience of overcoming obstacles. They hear from the leaders about ways of improving their communication, of resolving conflict creatively. They even have opportunities during the retreat of trying out new ways of interacting and realizing how much better they are than the old self-defeating patterns.

Over the years, we have observed couple groups in action. We have tried to identify some of the processes which occur. First in order is a sense of *reassurance*. As the couples share their experiences of marriage, they begin to realize how much they have in common. "We thought our marital difficulties were unique, that there were no others like us. Now we realize that every other couple in the group has been through, or are going through, what we're struggling with. It sure is good to know that we're not freaks."

Another important process is *cross-identification*. As one couple share a particular area of their experience, other couples begin to feel "in tune" with them. They may express this openly in the group or get together with the other couple between sessions. What we encounter here is the classical process by which we all learn the art of living—not through books or lectures, but by observing how others behave and following their example. The trouble is that our culture, by imposing what we have called the "intermarital taboo," has denied couples the possibility of this kind of learning. By relaxing this taboo in our growth groups, we open up rich possibilities of stimulating the dynamic learning process.

Closely allied with this is *modeling*. We know that one of the most powerful incentives for growth and change is to have the active help of people who have already moved from where we are to where we want to be. An excellent example of this process is Alcoholics Anonymous.

Success encourages success by saying, "What I have done, you also can do." The leader couple tend to be regarded as models—not of the perfect marriage, but of a couple who are obviously working on their relationship and making real progress. This is true not only of the leader couple, however. It turns out that almost every couple in the group can provide a model worthy of emulation to at least one other couple.

Another powerful process that takes place is *support*. It is always moving to see the encouragement the group offers to any couple who honestly admit that they are in trouble and the loving way in which helping hands are stretched out to them. Most groups, as the hours pass, develop great warmth and trust, and this creates a very helpful atmosphere for the couple who need to develop faith and confidence in their power to change and grow. Although marriage enrichment groups are expressly designed for couples whose relationship is stable and who are not in need of professional therapy, actually something very therapeutic takes place in the supportive atmosphere which invariably develops. We often hear a couple say in amazement, "A matter of hours ago we had never met you people; and yet we feel closer to you now than we do to couples back home whom we have known all our lives."

Comparison with Other Forms of Group Interaction

A question often asked is, "How would you compare a marriage enrichment retreat to other forms of group process?" In general, there are obvious similarities, but there are also important differences.

A growth group differs sharply from a *discussion group* in that we strongly discourage the exchanging of opinions and focus firmly on the sharing of experiences. If the group drifts away from this focus, the leaders will intervene to get it back on course. A growth group also differs from a *therapy group* in that we discourage the diagnosing or analyzing of the experiments of others; and the leader couple do not stand outside or above the group in the role of experts or authority figures—they are participating members of the group in every sense. A growth group differs from an *encounter or sensitivity training group* in that we strongly discourage the use of confrontation tactics—our emphasis is on positive encouragement and support, and we at once "take the heat off" anyone who shows signs of beginning to feel uncomfortable. One gratifying result of this policy is that in 14 years of leading marriage enrichment retreats we are not aware of a single "casualty" that has resulted from participation in a group led either by ourselves or by any leader couple trained by us.

A group of couples differs also from a group of individuals, and the group dynamics of each must be clearly differentiated. Experience shows that people who are highly skilled in leading individual groups can become incompetent in leading couple groups. They tend to break up the couple formation and shift the focus from couple growth to individual growth. A group of married couples is actually a group of subgroups of established social units each with a past history and an ongoing future. The dynamics are not only different, but also more complex.

The Importance of Support Systems

Under favorable conditions and with skilled leadership, marriage enrichment groups can be powerfully effective. Some significant recent studies of marriage counseling have shown that relatively short-term therapy can be just as effective, and in some cases even *more* effective, than long-term therapy (Reid and Shyne, 1969 and Gurman, 1975). Our experience bears this out. The total time spent in sessions during an average weekend retreat is approximately 15 to 16 h; and several studies have confirmed our observation that in that short period a marriage relationship can undergo basic reorientation which is sustained and extended in the following months and years. This does not happen to all couples — some are not prepared, or not motivated, to reap the full benefits which the experience offers. Yet it does happen often enough to be impressive and highly gratifying.

What follow-up studies have shown, however, is that many couples need further help if they are to make the best use of what the weekend makes possible for them (Swicegood, 1974 and less formal investigations). We have, therefore, seen clearly the need to provide what we call "support systems" for the couples who participate. ACME seeks to do this by establishing chapters in local communities which provide ongoing growth groups, couple communication courses, support groups, meetings, conferences, and the like. The chapter also makes referrals to professional help when this is indicated. It may also provide other related services such as parent effectiveness training and natural childbirth training. The aim is to give the couples all possible aid as they seek to extend their own personal and marital growth into all areas of their family life. The other major marriage enrichment organizations likewise seek to give continued support to their couples.

In some ACME chapters, the support system is being extended into experiments with what are called "extension growth groups." This stems from our increasing awareness of the fact that growing married couples are very good for each other, and the hypothesis that they may prove to be equally good for certain other groups in the community. So far, we have tried this out in four different situations — with unmarried young people, with engaged couples, with couples in marriage counseling, and with recently divorced persons. The idea is to form a growth group consisting of three mature ACME couples teamed up with an equal number of other persons in any one of the above categories.

Not enough experience has yet been gained to allow us to arrive at firm conclusions. But already we have reason for cautious optimism. Experiments with all four types of extension growth groups have raised the possibility that in couples with enriched marriages, who in order to help others are ready to be open in showing their own experience of marital growth, we may have a dynamic new resource that could become available to professional workers in the family field.

Marriage Enrichment and Marriage Counseling

An important question for readers of this book is "What is the relationship between marriage enrichment and marriage counseling? Must they be considered as quite separate operations? Do they have some common ground on which they meet? Can they be integrated in some degree?"

We might begin this discussion by saying that marriage enrichment is beginning to do what marriage counselors have always wanted to do, but didn't know how. The constantly recurring frustration of the marriage counselor is, "Why did these people wait so long before they came for help? A year ago, or 3 years ago, or 10 years ago, I could really have done something for them. But now they are hurt, embittered, and alienated, and there is so little left on which to rebuild their relationship. I will do my best, but my knowledge and skill could have achieved so much more if only they had come earlier!"

In other words, marriage counseling tends to be a remedial, corrective operation, whereas marriage enrichment is *preventive*. The counselor tries to extricate the couple from the trouble they are already in, while marriage enrichment tries to keep them out of trouble by enabling them to build their relationship on firm foundations.

Marriage counselors have always believed in prevention and longed to be involved in it. But until now, there has been no known way of achieving this goal. Even now, a marriage counselor who set up an exclusively preventive private practice would soon be out of business. The grim fact is that pathology pays, and prevention doesn't.

This situation will probably continue with us for a long time. Planning ahead intelligently has never been a highly developed human attribute. Yet real progress is now being made. Today more and more people recognize the wisdom of regular medical and dental check-ups, and more and more people buy life insurance and plan their financial future. While the message of marriage enrichment is resisted by many, its inescapable logic begins to make sense to a growing segment of the more thoughtful members of our community. And as the number of couples who have been through such an experience steadily increases, the volume of testimony swells and is heard by more and more people.

How can marriage counselors link up with the marriage enrichment movement and cooperate with it?

One obvious way is to get in and help. Herbert Otto recently told us that he is challenging professionals to spend from 10 to 15% of their time in preventive work, *whether they get paid for it or not,* as a contribution toward swinging the emphasis away from our pervasive remedial emphasis.

Many marriage counselors and their spouses have joined ACME and are working with us. Some of them have had to meet the challenge of laying their own marriages on the line, and the result has been highly beneficial. For many, it was a new experience to work with their spouses, but they found that it added something meaningful to their *living* with their spouses.

Marriage counselors are beginning to see the value, when they have successfully completed counseling with a couple, of sending them to a retreat or growth group so that they can begin a new phase of relational development for which they are now ready. In one case, a counselor terminated her work with a couple by giving them a year's membership to ACME with the comment, "This is the best way I can provide you with ongoing support and help—these people will keep in touch with you in a way I can't."

We would welcome the cooperation of marriage counselors in our experiments with extension growth groups. There is evidence that couples in counseling gain increased motivation when, in parallel with the counseling sessions, they also participate in regular meetings with ACME couples (Brown, 1974 and Mace, 1974). What seems to happen is that they find models and thus are able to formulate their goals more clearly; and they are also motivated by the support of the group to make the best of their counseling opportunity.

Counselors may indeed use marriage enrichment procedures more directly. Some who undertake couple group therapy have improved their skills and learned new approaches through attending a training workshop for couple leaders. Others have sent couples in counseling to a couple communication training course and noticed the improvement in their interaction patterns. There is evidence that a shift in the focus of counseling, from the eradication of pathology to exploring unappropriated potential and promoting positive growth, can speed up the therapeutic process.

What about giving couples books to read or cassettes to listen to with a marriage enrichment emphasis? Such materials are available. It is possible, however, to put too much confidence in the effectiveness of self-help without the stimulus of supportive relationships with other couples. Our experience shows again and again that it takes more than a good book on marriage to bring about significant and sustained growth; especially in a couple already locked into self-defeating and destructive interaction patterns.

Conclusion

The marriage enrichment movement is without question the most exciting development that has taken place in my 40 years of working with married couples. It represents a new, positive, preventive approach which comes at a time when rates of marriage failure in our culture are at an all time high. It represents a genuinely new development; yet it can also be seen as the cumulative result of a great deal of devoted and creative work on the part of clinicians, teachers, and researchers who have constantly striven to provide better services to the married couples in our midst. It can be seen as a genuine grass roots movement in which lay couples are playing an important and exciting role; yet it could not have developed and been sustained without the knowledge and skill of the family specialists. At this early stage we cannot be sure what new directions it will take or what power and influence it will wield. It has already achieved enough, however, to be entitled to all the encouragement, support, and practical help we can give to it. (See Otto, 1976.)

REFERENCES

Brown, R.J.: Unpublished report in Winston-Salem, North Carolina, 1974.

Brudes, A. H.: Ph.D. dissertation, Purdue University, Indiana, 1972.

Gurman, A. S.: In *The Effects and Effectiveness of Marital Therapy* (in Gurman and Rice, *Couples in Conflict*, Aronson, 1975), p. 397.

Mace, D. R.: Unpublished experiment, 1974.

Nadeau, K. G.: Ph.D. dissertation, University of Florida, 1971.

Otto, H. A.: *Marriage and Family Enrichment: New Perspectives and Programs*, Abingdon, Nashville, Tennessee, 1976.

Reid, W. J., and Shyne, A.W.: *Brief and Extended Casework*, Columbia University Press, New York, 1969.

Swicegood, M.: Ph.D. dissertation, University of North Carolina, Greensboro, 1974.

Wittrup, R. G.: Ph.D. dissertation, Western Michigan University, 1973.

NANCY C. ANDREASEN, M.D.

13

Deciding Who Must See a Psychiatrist

People who seek help from a marriage counselor may sometimes have an underlying psychiatric disorder which is complicating the marital situation. The term "counselor" is less frightening than "psychiatrist," and, therefore, a couple who know they are having problems are often likely to seek help from a marriage counselor as a first step in solving their problems. Most will be correct in having identified their primary problem as the relationship between themselves, but sometimes the problem is instead the existence of significant psychopathology in one of the partners. A counselor should be alert for this possibility both on initial evaluation and during the course of therapy.

Table 13.1 summarizes the major types of psychiatric diagnoses currently recognized. Any of these types of conditions may complicate marital or sexual counseling or require referral to a psychiatrist.

Individuals doing marital counseling should have a broad overview of these major types as part of their conceptual framework in order to recognize patients who may need referrals to a psychiatrist or patients suffering from psychiatric disorders which may complicate the course of marital counseling.

Organic Mental Disorders

As the name implies, an organic mental disorder occurs when brain function is impaired by some type of physical problem. The term "organic" means that the cause of this type of disorder is physical rather than emotional. Some common causes of organic mental disorder include: head injury, infection such as meningitis, or brain tumor. The most common cause of all is the aging process. Symptoms of organic mental disorder are quite common among elderly individuals

TABLE 13.1
Major types of psychiatric disorders

1. Organic mental disorders
2. Chemical dependency
   A. Alcohol abuse
   B. Drug abuse
3. Schizophrenias and paranoid disorders
4. Mood disorders
   A. Depression
   B. Mania
5. Anxiety disorders
6. Personality disorders

because blood flow to the brain is often cut down through the diffuse arteriosclerotic process which occurs in many older people.

The characteristic symptoms of organic mental disorder include: memory disturbance, cognitive impairment in other areas such as ability to calculate or to learn new material, occasional confusion about time or place, poor judgment, and emotional lability. Recent memory is usually disturbed more than long-term memory, and consequently the individual with an organic mental disorder may enjoy reminiscing about the past but be unable to describe what he ate for breakfast or what day of the week it is. People with organic mental disorders often become depressed and irritable, particularly with members of their own family. Personality changes in people with organic mental disorders may be quite striking: a person who was kindly and easy going in his 50's may be surprisingly disagreeable, inflexible, and even hostile when in his 70's. A person meticulous about his personal appearance and surroundings may become sloppy and careless.

Organic mental disorders are often described as acute or chronic. Those which are acute usually begin suddenly, often as a result of some abrupt insult such as a drug intoxication or a massive infection. If the underlying cause is cured, the organic brain disorder usually clears. Chronic organic mental disorders, on the other hand, usually begin slowly, particularly when they are due to arteriosclerotic processes. The chronic disorders tend to be slowly but steadily progressive, with gradual inexorable worsening of symptoms. No good treatment for the chronic conditions is available, although small doses of tranquilizing medication or environmental modifications may be somewhat helpful. Since organic mental disorders are most common among the elderly, these conditions are not as frequently seen among clients who come for marital counseling.

Chemical Dependencies

Chemical dependencies may be broadly divided into two categories: alcoholism and drug abuse. Either of these conditions may complicate marital or sexual counseling (see Chap. 10).

Alcoholism

Alcoholism is a somewhat global term, and authorities disagree concerning its boundaries. Perhaps the most widely accepted moderate position is that an individual suffers from alcoholism either if he is physically dependent on alcohol (*i.e.*, shows signs of withdrawal when he stops drinking) or if he has had significant personal difficulties due to drinking. One widely used set of criteria for alcohol abuse indicates that if an individual has problems in two out of the following four areas, he should be considered to have a problem with alcohol abuse.

1. *Legal:* arrested more than once as a result of drinking; had more than one traffic accident while drinking.

2. *Job:* missed work more than once because of drinking or hangover; fired from work because of drinking; trouble on job because of drinking.

3. *Interpersonal:* fighting when drinking; hitting spouse when drinking; child abuse when drinking; complaints or comments by family, friends, or acquaintances that drinking is excessive.

4, *Abnormal drinking pattern:* Drinks nonbeverage alcohol; binges (remains intoxicated during waking hours over more than 48 h with default of obligations); drinks a fifth of liquor daily (or its equivalent in beer or wine); has had frequent black-outs (amnesic periods while drinking heavily without injury or coma).

Indications of a significant physiological dependence on alcohol include: withdrawal, tolerance, and medical complications. Withdrawal symptoms usually begin within 8 to 72 h after the last drink was consumed. They include "shakes" relieved by morning drinking, hallucinations, convulsions, and delirium. A high tolerance to alcohol has developed when an individual regularly drinks 10 or more drinks (or bottles of beer) within a period of 3 or 4 h without becoming intoxicated. Common medical complications include a variety of gastrointestinal disorders, such as cirrhosis of the liver, inflammation of the pancreas, and inflammation of the stomach. Alcohol is also very toxic to the nervous system, and people who have drunk heavily for a number of years often have symptoms of nerve damage or paralysis or symptoms of an organic mental disorder. Patients who know they are dependent on alcohol may try to cut down or stop drinking, but their repeated attempts tend to meet with failure unless completed under medical supervision in a hospital. People dependent on alcohol also tend to feel guilty about their problem and frequently hide their bottles or drink secretly.

Alcoholism is notoriously difficult to treat. Alcoholics Anonymous, or other related forms of "group therapy," probably has the highest success rate. Referral to a psychiatrist or other physician may be required, however, for treatment of medical complications, withdrawal symptoms, or maintenance on Antabuse. Withdrawal symptoms can be quite dangerous and even life threatening. Whenever possible, withdrawal symptoms should be managed in a hospital setting under medical care. Antabuse maintenance involves giving the individual a drug which produces unpleasant symptoms (flushing, sweating, nausea, vomiting, and faintness) if he drinks while taking it. Although this drug does not necessarily diminish his craving, it prevents him from drinking impulsively and, therefore, may be helpful to the highly motivated alcoholic by diminishing the temptation to go on a binge or begin drinking again.

Drug Abuse

Drug abuse comes in many forms, each somewhat different in terms of symptoms and complications. The most common types of drug abuse include barbiturate dependence, amphetamine dependence, and dependence on heroin and other narcotics.

Dependence on barbiturates or tranquilizers usually begins innocently when a family doctor prescribes sleeping pills or tranquilizers in order to help a patient quiet his nerves. Since tolerance develops rather rapidly to all medications of this type, the patient may find himself taking more and more in order to get the desired relaxing effect. Tolerance to barbiturates develops more rapidly, but medical people are becoming increasingly more alarmed about similar risks developing more slowly among patients who take tranquilizers. One should begin to worry if he learns that a client is taking any sleeping medication regularly, particularly if he takes more than one pill at bedtime, or if a client is taking more than three or four tranquilizers per day. Symptoms of dependence on such drugs include slurring of speech, periods of inappropriate drowsiness or sleeping during the day, frequent falling, auto accidents, etc. The middle class housewife is the type of barbiturate or tranquilizer-dependent individual whom the marital counselor is most likely to see, but of course these drugs are also popular among high school and college students, who use them as "downers," often along with amphetamines. People dependent on drugs of this type can have significant and life-threatening withdrawal symptoms, which should always be managed in a hospital under the supervision of a physician.

Amphetamine dependence is dangerous primarily because of the psychological complications. Amphetamines produce increased energy, euphoria, and greater self-confidence. Consequently, they are very pleasant drugs for most people to take. Younger people take them for an "upper," and "tired housewives" take them to increase their energy, relieve boredom, and help in weight reduction. Sometimes an individual may begin to take them as diet pills and find himself continuing to take them for the psychological effect. Unfortunately, however, tolerance to the pleasant effects of amphetamines also develops rapidly, and so a person must take more and more to obtain these desired effects. When the dosage becomes high, people may develop an "amphetamine psychosis." This disorder is quite similar to schizophrenia or paranoia. Symptoms include increased suspiciousness, a preoccupied repetition of simple tasks, difficulty sleeping, unexplained outbursts of irritability or anger, and sometimes paranoid delusions. Withdrawal from amphetamines is not physically dangerous. If they are discontinued abruptly, an individual will simply sleep for a period of time. The primary danger after amphetamines are discontinued is the development of depressive symptoms, and of course an amphetamine psychosis requires medical or psychiatric treatment.

Dependency on heroin and dependency on other narcotic pain relievers tend to have different origins and outcomes, although the actual nature of the chemical dependency is quite similar. People begin to use heroin primarily for the pleasurable sensation it provides and, once begun, the dependency is extremely difficult to terminate. Most heroin addicts die relatively young because of the physical and social problems related to heroin addiction. Dependency on other pain-relieving narcotics, however, often begins under medical supervision when they are given for pain relief. Particularly when a person must confront chronic pain, a physical dependency may develop because of repeated usage. Patients who become dependent on narcotics in this manner tend to have fewer social problems than heroin addicts, but they have identical problems of developing tolerance, increasing need, and ultimately, difficulty in obtaining enough drugs to meet their needs. Treatment of either kind of patient must begin with carefully supervised withdrawal from the narcotic drug in a hospital setting. Follow-up treatment may involve methadone maintenance for the heroin addict.

Schizophrenia and Paranoid Disorders

Considered by most psychiatrists to be the most severe and handicapping of all psychiatric illnesses, schizophrenia nevertheless is relatively common. Approximately 1 person out of 100 throughout the world probably suffers from schizophrenia. Schizophrenia has been variously defined, but perhaps the most common prevailing characterization is that schizophrenia consists of a group of disorders all of which are characterized by a disorganization from a previous level of functioning involving multiple aspects of an individual's life, such as emotion, thinking, perception, and interpersonal relationships. The boundaries of the disorder are somewhat controversial, but probably at sometime during the illness a schizophrenic disorder always involves one of the following: delusions, hallucinations, disorder in thinking, or severe motor symptoms (catatonic stupor).

Perhaps the most common misconception about schizophrenia is that the "split mind" referred to in its name describes a split personality, such as that portrayed in *The Three Faces of Eve* or *Dr. Jekyll and Mr. Hyde*. In fact, the splitting of the mind in schizophrenia refers to the fact that many aspects of the patient's intellectual and emotional life appear torn up, cracked, split, or shattered.

Symptoms typically begin during adolescence or early adult life. Frequently, prior to the development of the full-blown syndrome there are such difficulties as social withdrawal, diminished effectiveness at school or work, or inappropriate behavior. People showing such early symptoms of schizophrenia are often referred to as "schizoid." The actual diagnosis of schizophrenia should not be made, however, unless some of the severe symptoms of a psychotic disorder appear. These are usually considered to be delusions, hallucinations, or disordered thinking. Delusions are usually defined as "fixed false beliefs." They include such simple paranoid delusions as the belief that others are spying or surveilling, spreading false rumors, or planning harm. Delusions of reference, in which unrelated events are given personal significance, are also common. For example, a newspaper article may be interpreted as giving a special personal message, usually of a negative or pejorative character. The hallucinations which occur in schizophrenia are usually auditory. Most typically, the patient hears voices talking to him which appear to come from outside his head. The voices may be familiar, may be responded to, and commonly make insulting statements. Bodily hallucinations (haptic) may be present and typically involve electrical, tingling, or burning sensations. Visual hallucinations are rare in schizophrenia and usually raise the question of either a drug problem or an organic mental disorder.

The disordered thinking in schizophrenia manifests itself in a variety of ways. Sometimes the thinking seems impoverished, so that speech is adequate in amount but conveys little information because of vagueness or empty repetition. Thinking may be extremely illogical, in that facts are obscured, distorted, or excluded, without any apparent conscious attempt to distort on the part of the patient. Or, thinking may be quite loose and circumstantial, so that sentences or phrases are said in juxtaposition without any apparent relationship to one another. Patients with schizophrenia also tend to have either inappropriate emotional responses or impoverished emotional responses. When inappropriate, the emotional response usually involves a marked difference between the content of speech and the emotion with which it is expressed, such as a person laughing as he describes his mother's death. Emotional impoverishment usually occurs in people who have had symptoms of schizophrenia for a number of years. They appear to have lost the ability to feel and respond normally to either happiness or sorrow.

Paranoid disorders may be a type of schizophrenia or they may be a separate group of illnesses. People in whom paranoia, or extreme suspiciousness and marked delusional beliefs, is the prominent symptom tend to have a somewhat older age of onset, less disturbance in thinking, less poverty of emotion, and somewhat less social impairment than occurs in typical schizophrenia. Paranoid disorders are characterized by a fairly well-circumscribed set of delusional beliefs which are often acted upon. For example, an individual may believe he is being surveilled, harrassed, plotted against, or obstructed in the pursuit of personal goals. One specific type of paranoid disorder, "conjugal paranoia," may become a particular problem in marital counseling. In this form of paranoia, one partner, on the basis of little or no evidence, becomes convinced that the spouse is being unfaithful. Small bits of "evidence," such as disarrayed clothing or spots on the sheets, will be collected and used to justify the delusions.

Schizophrenic and paranoid disorders are usually treated with medication. Acute forms of these disorders may respond quite well to treatment, but the more chronic forms tend to have a relatively poor prognosis. Most patients with these disorders should be referred to a psychiatrist for treatment as soon as the symptoms are recognized. Marital counseling should probably never be attempted when one of the partners suffers from paranoia (as rigorously defined above), and counseling should only be attempted in patients suffering from schizophrenia when their symptoms are in remission.

Mood Disorders

The term "mood" refers to a prolonged emotion which colors the whole psychic life. Mood disorders are thus those characterized by a primary disturbance in emotion. The two major types of mood disorders are depression and mania.

Depressive Disorders

The essential feature of a depressive disorder is a depressed or sad mood in combination with a group of associated symptoms. These symptoms may include loss of interest or pleasure, sleep disturbance, diminished appetite, weight loss, decreased energy, feelings of worthlessness or guilt, and thoughts of death or suicide. A person suffering from depression will describe himself as feeling sad, hopeless, discouraged, down in the dumps, or some other colloquial variant. Most people experience sadness from time to time, and consequently it is difficult to separate the normal experience of feeling discouraged from actual depressive illness. As a simple rule of thumb, most psychiatrists feel that a person probably suffers from depressive illness if that person experiences depressed mood and at least four associated symptoms for at least 2 weeks.

Depressive illness may begin at any age. A person may or may not associate its onset with precipitating factors, such as personal disappointment or misfortune. The degree of impairment varies, but there is usually some interference in social or occupational functioning. If the depression is severe, incapacity may be marked and pervade all areas of a person's life. The most serious complication is suicide, which occurs in approximately 15% of patients.

Depression is an episodic illness. It usually responds quite well to antidepressant medication, although depressive episodes typically cleared spontaneously within 6 months before such medications became available 20 years ago. Patients with significant depression should always be referred to a psychiatrist for treatment, and marital counseling should usually be delayed until the depression has remitted. People suffering from depression should be counseled to make no major decisions about their life or life style while they are depressed. Sexual disinterest or impotence is a common depressive symptom which may bring a depressed patient into marital counseling. Unfortunately, a few male patients may also have some difficulty obtaining or sustaining an erection as a side effect when taking tricyclic antidepressants. Patients having a problem with this side effect should be reassured that it tends to be transient and usually clears spontaneously, even while they are still taking the medication.

Manic Disorder

Depressive disorders are relatively common. Approximely 10 people out of 100 will have a depressive episode requiring treatment at some time during their life. Manic disorder, on the other hand, is relatively rare. Only about 0.05% of the population suffers from manic disorder. Most people who have mania also experience depressive episodes at some time. These people are usually referred to as "bipolar," since their disordered mood appears to swing between the two poles of feeling high and feeling low.

The essential feature of manic disorder is a distinct period when the predominant mood is elevated, expansive, or irritable in association with other symptoms of a manic syndrome. These symptoms include hyperactivity, excessive involvement in activities without recognizing the high potential for painful consequences, excessive talkativeness, racing thoughts, inflated self-esteem, decreased need for sleep, and distractability. The manic usually describes himself as feeling "wonderful," and his euphoric mood often has an infectious quality to the uninvolved observer but is recognized as excessive by those who know the patient well. Although euphoria is more typical, a few people experiencing mania are irritable instead. The irritability may become particularly apparent if the person is prevented from doing something he wants. Almost invariably there is increased sociability, such as renewing old acquaintances or calling friends at all hours of the night. Frequently the patient's expansiveness, grandiosity, and lack of judgment lead to activities such as buying sprees, reckless driving, foolish business investments, and sexual behavior unusual for the person. Behavior may have a disorganized, flamboyant, or bizarre quality: for example, dressing up in colorful and strange garments, wearing excessive or poorly applied make-up, and distributing bread, candy, money, and advice to passing strangers. Manic speech tends to be loud, rapid, and difficult to understand. Often it is full of jokes, puns, and amusing irrelevancies, and it can become theatrical with singing and rhetorical mannerisms. Manics are usually distractable. They begin tasks but rarely complete them. Their inflated self-esteem ranges from uncritical self-confidence to marked grandiosity which may approach delusional proportions. Common grandiose delusions involve a special relationship to God or some well-known figure from the political, religious, or entertainment world. Almost invariably there is a decreased need for sleep, so that the person awakens several hours before his usual time and is full of energy. When the sleep disturbance is severe, a person may go for days without any sleep at all and yet feel well rested.

Manic episodes usually begin rather suddenly and usually last from a few days to several months. Manic symptoms usually respond quite well to medications such as lithium or major tranquilizers such as Thorazine. Because he feels so wonderful, however, a person experiencing mania is often reluctant to obtain treatment. Impairment may be quite severe, in that the person requires protection either from the consequences of his poor judgment or hyperactivity. Prior to the development of appropriate treatment approximately 15% of manic patients died from physical exhaustion. The spouse of a manic patient may be placed in a difficult bind, recognizing the manic's need for treatment and also his potential anger if forced to seek it. Most manics are, however, glad that they were forced to seek treatment after recovery, since they then recognize the potential bad consequences of their previously impaired judgment. Marital counseling should never be attempted with people while in a manic episode.

Anxiety

This group of disorders shares the common feature of anxiety. Anxiety is either expressed directly in the presenting symptoms (for example, phobias and panic attacks), or anxiety appears if the symptom is interfered with (for example, resisting the impulse to perform a compulsive act). These disorders are divided into three basic subtypes: anxiety disorder, phobic disorder, and obsessive-compulsive disorder.

Anxiety Disorder

Many people are mildly anxious or tense, and most such individuals rarely seek or need treatment. Referral and treatment are only appropriate when problems with anxiety are severe enough to become handicapping. Often the stimulus to seek treatment is an experience which psychiatrists call an "anxiety attack." This consists of a subjective feeling of irrational fear or panic, a sense of impending doom, and such physical sensations as shortness of breath, pounding heart, sweaty palms, and queaziness in the stomach. These symptoms may be brought on by a realistically fear-provoking situation, such as when a student is called on in class or giving a recital, when a person is unable to perform satisfactorily sexually, or when a person is called on the carpet by his boss. But often severe anxiety attacks occur without any precipitating stimulus. Anxiety disorder becomes handicapping when it prevents a person from accomplishing desired goals or seeking new experiences. People suffering from severe anxiety disorder can be quite unhappy since their basic problem is irrational fear and emotional tenseness, which are subjectively unpleasant. Various treatments have been used with anxiety disorder, many of them with relatively good results. Psychotherapy usually aims at helping the individual understand the sources of his anxiety. Tranquilizing medications help relieve the subjective sense of tenseness and may help prevent or terminate anxiety attacks. Behavioral techniques, such as relaxation therapy, are also useful.

Phobic Disorders

The major feature of phobic disorder is a persistent and recurring irrational fear of a specific object, activity, or situation which the patient tends to avoid. Usually the avoidance is recognized by the patient as unreasonable. Avoidance of objects, activities, or situations which have only a trivial effect on the life pattern is not sufficient to warrant this diagnosis. However, when a change in life circumstance causes the avoidance to have a significant effect on the person's life, then that person probably has a phobic disorder.

Phobias may take several different forms. One of the most common is the fear of leaving the familiar setting of the home, with associated multiple fears of travel, crowds, close spaces, stores, and heights. In its severe form, a person may progressively restrict his activities until he becomes "housebound." Social phobias are defined as a fear of situations involving other people that are not associated with leaving home. The most common social phobias are fears of public speaking, eating in public, or using public lavatories. Social phobias tend to be less incapacitating than the fear of leaving home. Some experts consider phobic disorderto be simply a more specific form of anxiety disorder. A similar range of treatment is appropriate, including tranquilizing medication, psychotherapy, and relaxation or behavioral therapy.

Obsessive-Compulsive Disorder

Obsessive-compulsive disorder is a more severe manifestation of an underlying compulsive personality. A person with this disorder has either obsessions (which are recurrent or persistent ideas, thoughts, images, and impulses) or compulsions (which are recurrent behaviors generally accompanied by a sense of subjective compulsion and a simultaneous desire to resist). Usually the obsessions or compulsions are recognized by the person as foreign to his personality or excessive in degree. The most common forms of obsessions are senseless and repetitive thoughts of violence, contamination, and doubt. The most common forms of compulsions involve handwashing, counting, checking, and touching.

Obsessions and compulsions can be quite handicapping. Obsessional ideas are usually painful, unpleasant, and frightening. The person recognizes them as foreign or alien thoughts and wishes to be rid of them. Compulsive behaviors may become severe enough to prevent the accomplishment of ordinary daily routine. For example, a pharmacist may find himself unable to fill a prescription because he has to recheck continually to make sure he has counted out the right number of pills.

A variety of treatments has been tried for severe obsessive-compulsive disorder. These include psychotherapy, behavior therapy, medications, and even surgery. No treatment has emerged as strikingly successful.

Personality Disorders

Personality disorders are relatively enduring, habitual, and apparently ingrained ways of functioning, usually recognizable by the time of adolescence and continuing well into adult life. They represent pervasive character traits rather than isolated or circumscribed symptoms, and they tend to be manifest in a wide range of social and personal contacts. One should distinguish between personality traits and personality disorders. A personality trait, such as being meticulous or histrionic, is considered to represent a personality disorder only when it either causes personal distress or significantly interferes with social functioning.

A variety of personality disorders has been described and discussed. There is perhaps more debate about the nature and definition of personality disorders than any other aspect of psychiatry. Some experts consider them to be only mild variations from norm or simple examples of conscious, willful, or misguided behavior. Other experts consider them to be a real and significant subtype of mental disorder since they can cause considerable impairment. Perhaps the most widely agreed upon subtypes are antisocial personality disorder, hysterical personality disorder, and compulsive personality disorder.

Compulsive Personality

Compulsive personality is a milder form of obsessive-compulsive disorder. This type of person is conscientious, hard working, punctual, tidy, perfectionistic, and often quite intellectual. The housewife whose home is never messed up, the executive who is a stickler for details, or the conscientious and overworked minister or minister's wife are common prototypes. Although people with compulsive personalities are pleasant to deal with because they tend to be prompt and orderly, they are often hard to live with. Nagging about various details, based on compulsive personality traits, may be a significant source of irritation within a marriage. Such mild forms do not warrant referral to a psychiatrist and can usually be handled within the context of marital counseling.

Antisocial Personality Disorder

Antisocial personality disorder refers to individuals whose behavior brings them repeatedly into conflict with society. Many people who fall into this category have committed criminal or civil offenses, such as assault, major traffic violations, or theft. Symptoms of this personality type begin early in life, with such prodromal indications as running away from home overnight, fighting on the school grounds, or excessively early drinking or sexual activity. Such behavior often leads eventually to conflict with the law and almost inevitably leads to confrontation with authorities of some type. Some experts believe that the primary underlying symptom is a gross selfishness and irresponsibility which makes such individuals incapable of feeling significant loyalty to individuals, groups, or social values. People with this personality problem typically feel little guilt for their behavior and tend to blame others for their problem or offer plausible rationalizations. Apparently unable to learn from experience or punishment, they tend to repeat the same self-defeating behavior over and over. Because of their gross selfishness and irresponsibility, the marital relationship of such individuals tends to be fraught with discord.

Hysterical Personality

Like the compulsive disorders, the hysterical disorders range from mild to severe. This disorder occurs primarily among women. A woman with an hysterical personality tends to be rather immature, extremely dependent on others, sexually seductive but often anorgasmic during intercourse, histrionic and self-dramatizing, attention seeking, and emotionally labile. Her relationship to her marital partner is often one of making continual demands which can never be satisfied and expecting much in return for little. Some experts consider the hysteric to be the female equivalent of the male antisocial. Because such behavior is so demanding and maladaptive, it also leads to significant marital discord.

A more severe form of this syndrome is sometimes referred to simply as hysteria, hysterical neurosis, or Briquet's disorder. In this more incapacitating form of the disorder, the person tends to focus specifically on physical complaints as a method of gaining attention and establishing dependency. If asked about physical symptoms, the person will describe multiple complaints covering a variety of bodily systems, such as brief periods of blindness, paralysis, nausea, vomiting, pelvic pain, diarrhea, marked fluctuations in weight, etc. Usually the patient indicates that she has been "sickly" all her life and has a complex medical history involving repeated visits to physicians and often multiple surgeries. This maladaptive life style tends to be rather chronic. Excessive use of pain-relieving or tranquilizing drugs may be a significant complication, as may excessive or repeated surgical procedures.

Guidelines for Referral

The above brief descriptions of the major types of psychiatric disorders should permit recognition of the different specific disorders which may occur in people who seek marital or sexual counseling. Recognition of a specific disorder in a client does not necessarily mean, however, that the client should be referred to a psychiatrist. The need for referral depends on the nature of the disorder. The major purpose of referral is to permit management or treatment of conditions which the counselor cannot handle. Table 13.2 summarizes the types of problems in clients which may be indications for referral.

TABLE 13.2
Guidelines for referral

1. Clients requiring various types of somatic therapy such as medication.
2. Clients with a significant suicidal risk.
3. Clients suffering from chemical dependencies.
4. Clients needing intensive long-term individual psychotherapy.

Psychiatric referral may be combined with marital and sexual counseling in a variety of ways. In some cases psychiatric treatment should be done before marital counseling, while in other cases psychiatric treatment and marital counseling may be done concurrently. In a few cases, psychiatric treatment should be done instead, and marital counseling is contraindicated. These various situations, and their relationship to the above guidelines and to the various specific psychiatric diagnoses, may be treated in the following ways.

Psychiatric Referral before Marital Counseling

Three of the disorders previously described are characterized by behavior which tends to lead to marital discord: mania, depression, and chemical dependency. When in an episode of mania or depression, or when dependent on alcohol or drugs, patients tend to do a variety of things which are quite disruptive of the marital relationship. Often residual marital problems remain even after the acute episode of mania or depression has cleared or after the patient has been withdrawn from drugs or alcohol. During an episode, particularly of depression or mania, counseling is virtually impossible, since the client's perception and behavior is completely distorted by his abnormal mood. Consequently, each of these disorders should be adequately treated by a psychiatrist before the couple begins marital counseling.

Since depression is such a common condition, the marital counselor should be particularly alert to recognizing it and referring clients for evaluation and treatment when he suspects depression. Depressive disorder disrupts marriage in a variety of ways, any of which may lead a couple to conclude that they have a marital problem and to seek help from a counselor. The depressed person's lack of interest and energy almost always extends to include a lack of interest in sex, leading to feelings of rejection or anger in the spouse. People who are depressed also tend to be quite uninterested in most social activities, so the spouse may complain about his or her partner's unwillingness to invite people in, to go out to parties, etc. A depressed housewife tends to neglect tasks such as doing the laundry, preparing meals, or looking after the children. Depressed people with jobs may miss work because they feel inadequate or are unable to face the responsibilities of the day. In short, depression may make a person appear lazy, irresponsible, or unaffectionate.

When these complaints exist, the counselor should inquire about the associated physical symptoms of depression, such as poor appetite, weight loss, and sleep disturbance. He should also determine whether the apathy and disinterest represent a change from earlier patterns of behavior. If the client admits to the physical symptoms, or if there is a clear change in behavior, referral should be initiated. Most depressive episodes respond to treatment within a month or two, and sometimes the marital problem disappears when the depression clears. A number of people who experience depressive episodes, however, also have underlying problems with low self-confidence, excessive rigidity, or other traits which may complicate the marital relationship, and many of these will wish to return to the marital counselor for help after the depressive symptoms have lifted.

Patients with manic disorder are much less likely to present as a marital problem, but this may happen occasionally, particularly early in an episode of mania or in people having mild forms of the disorder. Manic symptoms which may complicate the marital relationship include financial extravagance, poor judgment in business matters, sexual indiscretions, or excessive sociability. Many people who develop mania are extroverted and outgoing anyway, and a person with an early mild mania may appear to have only a slight exaggeration of behavior which has always been present. Without recognizing that the problem is mania, a couple may come in because one of the partners has suddenly spent a substantial sum of money for items which they would normally consider an extravagance, such as expensive clothing, gadgetry, or vacation trips. Apparently with good justification initially, a mildly manic individual may take on extensive business responsibilities or financial responsibilities and then find himself painfully overextended. A previously faithful spouse may suddenly begin to seek sexual intercourse with a variety of different partners. A previously pleasant spouse may become insomniac, rude, and irritable. A man may begin bringing home large numbers of friends and acquaintances for spur-of-the-moment dinner or cocktail parties.

Because manics tend to deny that any problems exist, counseling can almost never be done during a manic episode. As in the case of depression, the problems may clear after the episode passes, but, on the other hand, manic disorder may also lead to marital problems when the florid symptoms are in remission. Particularly when manias are recurrent (as they often are) the spouse can become quite displeased. The economic and social consequences of recurrent mania can become a problem, in that manics often require hospitalization, may run up large bills in a period of extravagance, and may show poor judgment at work and therefore lose their jobs. The marital counselor can be quite helpful to a couple who must deal with these residual effects of manic episodes.

Of all the psychiatric disorders, the chemical dependencies are perhaps the most destructive of marital and family harmony (see Chap. 10). People under the influence of alcohol or drugs become uninhibited and therefore say and do things which they later regret. Unfortunately, however, the damage has often been done already from the perspective of the "wronged" spouse. Marital problems which result from chemical dependency include coming home at inappropriate hours, inappropriate behavior while under the influence of alcohol or drugs, inappropriate temper outbursts, losing jobs, and spending excessive amounts of money for alcohol or drugs. Most of these problems are likely to remain as long as the individual continues to abuse alcohol or drugs. Consequently, the counselor should probably recommend that the spouse with a chemical dependency seek psychiatric help and be withdrawn from alcohol or drugs before counseling is undertaken. If the dependent spouse refuses, the marital counselor may wish to try to help the couple deal with the results of the chemical dependency. The energy may be better spent in supportive efforts with the nondependent spouse.

Conditions Requiring Referral Instead of Marital Counseling

Marital counseling is likely to be ill-advised or impossible with a few particular psychiatric disorders. When one of the partners suffers from a paranoid disorder, efforts at counseling will be sabotaged by that spouse's suspiciousness and tendency to project. Paranoid suspiciousness will lead the person to believe that the counselor is continually undermining him in his relationship with his wife. Paranoid projection will lead the individual to believe firmly that the blame for whatever is going on falls anywhere except on his own shoulders. Since people with paranoid disorders can become quite angry and are potentially dangerous, such people should be under careful medical supervision if they are willing to accept it. Although schizophrenia can be quite disruptive of marital relationships, in that the schizophrenics tend to be withdrawn and often unable to work, patients with schizophrenia are typically too severely impaired in their thinking processes or emotional responsiveness in order to be able to cooperate adequately with marital counseling. In both the case of paranoia and of schizophrenia, efforts will usually be better spent supporting the healthy spouse and assisting him or her in coping with the consequences of the partner's illness.

Concurrent Psychiatric Treatment in Marital Counseling

In a few cases, it may be appropriate to refer a patient to a psychiatrist for specific treatment and to do marital counseling at the same time. In such cases, ideally the marital counselor and the psychiatrist should have good lines of communication with one another and a working understanding of mutual goals.

In general, the disorders for which concurrent treatment may be appropriate are the milder ones. They include some forms of anxiety disorder and some forms of personality disorder. For example, an individual experiencing anxiety or phobias may see a psychiatrist for tranquilizing medication, individual psychotherapy, relaxation therapy, or some other form of behavioral therapy. A person with a compulsive personality disorder may benefit from individual psychotherapy directed at helping him achieve insight about the sources and consequences of his compulsive behavior. Patients in whom depressive symptoms have remitted only partially may continue to need psychiatric supervision both for medication and for individual emotional support. In situations where there are two different therapists, the person seeing both an individual therapist and a marriage counselor may try to use his experience in individual therapy as a lever to manipulate marital counseling. Firm guidelines concerning this potential problem should be initially agreed upon by all involved: the marital counselor, the psychiatrist, and the marital couple.

How to Recommend Referral to a Psychiatrist

Ideally, the marital counselor should try to establish familiarity with the psychiatric facilities available in the area where he works. He then will be able to recommend referral to a particular psychiatrist wih some sincerity and confidence.

If a counselor sees that a particular client requires referral, ordinarily he should begin by bringing the possibility up gently and directly in front of both marital partners. He should tactfully identify the symptoms suggestive of the particular disorder which the client has and indicate that these respond best to medical care instead of or concurrently with counseling. Depending on the particular type of problem, the recommendations for psychiatric referral may be handled somewhat differently. For example, the paranoid patient should never be characterized as paranoid, but should be told sympathetically that he is unhappy and uncomfortable about the rebuffs which he feels he has experienced and that a medical doctor may be able to provide a medication which will help him feel less painful and unhappy. A patient suffering from depression, on the other hand, can be told that much of his unhappiness is probably due to the fact that he suffers from depression, that such conditions tend to respond quite well to medical treatment, and that after or along with such treatment marital counseling can be undertaken or continued as necessary. The counselor can indicate that the psychiatrist is the type of medical doctor most experienced in handling emotional problems and that, therefore, a referral of that type is recommended. In short, the patient should eventually be told directly that he needs to see a psychiatrist, but that should never be the opening statement in any recommendation for referral.

Disorders Which May Complicate Counseling But Not Require Referral

Some patients seen in marital counseling may have a recognizable psychiatric disorder, but referrals may nevertheless be inappropriate. As indicated above, the primary reason for referring a patient to a psychiatrist includes the need for hospitalization, the need for psychotropic medication, significant risk to the patient as in the case of the suicidal patient or the person undergoing alcohol withdrawal, and a few patients requiring intensive long-term psychotherapy or briefer individual supportive therapy. Some psychiatric disorders, notably many of the various personality disorders, may significantly complicate marital relationships but be inappropriate for referral because no acceptable treatment is available.

The marital counselor who observes that one of the partners appears to have a severe personality disorder should attempt to assess whether that person might respond to psychiatric referral or individual psychotherapy. Clues that the individual may benefit include good intelligence, the ability to feel anxiety and guilt, and a willingness to assume responsibility for his or her own behavior. Nevertheless, most patients with a personality disorder tend to be dependent and manipulative. They are most likely to use individual therapy and "the sick role" as a means of assuming leverage and domination in the marital relationship. Futhermore, since psychiatric treatment of most personality disorders tends to be unsuccessful, in most couples with personality disorder the potential risks are likely to outweigh the potential benefits.

Summary

Various specific psychiatric disorders may complicate marital and sexual counseling. The counselor should be familiar with the common symptoms of the major types of psychiatric disorders so that he can recognize them and make referrals when appropriate. In general, only the more serious types of disorders will require referral. In some cases, the counselor's major role may be to provide support for the spouse of a person suffering from a serious disorder. In many other cases, particularly the mood disorders, the outcome of marital counseling may be quite good if the basic psychiatric disorder is treated prior to counseling.

REFERENCES

Andreasen, N. C.: *Understanding Mental Illness: A Layman's Guide.* Augsburg Publishing House, Minneapolis, Minnesota, 1974.

Cadoret, R. J., and King, L. J.: *Psychiatry in Primary Care.* The C. V. Mosby Co., St. Louis, Missouri, 1974.

Woodruff, R. A., Goodwin, D. W., and Guze, S. B.: *Psychiatric Diagnosis.* Oxford University Press, New York, 1974.

Part III
Counseling in Sexual Problems

DAVID M. REED, Ph.D.

14

Male Sexual Conditioning

Sex is the only innate human function which can respond almost entirely to external conditioning. Whatever the stimuli—the passion of a relationship, a fantasy, the learned socialization within the family and peer group, or a committed value system—the human is able to have his sexual behavior shaped so as to present a remarkable variety. This is particularly true of males. Kinsey found it impossible to predict, from independent sociological variables, how a man's sexual response would develop. Variety in attitudes and behavior crosses all class lines. And these responses may change profoundly within the span of one lifetime. As a result, men range from Don Juans to saints and are scattered throughout society without regard to social class, age, education, religion, or health needs.

In exploring conditioning factors a few assumptions will be made. First, it will be assumed that each stimuli described as a conditioning factor does not stand alone, but is related to others. For the sake of clarity each will be approached differentially. Second, it will be assumed that to identify one stimulus or conditioning experience as a primary cause is probably inaccurate. While the language here may imply straight line causality, a closed loop relationship is close to the fact, and one can only speak of probable motivating factors, not ultimate ones.

The theoretical approach which the therapist should use here is based on adaptational psychodynamics, whereby behavior is interpreted as to its adaptive qualities for the survival and satisfaction (whatever that may be) of the individual. The individual is viewed as a composite of inherited physiological endowments and psychosocial experiences whereby adaptive skills are learned. A man thereby responds to his world through the equipment he has been given. This world, of course, includes family and society. The equipment refers to his psychological and physiological characteristics. The sum total of the interaction between the psychosocial and the physiological, in this area of sexual function, is what may be termed the *sexual self-image*.

As is the case with most human behavior, it may be said that experience precedes metaphor. So it is with sex. The male experiences which shape his sexual self-image wander from physiological adventures within his own body to emotional odysseys within the mind to interpersonal tasks over the life cycle. His self-image is a system of perceptions built from these factors. His *sexual* self-image is that portion of perceptions which are involved in and respond to the sexual motive state. In the colloquial sense, we all go a little mad over sex. The orgasmic excitement demands passion in even the coolest of lovers—at some level of awareness. It is how the male sees himself in the embrace of this involuntary state that his sexual self-image comes into play. It is here that sex counseling should focus, where the male "actually" perceives himself during the sex act. The same man may always be the same romantic lover no matter whom he beds. Or the same man may be many others within his sexual self-image at different times, a Don Juan, a Casper Milquetoast, a rapist, or a father figure.

The counseling problems are as follows. (1) What is the sexual self-image? (2) What motivates it? (3) Is it adaptive to the interpersonal context at hand? Male patients with dysfunction invariably live within defeatist, depressed, failure-ridden sexual self-images. To treat them, it is necessary to explore the physiological and psychosocial components in order to assess how the conditioning or shaping of these responses developed.

The following discussion will develop along these lines. First, it will be inferred that psychosocial conditioning can be subdivided into psychological and sociological components. The family will be described as the source of psychological conditioning and society as the source of sociological shaping. The former creates sexual identity; the latter shapes sexual role behavior. Physiological conditioning will be treated separately and its output identified as the sexual response cycle.

Psychological Conditioning: The Family

Sexual identity begins at home. The idea of the young boy made aware that he has a penis and is different from his sister becomes "I am a male." This is the early curious phase of exploration of his own genitals, often masturbatory, and brings about a dim awareness that he has something specific about him. This is a sense of identity about his gender. It is followed by expectations as to how a male acts, what he does, how he is held or touched, and where he is different from peers without penises. Often the male is asked, "What are you going to be when you grow up?" in the midst of being told to be tough, not to cry when he hurts, and to fight his own fights. He then senses, "I am a man." His sexual identity is under way. It includes self-assertion and competition acted out in play and sports. While his sister plays house he plays ball; and while she is cuddled when she hurts or just wants to be held, he is dismissed sooner from the parental embrace although he has the same needs.

It goes without saying that the boy is imitating the man. He watches his father figures and copies their nonverbal cues. As Freud and others describe it, he also encounters sexual feelings from the very start and with them knows the conflicting experience of excitement and guilt. He has some awareness of sexual excitement due to self-stimulation either accidental or intended. He has natural curiosity about his body, its openings, and those of the bodies around him. He wonders about babies and how they get here. But there are rules. He cannot get too excited; and he cannot get too nosy. So sex play is sporadic, sometimes obvious and sometimes covert. What he learns is a combination of factors. (Sadock, 1976.)

First the boy learns that having your plumbing on the outside is pretty neat: it is efficient and feels good. As the little boy said when arriving at a camp-out and learning that he could take off his clothes and go for a skinny dip, "Great! My penis needs a breath of fresh air!" But immediately following on this the boy also learns that people react differently to his sexual moods. Some like them, some are excited, some are bored, and some think they are distinctly out of place. Most of the parent figures who are concerned about his maturity and self-restraint have ambivalent feelings. They usually react with the "forbidden fruit" attitude: it is alright to enjoy as long as you keep it quiet and do not get caught. At the same time, there is a hidden danger to your passions, so watch out.

The young man thus learns self-restraint from experiences of rejection or punishment; and he learns self-gratification on his own. This is an imbalance, a flaw in the conscience which all too many families perpetuate, for without some positive regard for his sexuality the boy unconsciously starts to avoid his inner sexual feelings. He stops asking questions about the birds and the bees, about how adults feel, how they decided about sex at his age. Just when directions are needed the most at home, the boy has learned there is too much discomfort there to talk about such things. So he internalizes the ability not to talk and then pretends to learn from his peers. Meanwhile most of his peers have undergone the same ambivalence, and it becomes in early adolescence a case of the blind leading the blind in sexual matters. A few more enlightened friends may arrive to save the day. But the period of anxiety in the young regarding sexual wisdom is the source of later pathology.

Sex play for boys is uneven and unpredictable, based on personal appetite and available options. All experience masturbation. It is, however, the don't get caught type which starts an invidious trend. On the one hand, the child begins to repeat riddance behavior. He hurries through an experience in order to get it over. One must wonder whether this is another conditioning toward an avoidance of sexual feelings. At the physical level, it does seem to be conditioning toward premature ejaculation. On the other hand, the boy learns to create fantasies of instant attraction and seduction with women in his mind, a pattern which meets with a rude awakening when he meets the real thing. At the positive side, however, the boy at least receives permission to be sexual somewhere and somehow. As he begins to date and socialize there is positive reinforcement both from parents and peers, for to be a loner in teen years is a strike against one.

Most families express fears of homosexuality in their sons where there is not active heterosexual play and later dating. Peer groups apply the same pressure with no mercy. Kinsey pointed out fully two-thirds of boys have some kind of homosexual play in youth, with no predictable outcome. Many observers note same sex affection as a normal phase in learning to express affection and undergo individuation. From the conditioning perspective it is an important learning experience for the male to know his feelings about homosexuality. This usually occurs in early adolescence for nonspecific motives, going from curiosity to confusion about one's sexual identity. Perhaps 10% of the total adult population confirm their homosexual choices in adult life. For the great majority it is a phase only. (Udry, 1974.)

Stereotypes of the homosexual in family reactions seem to emphasize that too much feeling among men is effeminate—except aggression. Sons who turn gay are typically seen as failures by one or the other parent; and most (heterosexual) parents also blame themselves.

The teen-age child dates within a typical point of reference: will he marry this girl? Pairing off of the young in dating seems to be a preparation for mating. (Broderick, 1969.) With it comes another surge of ambivalence in most parent-child relationships: premarital intercourse. While the boy has been encouraged to gain experience, he must also now deal with responsibility for his actions, and most families in middle and upper America view premarital intercourse as a "rite of passage." It is not only girls who lose their virginity.

The young man has two problems: physical desire and emotional attitudes. For the first time he must begin to discriminate between an object and a person. He also knows there are different stakes being played between him and the girl. It is unlikely the motives of both are identical.

His sexual identity has been shaped by the time of entrance into adolescence, and he knows whether or not he values "being a man." He has tested—and been tested by—his parent figures. At the unconscious level, as seen by Freud, the male may develop oedipal anxiety, castration fears about intimacy with women due to an imbalanced relationship with his mother. She may have been covertly seductive. Or father may have been too distant. Whatever the cause, his internal sexual energies, within him since infancy and striving for expression, respond to the parent-child dynamics in an unconscious selection of a mate. As it is said, a man marries his mother. . . .

The family prepares the male to enter the sexual arena by satisfying what Kardiner describes as the "affectivity potential" (1945). This means the ability of the youngster to express sexual and assertive needs so as to achieve healthy intimacy. It has its roots in the quality of the emotional exchange between mother and child, especially around the early years of weaning. This is usually uncovered in the sexual history by describing the psychological atmosphere of the home and the son's relationship with his mother.

Of course the son reacts to more than this. He also responds to the marital interplay between mother and father, observing how each handles the other, imitating them, and then internalizing aspects of this behavior as he perceived it.

From the viewpoint of counseling, most male clients show a low affectivity potential. They are out of touch with feelings, either within themselves or others. Their approach to sex is far more stereotyped than intuitive. The usual reaction to a request to express emotions is one of embarrassment. More than this, there is also a lack of technique: no one ever showed them how to express the affective side of life.

> M, 26, was a medical student whose wife was anorgasmic with him. For awhile the therapy focused on her own anxieties about letting go, being able to enjoy. It was unclear where there was any irritation within the relationship, as both demonstrated great affection for the other. After several sessions it began to be clear that the husband never really let his emotional guard down. He was always "doctoring" his expressive wife and showing only a fatherly sympathy, nothing else. Confrontation of this revealed that he did not know how to express the feelings he felt. He only panicked at her intensity and covertly withdrew in confusion. The bind was broken through sessions which focused on "M's turn to feel"—during which the wife discovered that she had always neglected to be a good listener.

If the family does not suppress the ability of the son to express feelings effectively, he develops good comfort with his sexual self-image. The other detour to health here is also common, where the male is urged to express himself, but always through aggression. Tremendous urging to be a winner, an extrovert, to look good and compete is the chronic message for the American son. Parents fear the phase of introversion, where he may not want to date or play but simply to daydream and be left alone. And if he is not interested in girls. . . .

One result is the hard driving male adult who has to win in bed as everywhere else. Sex is an executive action, and something that a guy does to a gal. The son that absorbs this conditioning may be overaggressive in sex. His wife finds him unable to treat her as an equal or so mechanical in bed that she cannot react. Here the male is compensating usually for fears of his own dependency needs, keeping a tough exterior to cover a vulnerable interior. Some compensate by moving toward homosexuality out of fear of failing with anything else.

The goal of counseling here is to separate out the feelings of sexuality from those rooted in aggression. Does he take part in making love or does he direct it? Is he competing with some standard his peers imparted to him? Can he learn to feel sensual simply for its own sake? Or does he have to have coitus or at least some kind of genital success in order to validate the experience?

Family conditioning is basic sex education prior to that imparted by society. The output is nonspecific. Not so much a body of facts as a cluster of attitudes about being sexual . . . and about feeling sensual. Relatively few families ever reinforce the positive side of sensuality for boys. They are not hugged as much as girls, as will be noted below. The substitute for sensuality tends to be genitality with males. This begins in the family and is repeated endlessly in society as will be seen.

Sociological Conditioning: Society

Society builds on sexual identity to create and maintain sexual roles. Role behavior is determined by how the individual sees his peer group and the culture around it and how that group in turn transmits expectations to the individual as to the rules for group membership. (Shope, 1975.)

Today society presents constant sex education. There is constant bombardment about sensuality (being sexy) and sexuality (being a man or woman) to an extent never before experienced. The client who says he never had any sex education refers to formal types, such as books, school, or church. His true sex education comes from peers.

The major message today is one of sexual performance by the male. In every form of communication, books, magazines, and the all present TV monitor, the male is expected to perform. This cannot be underestimated. Male patients as well as counselors must be made aware of this, for there is no immunity. Everything the male sees or reads implies how important it is to be sexual and to perform well in this sphere. Our culture is renowned for its emphasis on romantic love (Reed, 1976) and for the sanction given sex and marriage in the name of love.

The glut of sex manuals on the market indicates our fascination with sex, our voyeuristic impulses seeking gratification through reading or seeing how others act in bed, and for the male the subconscious opportunity to compete. There is a cult of the "Big O," where couples are in search of bigger and better orgasms which are to be delivered to liberated women by dedicated men.

The average man is thus expected to be an instant sex expert in his sex role. Peer behavior among young boys shows much bravado as to sexual conquests. Girls are divided into nice and otherwise, with those willing to engage in coitus or genital sex play being quickly identified as "hot," and the boys in turn rating themselves as to their ability to make it with them. So the boy pretends to know. As dating experience continues, he discovers that the girls generally expect him to know and, having this knowledge, to be an expert in the clinches, the backseat, or the bed. Men seeking counseling constantly show the impact of this conditioning.

> Bert, 39, is a hard driving young executive determined to make it big in the market. He has a history of many girl friends and is not going to marry until he is through sowing his oats. He had too much to drink last week, had been working several days in a row, wanted to have sex with his latest friend, and was appalled to find himself unable to sustain an erection. He cannot sleep now and is haunted by the fear that he is now over the hill and will fail the next time.

Once the assertive male fails by his own standards, he expects to fail again the next time. This fear of failure makes matters worse and undermines his sexual self-esteem even more. So he withdraws in a depression, usually tries more alcohol to loosen up, but this also fails to help. The performance demand never leaves him, for it appears also in nonsexual spheres. Happiness for the male, by the tradition of our Protestant work ethic, is related to his industriousness. Peer group acceptance is closely allied to the demonstration of upward mobility and to the implication that the man is a cool lover—or hot one, depending on the rhetoric of the group.

Society also tells the man that sex is for the young and virile. If you don't use it you will lose it goes the myth. So many men act as if they will lose function over 50, certainly over 60, that they are doubly pressed to make the scene actively when they are younger. Implied here also is the code of sex appeal according to certain hair length, clothing, and body build. The male is shown role models in the media that emphasize athletic ability, intellectual quickness, and romantic expertise. If he is not expected to look a certain way, the objects for his sexual choice are, so the fashion industry affects women to equate beauty and sex appeal to an unfortunate degree.

Our culture also tells the male, by inference, that sex is a physical act. When one thinks of sex one is expected to think of coitus or genital excitement. The entire spectrum of the emotional aspects of sexuality are omitted. When this goes hand in hand with the performance pressure, one can see how the male develops the image of the sexual animal, the "rapist" in the minds of many women.

Today's world is in the midst of a renaissance of sexual attitudes, as has been pointed out by several observers. With the advent of the Pill, a liberalizing of divorce laws, and a generation of political restlessness and challenge to authority, the modern woman's liberation movement is a special challenge to the modern man. Not only is he expected to be a sexual expert with women, he is also now expected to deal with their new self-awareness. It was difficult enough when sex was something one did *to* a woman or *for* a woman; it is even more apprehensive when it is *with* a woman. The lines for the perennial battle of the sexes have been drawn anew. A new role relationship for men and women is underway, characterized by a new equality. (Janeway, 1971.) The male today is in a period of flux. His father and grandfather demonstrated that a man has certain rights simply as a man. The historic double standard for the sexes was built on this, so that the male could expect applause for his sexual exploits, while the woman could only be booed off the stage. In many areas this has changed. Women do not give the male ascribed rights; he must achieve them. Thus, the male is expected to negotiate with women. His forebears never had to do this, and he lacks an effective model upon which to rely. In this dilemma he encounters another condition of society about sex: secretiveness. The ability to communicate comfortably about sexual feelings, needs, and wants is quite rare.

> The Jacksons have been married for 17 years, with three fine children. Mildred has confessed, after reading her magazines about sex in this world, that she has been pretending orgasm. Jack, as in response to this, admitted that he has seen himself as a premature ejaculator all these years, but he was too embarrassed to mention it. The counseling started by encouraging them to discuss frankly their sexual needs, hopes, and feelings.

Perhaps the most common cultural stereotype which affects love-making in our culture is related both to the mystique of the male lover bringing his woman to climax and to the "let's not talk about it and hope for the best" approach which is so universal. This is the romantic idea about love as the panacea and fount of happiness in our society. It is the theme of adolescence and the proper reason for marriage according to the code. Part of love is the romantic, rather mystical notion, embedded in countless romances and fairy stories, that love is a form of knowledge. The saying goes, "If you really love me, you can read my mind." Under the impact of this perception, many couples abandon effective communication—also avoiding guilt and embarrassment—just when they need it the most, in bed. They also avoid the opportunity to learn from each other, thereby remaining vulnerable to simple ignorance about sex, another condition in our culture. We have created a problem about learning creatively about sexuality due to our equating knowing with doing. As a result, many men and women choose subconsciously not to know, relying once more on the magical thought that loving is all one has to try in order to be wise.

Counselors should view their clients as traumatized and secretive and ignorant about sex as a result of these cultural conditions. The diagnostic process should explore how the male and his partner have learned about sex, what kind of attitudes have occurred, and how these have affected performance. The problem areas derived from this portion of socialization are the following.

1. *Machismo:* refers to the performance ethic under which most males try to thrive and includes the double standard known as "sex is for men, babies are for women."

2. *Masturbatory guilt:* built into our culture as part of the emphasis on sex for procreation only and on the view that passions are dangerous; and it makes many men avoid inner feelings and fantasies about sex which should be more expressed than suppressed for the sake of growth.

3. *Myths:* which take the place of knowledge since the male usually chooses someone a little older and smoother with the tall tales as his sex educator. Two such myths are—if a woman does not climax in coitus it is the man's fault, and age withers.

Finally, perhaps the ultimate damage our culture seems to do in sexual conditioning is to separate the male from an awareness of his feelings. Thus, he takes on his sex role behavior with a limited ability to express affection. Since he has to be stoic at work and brave in sports, he is a combination of both in bed. The obsessive fear of losing control of one's feelings regarding sex seems to infect the ordinary male with sexual problems. Traditional psychotherapy has only made headway where this fear is attacked and men are enabled to change by trying to express themselves. Sex counseling often takes a shortcut by introducing the touching aspect of caress as a form of communication. The male is asked how he feels *during* the sexual experiences themselves (touching), since it is in the sexual motive state that the negative automatic response seems to recur. To express feelings while they are felt, both verbally and tactile (nonverbally), is the goal. When interlocked with the same behavior by his partner, a new dimension of communication begins and growth occurs as anxiety decreases.

The foregoing, either from family conditioning or that of society, depends on the physiological substrate within which the male responds.

Physiological Conditioning: Sexual Function

To paraphrase George Orwell, all men are sexual but some men are more sexual than others. Sex is a physiological experience if it is nothing else. It is characterized by the following overlapping features: desire for orgasmic release (sex drive), erotic pleasure response at the tactile and olfactory levels, and general health and body image.

First, the issue of innate sex drive refers to how great a demand for orgasmic pleasure the individual maintains regardless of external factors. Some husbands are described by their wives as "always" wanting sex. While there are several emotional motives for constant sex, one must also take into account that this man may indeed be born with his sexual accelerator glued to the floor.

> Gary, age 34, defended his high sex drive with an apparently airtight case. He had always had easy conquests with girls since teen-age years, as he had an easygoing manner and was physically attractive. He liked all sorts of sex play, yet was tolerant of his wife's more limited desires as to variety. He did not seem angry at women and determined to rape them all. His wife, also in her early 30's and herself a lovely and intelligent person, was flattered at his attentions but frustrated that he was an "instant turn-on" all the time. She was orgasmic most of the time and noted he was a good lover. She was troubled basically that she was always having to apologize for not being as eager as he—although she could be if she put her mind to it.

Many men depict a high sex drive with no underlying pathology or hidden agendas in the marital relationship. Their psychodynamics may imply a Don Juan syndrome, with a compensatory need to reassure oneself about one's own sexuality by constant conquest. But just as often they may not. A man at any age may simply like sex and have a more constant fascination for it than another man. By the same token, a man may have a low sex drive, to the frustration of his partner. Husbands have been reported by their spouses to do all the right things at the right time—but simply not often enough. Here again, while there are often, if not usually, other motivational factors contributing to this, such as the depressed, compulsive, and task-oriented man who is more gratified with things than with emotions, there are also men whose "normal" pace is to walk, not run.

The counseling task here is to aid in adjusting to the difference in sex drive between the partners. Most couples make the mistake of counting the number of times they have coitus and thereby creating a scorecard, with one winning and the other losing. Over a period of time they tend to revert to the needs of the lower driven partner, thereby producing a frustrated and irritable situation for the other.

> Bill, age 56, looks at his wife of 30 years with great longing. But she has never been that spontaneous, although she has done her best not to refuse him. He is nagged by her "surrender" mentality, where she presents herself as a receptacle for his needs. While he admits that she can be excellently responsive when she is in the mood, he also feels that she is basically in control of their sex life as to its quality.

The counselor can help here by providing each a chance to ventilate frustrations and concern and help them to re-evaluate the counting motif, which implies that more is better. They should also be guided to note the emphasis on coitus as sex, omitting most forms of noncoital sex play as of equal value. This is a common error. Couples with maximal sexual adjustment learn to prize all forms of sexual interaction, from a general massage to an orgy. Thus, in reference to sex drive conditioning, the only route to health is compromise in the midst of differences.

The second physiological factor for males is at the tactile level, referring to the degree of "skin hunger" he may possess for erogenous pleasure. Here we again see a physical factor shaped by subtle psychosocial forces. In our society young boys are expelled from the lap of the mother and put into aggressive play sooner than young girls. They thus undergo a nontouch conditioning which is reinforced later. Most families espouse a certain level of bravery and stoicism for the young male. The son is urged not to cry, to hold back the tears. This is typically translated into avoidance of one's feelings, which seems to be concomitant with lack of appreciation for erogenous pleasure at being held or caressed.

> George, age 44, is gregarious on the surface but his wife says it is like being married to a computer. He only rarely gets involved caressing her, and even if he does it to her, she is not permitted to fondle him. They sought to correct a case of secondary impotence and were instructed in therapy to experiment with nongenital caressing without intercourse in order to establish better tactile communication and comfort and to educate each other as to their physical desires. George was reluctant to "play around," as it was unmanly for him to be on the receiving end of caressing without him being in charge and moving toward intercourse. He tried it a few times and discovered—somewhat to his embarrassment—that he had deep desires to be held and touched. He came alive "for the first time in years."

The suppression of healthy skin hunger in our society does not seem to apply to females. It is the man who pays the price, who has to shake hands with his father as a teen-ager when he wants to kiss him or be held by him. And teen-agers tease each other unmercifully about being gay or homosexual where any same sex desires for touching are demonstrated.

The male is thus conditioned to undervalue his body as a sexually enriching factor. He either avoids caressing altogether, dispenses it mechanically, or overemphasizes genital sensations from caressing as the only legitimate ones. If he is being caressed directly through penile stimulation for an erection he usually accepts this as masculine and gives himself permission to enjoy this. The physical sensations are so directly pleasurable as to overcome learned ambivalence. Nongenital sensations are seen as unimportant, and the body is often quite out of tune for effective erotic or sensual pleasure. This is a serious breakdown in the sensual biofeedback pattern between the cortex which may hold the ideas for sex and the hypothalamus which may retain the orgastic sensations themselves. Elderly males in particular who have been literally as well as figuratively untouched over their bodies for years tend to suffer more erectile insufficiency. Therapy must begin with tactile awakening and then proceed to genital caressing, all within the context of increasing sexual self-esteem, in order to recapture lost abilities. The combination of underdeveloped skin hunger and overemphasis on genitality should be explored wherever males of any age and background seek to improve their sexual self-comfort. Obviously, there are implicit cultural taboos reinforcing the conditioning here. Our heterosexual culture, with its heavy flavoring of male "machismo," creates negative sanctions for fully developed tactile responsivity. So the male develops within the generic limits of his body at the tactile level and at the same time deals with the limits imposed by his world.

Related to this tactile deprivation is the use of the olfactory senses by the male to develop sexual potentiality. Here again he is shortchanged. Only in very recent years has the man been encouraged to use colognes as part of his sex appeal. Yet it is worth noting that the most sexually dormant of males, unable to be well-aroused for a long time, can have his erotic interests provoked by the use of attractive colognes. Masters and Johnson have informally reported that one of the best unobtrusive measures for outcome of their sex therapy with disinterested males was whether the couple purchased and used massage lotions—with scents chosen by the male.

> Harry, 52, was a butcher with a long-standing pattern of limited libido. The history showed that he was chronically fatigued, bored with his life, yet in love with his wife and embarrassed that he was so reluctant to make

love. He had periods of impotence as well as chronic premature ejaculation, indicating anxiety about his sexual abilities in addition to a confused erotic appeal. He had lost sight of what aroused him, and this added failure to failure. The therapy focused first on his depressed self-esteem, then his ambivalence about his wife (seeing her as too intense), and finally on the recovery of his libido. Getting him to create a massage lotion with a scent of his choice was the first breakthrough, and his sexual withdrawal later remitted successfully.

While we do not yet understand the chemistry involved here, it is well to note that the body itself can and will affect the sex response and be a source of conditioning both as a stimulus and as a response. The innate predilection a man has about sex must affect how he reacts to external stimuli, just as it must affect those same externals by its own characteristics.

The third physiological condition within which the male functions is the congenital factors which define his health. It is important to note these however briefly because too many counselors with training in the behavioral sciences tend to overlook the fact that where the male has a sex problem he may well have a medical problem. The literature is so emphatic about psychological aspects of sexuality—and these are obviously quite important—that the physical aspects are overlooked. This is problematic, especially regarding males. Attention should be paid to the following.

1. Nervous system diseases such as the scleroses, syphilis, Parkinson's disease, and lesions of the spinal cord.

2. Diabetes, often undetected, but showing that from 25 to 60% of males over 40 with diabetes suffer erectile insufficiency at times.

3. High blood pressure and heart disease, where the medication for these illnesses may impair effective blood flow to the penis and thereby reduce sexual effectiveness.

4. Obesity, where the male overeats and is also physically inactive. Everything slows down, including sexual desires. Fatigue becomes the excuse and it usually is, since sex demands at least as much exertion as climbing two flights of stairs.

5. Alcohol intake where there is an addictive pattern indicating not only a personality disorder and self-deflating life style, but where the chemicals themselves heighten the desire but threaten the performance.

There are congenital limits to all humans, and these affect the sexual ability of the male most significantly. The counselor can diagnose an underlying health problem rooted in these areas only by focusing on them. Most men, keeping their casual self-sustaining image intact, will not report disease entities in their history unless asked. And because this list also implies inherited characteristics, histories which do not look at family health items will also be incomplete. The most common telltale symptom of male sexual "nonhealth" is the report of fatigue. Wives can indicate how the fatigue element destroys romance and sexual pleasure in the male. If it is a catchword that the American wife avoids sex by claiming headaches, it is equally true that the American husband claims tiredness. And he often is, especially if he is hiding one of the subtle illnesses noted here.

The obvious fact is that each man is limited by his physical endowments. How these limits affect actual sexual behavior is a fairly predictable theme.

The sex drive response affects the sexual motive state and thereby how sex is used by the male. Physically, the male can expect an orgasm 95% of the time over his life cycle. Instead of dealing with the female's question of "If I have an orgasm . . .," the male deals with "When I have an orgasm. . . ." Thus, having sex can often include mixed agendas, for each partner is predicting a different phasing to their response. Of the two, the male also relies on the experience of having genitalia which are both external and comparatively simple in operation. Thus, the male can learn about his erotic response or sensate focus which takes him to climax at an earlier age and with much greater certainty than can the female. He cannot easily empathize with the female's vastly more complex response pattern. The fact that the same woman who responded to one's foreplay so well last night will likely not respond so predictably to the same approach and sequence tonight is a chronic source of bewilderment to most men, and of irritation to most women.

The touch factor also has impact on sexual life style and technique. Men who avoid touch are generally unable to maximize the opportunities for true intimacy in a relationship, or they tend to overemphasize the heterosexual machismo stereotype, interpreting male affection as homosexual and therefore sick or silly. With women they make love out of duty. Furthermore, the male often responds to his experience with specific genital pleasure from touch by striving always to have sex which is selectively genital and nothing else. One physical factor here is that as the male approaches climax, stimulation demand becomes intense not only in the genital area but also at the base of the penis, above the scrotum. This in turn produces a demand for deep thrust and penetration at orgasm and ejaculation. With it comes an automatic muscle contraction extending to fingers and toes, so that the touching experience moves dramatically from caressing to grabbing. This is often a difficulty for the female partner, for at this time she may seek light caressing in the clitoral-mons veneris area in order to enhance her own response. Just at the moment of truth, so to speak, where the sympathetic nervous system begins to take over one's decision making, a marked difference in tactile needs can develop. The male needs to be touched precisely during these crucial moments in a nongenital, body-oriented embrace; and if he is one of those with underdeveloped response here, both partners may lose a key dimension of sexual pleasure.

Finally, the component of general health affects the sex life in a variety of ways. Put most simply, sex demands a reasonable degree of physical fitness both to exist as an attractive partner and to generate the libido or erotic interest which must exist as a starting point. This is not to advertise for slimness and youth, as is done in our youth-oriented society, but to denote the difference between a healthy self-image and one which is deprecated by its owner. There is no perfect physical shape for sex, only the ability to be active within interesting limits. This is not to sell the cult of the sexual athlete as is done in our world, but it is to point out realistically the difference between not caring about one's nutrition and whether one drinks oneself to sleep to avoid the possibility of sexual embarrassment and taking reasonable care about diet, drink, and health. A good attitude can overcome any specific physical limitation.

Finally, the point where physiology meets psychology, so to speak, is at the point of *body image* in the male. The growing male responds to the changes in his own body both from within and from without. He knows his own energy level and compensates for this over his life cycle. He must also look at his own body and react to this. The typical male judges penis size and body build—athletic or not, thin or not etc.,—and makes an evaluation of his sex appeal. From this grows his approach to sexual encounters, his inner sexual motive state. Fisher (1973) studied female orgasms and noted the woman as seeing herself as curved receptivity. In other studies he also found the usual male self-image as *extended vulnerability*. This has profound psychological implications for the man, indicating as it does the consequences of phallic possession. A man troubled by his sexual performance feels vulnerable, yet in order to function sexually he must perforce extend himself. This is a preconscious paradox which interferes at every level of function. It usually worsens over the life cycle, for with age the body changes, and a man's view of his body as sexual-sensual is under stress. He is no longer young, he feels it, and he looks it. He has been living in a world which has implied all the time that sex is for the young. He also runs into mythology about the male menopause. What he usually does not know is that while his erectile ability may be delayed in a sexual state, he can obtain full erection by effective genital stimulation. And he will be able to avoid premature ejaculation far better than he could decades earlier.

As can be seen we thereby return to ideas related to the sexual self-image, which is built upon identity and role factors as well as physiological function. It is ultimately a toss-up: mind over matter most of the time, but never all of the time.

REFERENCES

Broderick, C. B. (ed): *The Individual, Sex, and Society,* Johns Hopkins University Press, Baltimore, 1969.

Cuber, J. F., and Harroff, P. B.: *Sex and the Significant American,* Appleton-Century, New York, 1966.

Fisher, S.: *The Female Orgasm,* Basic Books, New York, 1973.

Janeway, E.: *Man's World, Woman's Place,* Dell Publishing Co., New York, 1971.

Kardiner, A.: *Psychological Frontiers of Society,* Columbia University Press, New York, 1945.

Reed, D. M.: Traditional marriage, in *The Sexual Experience* (Sadock, B. J., Kaplan, H. I., and Freedman, A. M., eds), pp. 217–230, Williams & Wilkins Co., Baltimore, 1976.

Sadock, B. J., Kaplan, H. I., and Freedman, A. M. (eds): *The Sexual Experience,* Williams & Wilkins Co., Baltimore, 1976.

Shope, D. F.: *Interpersonal Sexuality,* W. B. Saunders, Philadelphia, 1975.

Udry, J. R.: *The Social Context of Marriage,* 3rd Ed, J. B. Lippincott, Philadelphia, 1974.

E. LEE DOYLE, Ph.D.

15

Female Sexual Conditioning

Since this book is designed for the counselor in marital and sexual counseling, I shall share in this chapter, based on my professional experience with many females who have sexual difficulties, many of the "learnings" that females have as an infant, young child, adolescent, and as an adult which contribute to their sexual satisfaction and dissatisfaction. Females who function satisfactorily in their sexual life are those who have sufficient awareness, knowledge, confidence, and high self-esteem to be accepting of their bodies, minds, feelings, and values.

When working with females who have sexual problems, I want to categorize very early in the history taking whether the difficulty seems to be inorgasmic response under certain conditions, psychological or physiological vaginismus, dyspareunia, irregularity in sexual desire, or differences in sexual desires of her and her partner. It is very important to me that I take a complete developmental history—medical, social, physiological, psychological, sexual, and role identification and role expectations for themselves and those expectations that have been "placed upon them" as a female by their religious beliefs, family, peer, and community group relationships.

When garnering information related to the woman, my preference is that she "spin and weave" her own story of historical data, which gives me an opportunity of seeing and hearing (1) what events she sees and feels to be most important to her, (2) those areas of her life which she feels most uncomfortable and most comfortable and those which cause her most pain or most pleasure and (3) the areas of her life which she is willing to discuss and those aspects which she is reticent to reveal. Sometimes all the woman patient needs is to have someone who is interested, warm, open, honest, candid, understanding, and accepting of her as a person for her to "spill" all the information that is relevant to her within a very short period of therapy time.

The method used when I take a history is what I call a "whipped cream" fashion or "flow type" of history taking. That is, I allow the woman to move from subject to subject, topic to topic, and I move with her flow in gathering informaton. If she moves from time period to time period in her life story, I feel that it is my responsibility to flow with her in order to be effective by not stopping her natural, normal process. I then have the opportunity to observe how she responds to herself, what her powers of concentration are, her rigidity, her acceptance of herself, her resistances, pressures, rambling tendencies, interests, anger, and motivation. In seeing, hearing, and feeling her process, I get to know her more as a total person rather than having a check-list type of information gathering. Also, relevant questions asked with appropriate timing can illicit more information which assists in the therapy process.

Conditioning factors which contribute to the enhancement of female sexuality or deter her sexual development are multifaceted, varied, and each individual has a unique set of conditioning factors or "learnings" with which to work, unlearn, and relearn in order to function satisfactorily according to her values. Any conditioning such as lack of information about the physiological development of her natural, normal developing body, psyche, and mind contributes a great deal to her lack of sexual development. Awareness, knowledge, and acceptance of the body, emotional feelings, mind, and values of an individual are very early influenced by parental attitudes toward the child.

Awareness, Knowledge, and Acceptance of Body

Awareness of one's physical body begins at a very early age. Parental attitudes toward natural secretions — tears, mucus, exudates, perspiration, vaginal fluids, blood, saliva, excretions, and/or appreciation for the natural secretions and odors of the body affect the woman's acceptance of hersef. Her positive or negative feelings toward her body and its functions begin from birth and are based on the attitudes of others.

When the baby girl is being diapered and touched, looked at, talked and listened to, and is reared by loving and accepting or disapproving parents, negative or positive feelings and beliefs about herself develop. Negative conditioning, such as frowning faces, when the parents and other adults look over into and on top of the child and negative, harsh, and uncomfortable noises and sounds like gagging sounds and "pew" or "shew" when diapering her all contribute to a negative attitude toward the genital area. Spanking or whacking the hands and/or bottom of the child and jerking or yanking the legs high into the air is an entirely different feel than stroking, rubbing, and caressing; therefore, sounds, looks, and appearance of adults and touch are all indicators to the perception of the child as to whether or not she is an acceptable human being.

Long before the woman can remember, she was learning whether she was acceptable to other people, those people who reared her as well as others who were around her. How she was handled, how she was touched, how she was talked to, the expressions on adult faces, how they touched, whether tight and jerky or smooth and soothing, whether warm and affectionate or brusk and hostile contribute to her perceptions and beliefs about her personhood. So many of the attitudes and learnings of the female occurred before she can consciously remember.

After she is old enough to consciously remember touch, sight, sounds, smells, and her parents' attitudes toward her in her exploring, investigating, and touching her own body contribute to either positive or negative attitudes toward her skin, eyes, hair, nose, mouth, hands, genitals, legs, and feet and her appreciation and acceptance of her body and its functions. The young child is naturally curious and will touch, feel, ask questions, and express her wants and needs early in life through crying, cooing, laughing, smiling, frowning, kicking, yelling, beating, and contractions of the total body unless this natural desire is squelched by fearful, frustrated adults.

Early learnings in body awareness, its appearance and function, will be those demonstrated by adults, such as warmth, touching, hugging, stroking, laughter, fun, and expression of affection through gentle squeezing. Physical warmth is created by holding of the child and *touch is taught*. Many times parents feel uncomfortable in the caressing and gentle squeezing of their children and create negative touching by jiggling the head, patting the head, "tweeking" the ears, "tweeking" the nose, "chinny-chin-chin" the chin, and jerky playful movements, which are playful and positive but do not include the smoothness of a caress. Also, the acceptance of the parents bodies and the physical closeness of the child provide physical warmth and is one way of teaching the child how to touch.

Since touch is taught, young women often have not been taught and do not know how to touch pets in a way in which to bring pleasure, or the ears of a parent so they do not hurt, or objects worn by parents such as beads, earrings, shirts, and garments in order to have pleasure for themselves and the person being touched. So many times, parents and/or other adults move away rapidly, creating the sense and feeling of rejection to the child when in reality it is a self-protective movement of the adults. Self-protection of one person and the feeling of rejection of the other person often go hand in hand. It is most important that the parent supply information and teaching to the child to show meaningful touching so that the child does not, early in life, learn the feelings of rejection based upon lack of knowledge.

Laughter also is a very important expression for the child to hear and to understand early in life. It is important that the parents share, explain, and clarify that laughter is *with* the child *not at the child* or *about the child*. Laughter can be perceived by the young child as a put down or negative expression rather than an accepting and loving expression; especially, when it pertains to the early physiological development of the child and her self-awareness.

Seemingly, in our culture, we live in what I call the "Comparison Syndrome." So, very early in life, the female learns to *compare* the growth of her body and what her body does in relationship to others bodies rather than accept the differences. Some of the areas in which parents and other adults compare a child to another are psychological and physical growth patterns, choice of toys and activities, play patterns, and types and amount of body activity. When she is toilet trained, when she loses her teeth, when she develops breasts, how she is compared with behavior of other young girls, whether she is accepted as an individual with individual interests, or whether she is compared with others affects her sexuality. Because sex and sexuality have been such "hush-hush" topics within our culture, there has been little talk about the differences in developmental stages of people. Similarities of physiological development and behavior to fulfill role and cultural expectations and comfort levels of adults are emphasized. Much comparison is done rather than the acceptance of differences that each young woman develops physiologically and psychologically at different ages which enhances or deters self-worth, which then affects sexual satisfaction.

Enuresis (bedwetting) and toilet training affect the child's comfort and acceptance of her vulva area. Nonaccepting, negating, shameful, and shaming parents and other adults who are ignorant of body and muscular development, sensory awareness, and the learning process of the child can create an atmosphere of guilt for the female. Because the genitalia and excretory orifices are so near in proximity, she very often associates the punishment, attitudinal, verbal, and/or physical, she received in toilet training with any sexual feelings, whether emotional or physical; therefore, she denies sexual feelings due to prior conditioning.

Body movement and language are very important to a child's physiological and psychological development. Acceptance of the child's patterns of movement from the parents and other adults in the child's life contribute to her self-esteem and ability to develop positive attitudes toward and about herself. Kinds and rhythms of body movement— jerkiness, fluidity, tenseness, smoothness, hesitancy, and other responses to feelings are aped and copied as well as specifically taught. Freedom, flow, and use of the body depend upon inherited physical characteristics, psychological traits, learned behavior, self-acceptance, and energy level of the child.

As the female child grows into adolescence, there are other factors regarding her body which are important for her to know and understand, such as the general health rules of nutrition, rest, and personal hygiene, all of which contribute to her self-value. Knowledge and acceptance from adults that she is aware and self-conscious about her "growth spurt," late or early development of breasts, pubic hair, underarm hair, change and shape of her body, and body movement contributes to her self-confidence.

When a young woman's body starts changing and developing, it is most important that she get approval with warmth and tenderness, from both the same-sexed parent and siblings and opposite-sexed parent and siblings. Her fathers and brothers' approval and acceptance of the naturalness of her body and its development will enhance her own comfort level. Positive recognition from them as well as female role models and peers without timidity, shyness, or discomfort will contribute to her feelings of competency and hopefully allay her feelings of inadequacy. Learning self-identification through experimentation with cosmetics, clothing, voice tone, word choice, and body movements can be encouraged and accepted by parents. Parents who are supportive of self-growth and individual differences can contribute to the young woman's feelings of self-hood for her concerns, worries, and interests in her body—skin, hair, and nails—are heard.

Due to the Comparison Syndrome of visual standards or ideals of physical appearance in our culture, the young woman's ability to meet her ideals with either enhance or negate her acceptance of herself and her sexuality. Standards are mental images of what she feels to be necessary and these fantasies keep her from accepting the realities of her own body and its behaviors with appreciation. Standards or ideals of physical appearance are often so high and rigid that there is a lack of acceptance of her body and abilities, which interfers with comfortable, satisfactory behavior in order to reach satisfactory sexual response in adult life. Sometimes excessive pride and vanity develop because of cultural expectations and promotion of how a female "should" look or act. Comparing her own self-image to her "ideal image" prevents the young woman from self-acceptance of reality and of the amount of time it takes to learn to be appreciative of her body and its functions. This female can often have physiological pathways open to expression of her sexuality, and not the psychological pathways.

Awareness, Knowledge, and Acceptance of Feelings

Very early in life young women are conditioned as to which emotional feelings are acceptable and unacceptable and what behavior responses to her feelings are expected and rejected by their family, religion, community, and peer groups. Having opportunities to hear, see, and participate in positive, effective communication with her family and other people is a contributory factor to the acceptance of her own feelings early in life as well as in young adulthood. Communication is a process which includes the ability to (1) be aware of emotional feelings which are felt in the body, (2) find words in the head that fit with the emotional feelings in the body, (3) express verbally and physically those feelings in a positive and constructive way to others, and (4) "checkout" with the person who is listening to see if *you* have been understood as you mean to communicate.

When parents do not express emotional feelings with self-responsibility and a specific, definitive vocabulary that is understood, she is confused, puzzled, and frustrated. When parents do not verbalize as well as physically respond to their feelings, they leave a child wanting for a vocabulary that fits her emotional or psychological feeings. With a lack of an emotional vocabulary and inadequacy of expression of the parents and adults within the child's life, there is a lack of clarity as to what the adult is expressing or meaning and with lack of clarity, the child begins to wonder, think, assume, imagine, guess, believe, and/or have hunches about what the adult is thinking and/or feeling. So at an early age, the female child learns assumptions and game playing such as "detective" and "watch, look, and listen" in order to discover what others are feeling and/or meaning by their actions and how others feelings are stimulated, created, or hindered by her. Hearing sentences such as "I feel sad, I feel empty, I feel hurt, I feel tired, warm, loving, explosive, excited, anger, tenderness, warmth, caring, cared for, concerned, mischievous, loving, loved, sneaky, displease, easy, and uncomfortable" give clarity, confidence, and trust in her and others' feelings and ability to communicate.

An adolescent female is often confused by her own feelings, especially when they are different from her parents' attitudes or feelings. Her own feelings may be quite different and so she has conflicts early in life in that she learns attitudes and behaviors from the parents. Frustrations over certain activities, curiosity over certain activities, ways of encouraging and enhancing a person's curiosity, ways of showing trust, ways of showing enthusiasm, and how the parent offers stimulation of sensory awareness, such as to sight, smell, touch, hearing, and taste, are developed by expressive and motivated parents in allowing children to investigate and explore their bodies and emotional feelings under safe and stimulating conditions.

Awareness, Knowledge, and Acceptance of Intellect

Many females have not been taught to recognize or appreciate their intellect, logic, and thinking ability. Often the female is unaware and unappreciative of her mind and of her abilities to make decisions and choices and to create alternative actions and reactions for herself and others in an open, positive, and constructive way. Because of the "role expectation" that others will "take care of her," "protect her," etc., many women become manipulative, cunning, conniving, skilled, and destructive to relationships in order to fulfill their needs. Often, she does not know and is not taught how to make decisions or that she has a choice in decision making, as to action and feelings, or that she can think, that she can use her brain for alternative solutions. She often does not have nor make the opportunity to experiment intellectually and learn responsibility for her decisions. Therefore, her fears of her intellectual limitations are fantasies, irrational and negative attitudes introduced by others which prevent her from experimentation and learning her own limitations in reality.

Skills of decision making are learned, and one of the simplest processes is:

1. State the concern.

2. Investigate and expore what others have done with the same concern both "pro" and "con."

3. List the many various alternatives of choice available.

4. Contemplate the consequences, both positive and negative, on a factual and feeling level for each of the alternatives.

5. Select the alternative which best fits your needs and wants at that time, knowing and feeling that other choices and changes can be made at a later time.

Since satisfactory sexual response includes the "head" and intellect of the person, it becomes very important that the female learn and know relevant information concerning her body and mind and actions and behavior necessary to create pleasurable sexual experiences.

Knowledge and factual information related to the female's sexual anatomy alleviate misconceptions she might have as to the voluntary and involuntary responses and actions her body may and can make during sexual activity. A female learns very early in life to fear her own thoughts and fantasies of actions that she might take in the area of her own sexuality. Sexual fantasies, originating in the mind, are fearful and she develops many negative and guilt-ridden feelings related to her sexual thoughts, fantasies, and feelings due to the lack of sufficient knowledge and freedom to discuss them with understanding and knowledgeable adults.

With lack of factual information, other fears and fantasies which can develop are exaggerated fears of: (1) performance or lack of performance; (2) punishment following pleasure; (3) body odors and secretions; (4) pain, either physical or emotional; (5) loss of control; (6) loss of life; (7) domination; (8) disintegration; (9) loss of power; (10) visual, auditory, and kinetic stimulation; (11) responsibility for her own emotional and physical feelings; (12) sharing emotional and physical pleasure; (13) acceptance; (14) being overwhelmed; (15) being "swallowed up"; (16) disoriented; (17) natural and involuntary and voluntary movements associated with orgasms; (18) disapproval of self, parents, partner, and others; (19) looking and seeing her own and her partner's genitalia; (20) sexual feelings in her body; (21) pregnancy; (22) menstruation; (23) veneral diseases; (24) seduction and flirtation; (25) entrapment with sexual release; (26) orgasmic responsibility; (27) her own or her partner's sexual sounds and facial expressions; (28) masturbation; (29) various choices of masturbatory pleasuring; (30) different sexual positions with the partner; and (31) experimentation with her and her partner's body to discover pleasures of each and together.

Fears of sexual activities and responses, acceptance of her personhood, and her abilities and self-value create dryness of all the natural flowing juices of her body, including thought processes and vaginal secretions. So eradication of "old wives tales" and irrational fears through education and learning will greatly assist the female in accepting her own sexuality to fulfillment of desire, expression, release, and pleasure.

Awareness, Knowledge, and Acceptance of Values

Values can be defined as tangible and intangible feelings, thoughts, and ideals held dear or cherished by an individual. Values of the female and her self-expectations are often affected by the role expectations placed on her by her parents, community, peer group, religious beliefs, and culture. The moment a female child "pops out" of her own mother's vagina, she is given a list of her role expectations by the doctors, nurses, other professionals, parents, and family as to what is expected from her as a girl child. Often, she is touched, talked to, and handled differently from boys and soon picks up that she is to be protected. These are generalizations of learnings and female conditioning that contribute to her lack of curiosity, initiation, motivation, active participation, sexual responsiveness, experimentation, and self-satisfaction. She is expected to not be "too active, not say too much, not say 'no' to anything except her sexuality, don't yell, don't scream, don't complain, don't be angry, and don't want or do too much." The "do's" in her life include: "keep her skirts down, keep her legs crossed, protect her vulva area at any cost, be seductive, be grateful, be sweet, be kind, be cooperative at all costs to herself, and be loving."

She receives very little instruction in the area of how to defend herself and how to develop a sensitivity and awareness in discerning and differentiating ways of when, how, and with whom for using her defenses. She is usually not encouraged to experiment and is not given self-protective methods, either physiologically or psychologically, to be utilized in a loving, caring way with others and as protection for herself.

Quite often young women learn behavior in extremes and either become overly dependent or overly independent in their role expectations of themselves based upon their own feelings and their perceptions of other people's feelings. Below is a list of characteristics of behavior in the extreme dependent and independent person.

Extreme Dependent — Receiving attitude (fear of giving, fear of rejection), acquiescence, helplessness, spectator role, maintenance role (detail person), overprotective of self and others, withdrawn, tense, fearful, underachieving, "big daddy attitude" ("men will take care of me"), "china doll-paper doll" attitude ("I cannot be mussed and I will break very easily"), relying on males and/or other authoritarian figures, lack of acceptance of female gender, and "goody-two-shoes" attitude (which means conditioned to please others in a passive way to gain acceptance, regardless of her personal feelings).

Extreme Independent — "Giver" attitude (fear of receiving or fear of being rejected), dominate or domineering attitude, initates from fear of rejection, physically active out of fear of nonacceptance, can be obnoxiously tenacious and persevering, tense, fearful, competitive, rebellious to men and/or authoritarian figures, "do-gooder" attitude (usually actively giving so as to look good), nonreceiving of males due to fears, and rejection of female gender.

I have listed several extreme traits of either the extreme dependent or extreme independent female due to the lack of teaching of negotiation. She is rarely taught what, when, and how to share or negotiate and techniques for defending herself and her rights. She is usually taught the skills of acquiescence or domination, not negotiation. Negotiation is a necessity in a sharing relationship whether in her same-sexed relationships or her opposite-sexed relationships. She learns at a very early age to shackle herself from physical activities that she would like to experience due to role expectations put upon her by culture, community, church, nuclear family, or special individuals in her life. She often develops the attitude of helplessness, spectatorism, sometimes called voyeurism ("look but don't participate," "look but don't feel worthy or valued enough to contribute"). Even if she develops comfort in the "looking and learning" phase of living, she often has trouble in initiating or requesting participation in activities, all of which can contribute to her feelings of sexual inadequacy.

Being taught to receive ideas and concepts from others, she often is encouraged to maintain a relationship by being the "detail person" and can show her assertiveness by carrying out others' wishes and desires. She is often overprotective of herself and others because of her role expectations. She is not usually taught tenacity, "stick-to-itiveness," and perseverence in learning and is often protected by members of her family and encouraged to stop if the job seems to be too difficult. She is often told of all of the negative or bad things that will happen to her if she reaches her physical or mental potential. In fact, rarely are female potentials even talked about except in a negative way. If you "out-play, out-do, or out-win with the boys, they won't like you and will be threatened by you." So usually, the extreme role of underachieving and/or overcompetition develops due to fears of lack of acceptance and self-identity. The fear of reaching or examining the extent of her potential usually creates situations in which she gives her personal power away to men and/or other perceived powerful or other perceived authoritarian people.

Often, females will develop a relationship with a male as a "trade-out" relationship, which is an unbalanced relationship. She can and will trade money for sex, companionship for financial security, or the social role of wife and sex partner for children. Women "trade-out" their skills and abilities to meet the complementary needs in their partners. This is an unbalanced relationship, rather than a sharing relationship in which each of the two people, male and female, have similar skills and abilities and are able to share and learn together and "take turns" in the varied responsibilities and skills of everyday living.

Many women, based upon the rule expectations of their culture, community group, religion, and others have what I call the "Big Daddy" syndrome in their expectations of men. They have role expectations that man knows all the answers, not only for himself, but for her and for their relationship. He is supposed to have the ability to take care of himself, her, and their relationship and should be knowledgeable about all things and all people. This is a description of a very dependent person who has very erroneous attitudes about people and who will become very disillusioned and hostile when the partner of her choice cannot meet her expectations.

Females who develop the "china and paper doll" attitude that they cannot be mussed and that they are easily broken and the "goody-two-shoes" attitude that they cannot ever question or have a difference of opinion in feeling or ideas from those of cultural expectations rarely have the statisfaction of being a total female being in which she initiates and maintains relationships in such a way that she has mutual satisfaction with her partner both in and out of the sexual areas of her and their lives.

Many times females learn or have the fantasy of the male being a "push-button animal" or "sexual robot" or "electronic device" as far as his expression of his sexuality and have erroneous ideas about men's attitudes and functioning ability in the sexual aspects of their relationship. Also, when the female is sexually frustrated, she sometimes develops the "sexual athlete" attitude by "bedhopping" from one bed to another, searching for the "magic penis," and looking for the "right man," and by "doing it more and enjoying it less" due to her lack of sensual and sexual awareness, knowledge, information, and acceptance of herself as well as her partner.

Often females have fantasies of having sexual intercourse at "the right time" which usually is in the evening, after dark, and with all lights out, in the "right way" which is usually in what I define as the "All American standard position" which a lot of other authors have called the "missionary" position, and with the "right partner," which usually means one who can create or give an orgasm to her. Lack of sexual information and acceptance of how her body functions and how her sexuality is the sum total of her personality traits inhibits her in *being* "the right partner" which necessitates learning for herself what pleases her, so that she can communicate and share with her partner what pleases her for the moment. Taking the responsibility for learning, communicating, and sharing takes emotional maturity.

Sometimes she has erroneous expectations of her body in regard to different time periods necessary for sensual/sexual arousal and response. She often has no earthly idea of the physical behavior and/or movement and/or activity involved or the mental and emotional feelings needed in order to have a satisfactory sensual/sexual response. Often she tries too hard mentally to learn too fast and/or to do too much in her eagerness to learn as well as in her fear in learning about her own sexuality. Again, these attitudes depend largely on what was learned from the feelings of the adults with whom she has lived and is living. When learning new activities, discovering new feelings, rearranging old thought patterns, these three sentences: "I can," "I will," and "I can and will stop whenever I am too uncomfortable" allow and give permission to her to learn new skills at her own speed and pace without the fear of being overwhelmed.

Often, she resists taking the responsibility for herself and her orgasmic response due to the fact that she has been "pushed" to learn too much, too soon in nonsexual areas and aspects of her life. She can become resistant, hostile, self-blaming, self-effacing, and other person blaming, and unwilling to take the responsibility for her own learnings and bodily responses. Another erroneous fantasy of sex is that being of "roses, champagne, and a little white house on the hill with a white picket fence, music, and with sex always being lovely and gentle." She does not realize or recognize the fact that sexuality can be expressed vigorously and actively and fulfills many needs other than those of romance.

When growing up, women often hear sexual jokes that are told about women who enjoy sex. Often the sexual material is taken personally and again they are living in conflict. That is, they hear through "sexual jokes" that they are allowed to be orgasmic and enjoy their sexuality, and then they also hear that if they enjoy their sexuality, they will be laughed at, ridiculed, or criticized. So on one hand, they feel that it is acceptable to be sexual, have sexual feelings, and express their sexuality, but due to their tenuous attitude about their own sexuality, identity, and acceptance of their own body, they are afraid to risk even with the partner that they care for the most their own open expressive sexual feelings and fantasies and activities, being very fearful of being "put down" by the partner as were the women in the "sexual stories."

Another conditioning factor in the life of the female, which enhances or deters her sexual response, is whether she accepts or rejects the female sex gender. Again, attitudes of adult males and females in her early life contribute to whether the female gender is one of respect, acceptance, worthiness, value, appreciation, and a contributing person to the lives of others, or that females are dumb, lifeless, boring, an unwanted necessity, a sex object, stupid, a "play pretty," and "cheap."

Very early in life the woman in our culture develops what I call a "serving" attitude in which men are to be waited on, cared for, catered to, and acquiesced to, due to the messages she hears such as "Men are supposed to make the decisions," "Women are supposed to play the role of maintenance," "Men are to be conceptual and intellectual," "Women are to be detail people," "Men are thinkers, women are doers." Under these role expectations and learnings, even though women feel and know differently, they sometimes feign orgasm and pleasure with their partner in order to support the indoctrinated role expectations of both the male and female, the male being assigned the role of aggressor and the female being assigned the role of receiver. They often hide their aggressiveness with passivity in activities other than those which are culturally assigned. They accept assertiveness in culturally assigned activities and accept assertive roles in areas in which the male feels inadequate. Therefore, the female has fulfilled her role expectations in some areas and displayed passivity in other aspects of living to support the role expectations started by culture many centuries ago.

Conflicts in role identification and role expectations develop when the young female realizes that her parents wanted a boy instead of a girl. She frantically tries to fulfill her father's expectations as well as her mother's expectations of her to be the male child.

Early birth tales of woe, pain, and fear of childbirth and the attitude of "look what all I had to go through in order to have you" all contribute to fear of mensturation, fear of pain, fear of sex, fear of pregnancy, and fear of sexual responsiveness which is associated with the pain of "birth tales."

Other early sexual experiences such as fondling of the genitalia by cousins, brothers, fathers, members of the family, or friends usually cause a great deal of conflict in eary childhood as well as in later life. Often, she has been told that sex is bad, touching genitalia is bad, rubbing, stroking, hunching, and rubbing on the mons are not acceptable; so, therefore, when someone for whom she cares, loves, appreciates, and admires begins sexual activities with her, she is confused. Often she finds the sexual activity pleasant, both physically and emotionally and the pleasing of her partner pleasant. So, therefore, she is in a double bind. On one hand, she is having pleasure and comfort, and on the other hand the stories either told directly or inferred to her by her parents and family are that sex play, having intercourse, and sexual feelings are all bad, therefore, she must be "bad." When working with the adult woman with sexual difficulties, the therapist needs to work with her double bind and conflicts which she is experiencing.

Early sexual games which children play, such as I can "dropsy drawers-sies," "feelsy upsies," "let me feel, let you feel," "let me looksie," "doctor and nurse," and "mother and father" games which allow children to touch, feel, look, and see and smell genitalia, sometimes are quite exciting in that they are pleasurable, satisfying, and rewarding. Because they are "no-no's" of our general cultural conditioning and "scary" for fear of being caught, females, sometimes, carry on the attitude in later life that sex has to be naughty, dirty, secretive, and under scary or adverse conditions before they are sexually responsive.

Generally, genitals of the body are the only area of the body that are covered with clothing practically at all times from birth to death, except in privacy—even while sleeping in private—whereas other parts of the body are exposed at different times based upon climatical temperatures and socially acceptable conditions. This cultural habit contributes to a nonaccepting feeling of looking, touching, smelling, and responding sexually.

Another factor which contributes to negative sexual conditioning is when children hear the noises initiated by their parents during sex and sex play. The noises are sometimes and frequently interpreted by the children as "hurting" sounds rather than pleasurable sounds, due to their being unable to see or talk to the parents about their sexual feelings and activities.

Talking about it helps is my slogan. "It" being a pronoun which can mean anything. In working with people who have sexual difficulties, "it" usually is sexuality, genitalia, sexual activity, sexual positioning, sexual feelings, and other parts of the body and is used to define many sexual feelings.

Early conditioning factors which can be a deterrent or enhancement to the development of female sexual development are multiple sex partners of the parents. When a child grows up in a home in which there is a frequency in change of sexual partners of her mother, the female sometimes gets confused as to what is her role as a sexual human being depending upon the type of men that her mother selects. If the men are exploitive, if sex is "performed" for money, if the child is approached sexually, is sexually molested, or is included in sexual feelings and activities, is overstimulated either mentally or physically prior to her psychological readiness, then she is sometimes confused and withdraws from her own sexual feelings due to her fears of exploitation and lack of respect. She can also develop the same attitudes of her mother and select partners who are exploitive or those whom she can exploit or use. Advantages of relating and being with many different men allow her to have experienced many more personalities and give her a broader base of selectivity in choice of her own partner.

Often extramarital affairs of either parent contribute to her attitudes toward herself and stereotypical attitudes toward other women and men. Extramarital sex of parents can create reserve and/or hostility which colors her thinking, feeling, and action and can prevent her from her own full sexual development. Hostility toward the mother and/or father's extramarital affairs can sometimes contribute to the attitude of becoming the "sexual athlete" in which she is physiologically open to having sex, but is closed to receiving emotional satisfaction for her own pleasure.

The family's friends are most important to the child's social and sexual development. Seeing her father with his friends, male and female, mother with her friends, male and female, and parents with their couple and single friends and having the opportunity to relate to other adults contribute to a child's acceptance of other people as being loving, trusting, and caring. Sharing of food, companionship, games, social activities, play, hostessing, hosting, and the giving and receiving of pleasure contribute to positive attitudes toward the opposite sex and same sex and the coupling of the opposite sex. Having a lack of adult friends, both social and intimate, within the home creates a void for the child to observe relationships from a positive perspective. Likewise, frequent contact and experience of hostile relationships — whether male and female, female-female, or male-male, be it parents, grandparents, friends, or neighbors — may also create the attitude of either "My relationship won't be like that" or "I don't want any kind of relationship, for *all* relationships are of a hurting nature."

Being allowed to invite and have her own friends, both male and female, into her home at an early age and feeling, seeing, and hearing her friends accepted by her parents contribute to her development of accepting both boys and girls as being people. She can learn that both male and female have similar feelings and that both have basic wishes and desires of being appreciated, loved, cared for, respected, admired, pleasing, and caring and that there are innumerable ways in which people choose to have their "wants" fulfilled. These observations give her more varied experience and allow her to be more creative in her relationships.

How and what she was told about menstruation prior to her own onset of menses is another important phase for the young woman in the acceptance of her own body and its natural functions. Often, negative statements are given in relationship to menstruation, such as "Oh, you'll be doing this for the next 50 years," or "Oh me, poor child, now you have to suffer like I have." Often the negative feelings, such as cramps, headaches, and discomforts associated with mensturation, are taught rather than the pleasure of the body functioning beautifully, naturally, normally with "child-like stories" of the hormones running around in the body like "little elves making her body tick, pound, pump, and work to develop and function beautifully which contributes to her womanhood."

Information related in a positive and accepting manner about young men's physical and sexual development such as nocturnal emissions, penile erections, ejaculation in intercourse, sperm, sensitivity and function of testicles, and others can dispel her fears of male anatomy, sexual desire, and the variety of responses which he may have. Receiving information about male's physiological, emotional, and sexual feelings from a caring, knowledgeable, and unbiassed male is very important to her acceptance of males' feelings and attitudes.

Also, her friend's, parents', neighbors', and other childrens' attitudes toward masturbation contribute to her positive feelings or toward her negative feelings or toward her unaccepting feelings about her body. When she begins to fondle her genitals or masturbate at several weeks, months, or years of age, she has an early acceptance of genitalia and their functioning and their "pleasure bringing". When a child is found masturbating in private, with neighborhood children, or with relatives, the attitude of the parents and/or other adults contributes to positive or negative development of her sexuality. The word "caught" is often used when relating masturbatory activity due to cultural and familial attitudes. Parents who recognize, accept, and express their knowledge of the child's masturbation as pleasurable can assist the child in finding an appropriate place, since touching the genitalia in public in our culture is unacceptable. Often, when I am making professional speeches or talks before lay groups, parents are very interested in how to communicate with their child in a positive way and have not been taught communication skills when related to sexual feelings and activities. I often say that there are other activities in our culture which are unacceptable in public, such as "picking the nose at the dining table, urinating in the vegetable bin at the grocery store, defecating in the street, and farting in church." This usually brings laughter from the adult groups. Laughter is expressed for rarely are natural body functions talked about in public, much less talked about openly with children. Yet parents help children find appropriate places for other normal, natural body activities, so why not assist the child in finding privacy for masturbation which also brings pleasure and release.

Early homosexual experiences which are also natural in the development of a child are sometimes perceived by the child as a "no-no" with a lot of fear-producing results. Playing strip-tease in their "garage-stage dramas," investigating genitalia and feeling breasts at slumber parties, playing "sneak-a-peek" in the dressing rooms at school, and looking at breast development and pubertal hair creates conflict for young women. It is of natural interest and curiosity to all human beings to see how other people look and develop. Yet young women are not told that looking and curiosity are natural and normal and beautiful. They develop all kinds of guilt feelings, shy feelings, and withdrawn feelings of wanting to look and see and yet not feeling that those activities and feelings are acceptable. Not receiving permission early in life to look, explore, and investigate aspects of their own sexuality and also being given the precaution and "no-no's" of others sexuality again create a double bind and conflict for self-acceptance and "other acceptance."

Often, the parental fears of the father's own sexual feelings for his own developing neophyte create a "cut-off" relationship between him and her even though there has been much tenderness, love, affection, touching, cuddling, and hugging prior to puberty. Often the father in his own discomfort withdraws before the child is ready for such a change within the relationship. His withdrawal, reservation, or changes in his behavior are very confusing to her and sometimes create the feelings of alienation and the fear of loss. Therefore, she often is afraid to create such a close, loving relationship with any other man for fear that sometime due to her lack of understanding and knowledge the relationship will stop. Again, I feel it is very important for parents and children to talk about what is going on between them as far as feelings, separate and apart from action.

Feeling, thinking, fantasy, and reality action are all different concepts. Sometimes also, the child's sexual coquettishness, her impishness, her seductiveness becomes quite obvious to the mother and creates disharmony between the mother and the father if the father is not willing to accept the mother's feelings and her discomfort with the girl's developing sexuality. Often the collusion of the female child with the father against the mother creates sexual hang-ups and disabilities for the young woman at a later time. In this type of family interaction, she sees sexual feelings and behavior as competitive, rather than shareable, negotiable, and loving. The mother's security and comfort level with her own sexuality are very important at this stage of development with the child, so the child is not seen as threatening—only developing, discovering, and expressing her new awarenesses of herself. If the mother feels secure with her own sexuality, her sexuality with her husband, his sexuality, and their sexuality together, and if they have a working relationship, which is of primary importance, then both parents can have an approving attitude of the child's development and yet not allow the seductive child to alienate them as a couple. So approval from both sexes, opposite-sexed and same-sexed parent, is given and received which is very important to the development of the young woman.

When taking the sexual history of the female, it is very important to find out about her and her friends rape and abortion experiences, whether these be fantasies or reality experiences and what attitudes she then developed about her sexuality. Sometimes in rape experiences, there has been no physiological pain, in fact, sometimes this is the first time that the female has ever reached orgasm. Again, the double bind and conflict of pleasure reality versus social acceptance occur. Rape is such a socially unacceptable activity and if she had physiological pleasure during a psychological and physical invasion of her body, then she "must be bad and unacceptable." Therefore, the attitude which sometimes develops is that she must have sex under forced conditions, under resisting conditions, under unacceptable social conditions, with perhaps socially unacceptable partners in order to have sexual response and release. Another fear that often develops during the rape scene is the fear of death and often there is a cut-off or shut down of breathing due to the rapists hand over the mouth and nose to prevent screaming. Fear of loss of life has more primary importance than fright of hurting the genitals. However, during this primary fright, the genitalia sometimes become anesthetized even though the anesthetization of the genitalia can occur from experiences other than rape.

Abortion experiences, either personal or those of family or friends, can either be positive or negative for the female depending on the attitudes of significant others as well as her own feelings. Sometimes in her own personal experience she has not had enough time and counseling assistance to make her own decision and has been told how, what, and when to do and act and then feels guilty about the loss of her child. At other times, she does want an abortion, does not want the child, and the feelings of other people influence her feelings of guilt, sadness, degradation, blaming others, and hostility. A double bind and conflict again develop in that her feelings are different from her parents, and/or her girlfriends, and/or her partner or her partner's family. Again, it's "her against the world"; at least her world and their worlds are different and in conflict. Feelings about abortion experiences of other family members, premarital sex, and/or pregnancies of other children within the family or friends affect the attitudes, both positive and negative, that she develops toward the expression of her sexuality and pregnancy.

Cultural and role expectations, socioeconomic background, knowledge and factual information, fears, education and learning communication skills, encouragement and freedom to explore and experiment with her feelings, mind and body all affect the female's physical, emotional, intellectual, and sexual growth. Balanced growth is most advantageous and is most difficult to achieve due to lack of positive feelings and accurate information in the area of sex and sexuality.

The female is often confused as to the meaning of her sexuality. She often questions herself and wonders if sex is for marriage, sex is for love, sex is for children, sex is for her own pleasure, sex is for acceptance, sex is for emotional security, sex is for physical release, or sex is for money. Rarely is she informed that her sexuality is an innate natural gift as are all other parts of her mind, body, and feelings. Like all other aspects of her total being—her eyes, ears, nose, fingers, and legs—her genitals feel, move, explore, and experiment as to what brings and creates pleasure for them. Her genitals, as her eyes and other parts of her body, must take time to learn to be definitive and sensitive as to what kinds of touch are loving, caring, and pleasurable and satisfying and which ones are displeasurable, physically or emotionally.

She rarely is informed that her sexuality is her own gift and is not given to her or that can be taken away from her unless she chooses. She can choose to enjoy her sexual feelings, fantasies, and actions alone and/or choose to share her gift of sexuality with a partner of her selection. Her sexuality, the total expression of herself, physiologically, psychologically, and intellectually, is hers alone and is learned based upon her experiences. Her sexuality can be relearned when she wants, is willing, and is open to new experiences or similar experiences with different attitudes, new information, and emotional support.

Sexual feelings and fantasies are natural gifts which do not have to be taught or learned. However, sexual behavior is learned in order to have satisfying responses and release.

Now is the time for females to stop playing games by denying their sexuality and to take responsibility for their sexual feelings and their needs for sexual expression. It is now appropriate and timely for women to develop positive attitudes toward their sexuality by being open and honest in their communication as to what sexual activities are pleasurable to them. It is past time for women to accept realistically a natural response which brings pleasure to her and eradicate the "old wives tales" and attitudes which negate pleasurable body and emotional experiences.

Women who seek and desire a satisfactory sexual relationship with themselves and their partners should continually remind themselves that (1) having open communication, (2) giving and receiving pleasure, (3) accepting the responsibility for their own responses, (4) being open for change, (5) allowing creativity, (6) having an exploratory acceptance of their own and their partner's uniqueness—physically, emotionally, psychologically, and sexually, and (7) developing attitudes which accept sex as fun and pleasurable, not work, duty, and an end in itself, will all contribute to her sexual acceptance and satisfaction.

It becomes important to impress upon women in our culture that knowledge, behavior, and emotional experience in sexual activity are three different concepts. A woman may have knowledge without overt behavior or an awareness of emotional feeling. She may have emotional experience without knowledge or action, and, she can take action without knowledge and awareness of her emotional feelings. All three concepts should be included in learning satisfactory sexual response—and the old adage, "practice makes perfect!" does not apply. The old adage should be stated, "perfect practice makes perfect," with the understanding that "perfection" varies from individual to individual and from situation to situation.

It is the responsibility and obligation of each person to become knowledgeable, trained, or retrained in human sexual response in order to eradicate negative attitudes which contribute to the frustration of sexually feeling, thinking, expressive, and responsive human beings. Therefore, warmth, caring, loving, giving, receiving, and sharing, with freedom from fear, will be the results.

16

Talking with Clients about Sexual Problems

Some counselors find it easy to talk with couples about anything. Others know that there are certain areas from which they ordinarily shy away or in which they are reluctant to become involved. The sexual experiences and problems of a couple is one such area.

Other chapters in this section on counseling in sexual problems will address special issues in sexuality and sexual counseling. These chapters will focus on special dynamics in sexuality which need to be explored and various treatment techniques for couples experiencing sexual problems.

This chapter, however, will focus on some of the fundamental principles which tend to improve counselor-couple communication about sexual matters. To put it in other words, this chapter will focus on *how* the counselor communicates rather than on the content of that communication.

While most of the material in this chapter will be addressed to couple counseling situations, much of it is equally applicable in premarital counseling, which will also be addressed in a separate section later in this chapter.

Counselor's Self-Confidence

The self-confidence of the counselor in discussing sexual material with couples will be one of the key factors in facilitating ease in communication. Counselor self-confidence is built and molded around three dimensions.

First, a counselor needs to be aware of his/her own sexual feelings, attitudes, and experiences. Self-awareness and understanding is built on a composite of rigorous self-analysis, interaction with professional peers, and supervised experiences. In order to facilitate couples talking about their sexual problems, the counselor needs to have adequately dealt with his own sexual-emotional feelings so that he/she can deal objectively with the variety of sexual experiences and behaviors encountered in working with human beings.

Some counselors will experience discomfort and distress in discussing sexual matters with couples. Sometimes the discomfort is caused by conflicts within themselves regarding their own sexual feelings and urges. Others will experience unusual curiosity about the behaviors of others, perhaps coming out in an unusually lengthy exploration of the details during the evaluation process. In either case, it would be well for such a counselor to make use of resources to confront and more adequately deal with his/her own sexual conflicts and unresolved feelings. Either a therapeutic experience or an intensive workshop on sexuality would be a helpful resource for removing the counselor's own sexual conflicts.

The second dimension in building counselor self-confidence pertains to sexual knowledge. Being knowledgeable about sexuality in all its aspects lends a feeling of competence to the counselor.

Self-assurance and competency can be built by securing a good background and understanding of the following four areas: (1) male and female physiology; (2) sexual psychology (see Chap. 14 and 15); (3) male and female physiological and psychological responses during sexual stimulation; and (4) contemporary social values.

A good background and understanding of the various aspects of sexuality is not only of value in building counselor self-confidence. It also has value for couples. Masters and Johnson have repeatedly commented on the fact that many couples experience sexual difficulty simply because they lack knowledge and information. It takes only one piece of misinformation to significantly affect a couple's interaction in their sexual relationship.

The third dimension shaping counselor self-confidence pertains to the counselor's knowledge of his/her clients.

Knowing where the couple is in regard to their own sexuality is of great importance. In order that the counseling process moves along with an appropriate sense of timing and rhythm, the counselor will need to know specific information regarding the couple's own sexual history. Among the areas the counselor will want to know something about are the following: (1) each partner's value system; (2) each partner's sexual conditioning; (3) each partner's cultural background; (4) the nature of each partner's sexual education; and (5) each partner's sexual experiences. By being sensitive to each partner's sexual history the counselor will be able to move the counseling process in a direction appropriate for each couple with a sense of self-confidence and competency.

Couple Expectations

Couples enter marriage counseling with a variety of expectations regarding that experience. Let us examine some of them.

First, there is much being written and said in the popular literature and in the news media on marriage counseling, sex therapy, and the importance of a good sexual relationship in maintaining a satisfying marriage. As such, millions of Americans are exposed via the popular literature and media regarding the importance of the sexual relationship. They come to the marriage counselor with the expectation that the counselor will in fact discuss their sexual relationship. The pump has already been primed.

Second, couples coming for marriage counseling generally have expectations and attitudes regarding counseling. They come because they are experiencing distress and pain in their relationship and are prepared to talk about it. Not only are they prepared, they usually want to talk about areas or activities which have specific reference to their own marital relationship. They come wanting to discuss those areas which have reference to their pain and dissatisfaction. Thus, if they are experiencing difficulty in their sexual area, they will want to talk about it, hoping to find some solution, some improvement in their own situation.

Third, couples coming for marriage counseling want information. Their very coming is a way of saying that they are looking for answers, that they are looking for some kind of solution to their pain. While clients, to be sure, can be cleverly resistive, one part of their personality is looking for growth, wants answers, and is looking for some kind of solution.

Counseling Style

Couples coming for marriage counseling usually expect to discuss their sexual relationship and/or sexual problems. Many will do so with little anxiety. Others will have a great deal of anxiety discussing their sexual relationship and/or sexual problems. Here are some techniques designed to facilitate communication regarding sexual material.

Warm Permissiveness

When couples have difficulty discussing sex, the first task of the counselor is to establish an atmosphere of warmth and permissiveness. In part that is established by the counselor's own security and comfort regarding sexual areas. If the counselor is accepting of all human feelings and behaviors, the counselor will lend an atmosphere of permissiveness to whatever the couple is saying. By being warm and permissive the counselor will establish a sense of security which will allow the couple to begin expressing themselves. Warmth and permissiveness is also communicated in subtle ways, many of which are listed next.

Encouraging Listening

Various verbal and nonverbal responses and behaviors are important in setting the tone and atmosphere for permissiveness and security. Among them are such behaviors as reassuring nods, patient pauses, understanding smiles, and gentle questioning.

Thoughtful Responses

Another technique for establishing a warm and accepting atmosphere concerns the nature of the counselor's responses. By summarizing and reflecting what the partners say in a careful and thoughtful manner, the counselor can encourage and facilitate talking about sexual matters.

Depersonalization

Another technique for facilitating sexual communication could be labeled depersonalization. This is a process whereby a piece of pertinent information is given, followed by a question. This has the effect of depersonalizing the situation, establishing a sense of naturalness and normalness to the area being explored and thereby enhancing client comfortableness. For example, suppose you decided it important that you know whether the partners have engaged in self-stimulation and whether they had experienced any guilt feelings about it. Suppose also that you felt a direct question would be experienced with pain by a couple. Then, the situation could be depersonalized by saying something like the following: "Almost everyone has stimulated themselves to the point of orgasm at sometime in their lives; some have had guilt feelings about it. Have such feelings of guilt troubled you?" This allows the information to be gathered in a greater context, placing their behavior in the context of what is usual and natural for other human beings.

Acceptance

All of this is a way of saying that the counselor's task is to establish an atmosphere that is accepting and secure. This is accomplished by a variety of means, including a nonjudgmental stance by the counselor. Not being surprised or alarmed at what couples describe in terms of their own sexual feelings and behaviors will enhance the communication. The use of ridicule or a judgmental attitude will obviously hinder communication. That does not mean that there are not times when it is necessary to point out misinformation and correct false ideas or attitudes, but that can be done in a helpful and healthful manner.

Level

It is important in facilitating sexual communication to meet the couple at their own level. On the one hand, it is important not to talk down to couples. Some partners have done extensive reading in sexual areas in an attempt to improve their own marriage. As such, they have some knowledge regarding sexuality and to speak with them as if they are illiterate in regard to sexual matters would be inappropriate. On the other hand, other couples are almost illiterate in regard to their own sexual knowledge. To assume that they are more knowledgeable than they are would be equally inappropriate. This obviously is a kind of dilemma for the counselor: being careful not to assume anything, but at the same time not speaking down.

Sexual Words

There has been some debate in recent years over the kinds of words counselors ought to use in discussing sexual material with couples. Some professionals have argued that only the scientific and medical words ought to be used. Other professionals have argued that earthy and four letter words ought to be used (Kinsey et al., 1948).

I am not sure, however, that the case for which words to use can be made so clearly and so simply. Rather, it seems to me that it depends upon where the counselor is and where the clients are. In other words, it has to do with the setting in which the counseling is being done, the sociocultural background and class of the counselor and the couple. In some settings the use of earthy and four letter words would be regarded as inappropriate or vulgar. In some settings the use of medical words would not lead to communication and understanding, rather, miscommunication and nonunderstanding.

There are several assets in making use of the scientific and medical words for sexual parts and sexual behavior. Let us look at some of them.

First, the use of the scientific and medical words creates an atmosphere that could best be described as professional. As such it creates a kind of confidence and a sense of expertise in the professional.

Second, the use of medical and scientific words allows for greater objectivity. The earthy and four letter words tend to be emotion-packed words. Since some couples already experience a great deal of emotion over sexual issues, the use of scientific and medical words which are less emotionalized will allow for a lessening of tension, anxiety, and feeling, and greater objectivity when discussing sexual matters.

Third, the use of scientific and medical terminology probably matches more closely the expectations of couples in regard to counseling. Many couples come with the expectation that the professional will make use of accurate medical terminology.

In spite of the assets involved in making use of medical words, there are some cautions or difficulties.

First, the use of accurate medical terminology will often require the professional to explain the meaning of the words. To use the terminology without explanation or illustration would not enhance couple-counselor communication.

Second, while medical terminology can enhance communication, it can also hinder communication if the professional making use of the medical words does so in a rather stuffy or condescending style. In other words, the medical words in and of themselves do not guarantee good communication; they must be used with an appropriate sense of explanation and naturalness.

Let us look briefly at the positives and negatives in regard to the use of four letter Anglo-Saxon words for sex.

The use of four letter words in some settings has a distinct advantage in that it aids communication. In some settings couples would be very ill at ease with medical terminology. Rather than enhancing the counselor-couple relationship, it probably would hinder it, creating a sense of stuffiness, a sense of being alien to their own life style.

As indicated earlier, the four letter sexual words tend to be emotionalized and carry an emotional impact. In many situations the counselor will be wanting to facilitate communication by finding ways to look at emotionalized issues in a nonemotional and more objective fashion. But there are some situations in which the counselor might wish to make use of a treatment technique which impacts couples, bombarding them with highly charged words. When the counselor chooses this treatment technique as appropriate, the use of four letter sexual words might be helpful.

All of this is a way of saying that the choice of words in communicating about sexual problems is important. But the issue does not rest with the words alone. It rests with the counselor's ability to project meaning and a sense of security in whichever way the counselor chooses to communicate in a given situation.

Normalcy

Some couples seek marriage counseling because of a struggle within the marriage regarding the issues of normalcy or rightness about their sexual behavior. They want the counselor to make a judgment, a statement about the normalcy/abnormalcy of a particular piece of behavior or of one of the partners.

Some couples seek marriage counseling because one or both partners are caught in a conflict about a particular sexual feeling or behavior. On the one hand, they want to feel that way or engage in a particular kind of behavior, but on the other hand fear the disapproval of other significant people in their lives or society if they knew about that feeling or behavior. They are looking for the counselor to grant approval or disapproval and thus solve the conflict.

Other couples enter marriage counseling for a sexual dispute because they are at odds with each other. There is a kind of war going on regarding some sexual feelings or sexual behavior. In that war the issues have been stacked up as good/bad and right/wrong. They attempt to engage the counselor in that struggle, wanting the counselor to take sides in the issue. They seek a judgment regarding the rightness/wrongness of a particular sexual feeling or act.

In such situations it is helpful to have a broad range of knowledge regarding how people experience their sexuality and the varieties of sexual behavior within human beings. This knowledge is built by clinical experience, familiarity with the research, and awareness of the literature in the field.

When counselors have a broad range of knowledge about the sexual behavior of human beings, they can be helpful in dispelling fear that certain sexual feelings or behaviors are bad or abnormal. Couples very rarely know much about what happens in other marriages, how other people experience their sexuality, or how other couples behave sexually with each other. In that sense, the counselor is strikingly different: he/she has a great deal of intimate knowledge about how other people experience their sexuality and behave sexually. For this reason the counselor needs to be viewed as a purveyor of information, a resource in regard to what is common and shared about sexual feelings and sexual behavior among married people in our society.

It should be noted, however, that what other people do only serves as a guide. Each couple is unique unto itself. Theirs is their own special case. What may be true for other couples is not necessarily true for them.

In order to be helpful to couples regarding their fears and inhibitions, it is important that the counselor be well-informed regarding the sexual behavior of married people. By being aware of the frequency of intercourse at various ages in life, by being aware of the kinds of sexual behavior the couples engage in, and by being aware of the sexual cycles within men and women, counselors can dispel fears about being abnormal by knowing something about the commonness of sexual feelings and behavior. Counselors desiring more knowledge in this area may wish to consult Gadpaille (1975), Goldstein (1971), Kaplan (1975), Kogan (1973), Lang (1972), Masters and Johnson (1970 and 1974), McCary (1973), and Rubin (1965). Other sources can be found at the end of the chapter.

Perhaps the abundance of sexual literature in our society is not always helpful. Sometimes such literature sets forth goals that are not attainable by a given couple, either in terms of frequency, positions of intercourse, or varieties of sexual behavior. Rather than enhancing the concept of uniqueness such literature sometimes supports the idea that, "Everybody else is doing it so there must be something wrong with you."

When counseling with couples caught in conflict about the rightness or wrongness of a given sexual feeling or behavior, it is important to remember that the counselor's task is not to take sides in the controversy over specific feelings and behavior, but rather to help the couple see that each partner's values are to be respected. As Blood (1962) well puts it, "In short, while marriage may encourage variety for variety's sake, respect for the partner's scruples is still fundamental." (Blood, 1962, p. 367.)

Margaret Meade summed up the discussion about what is normal well when she wrote,

"Perhaps most of all there is a need to individualize each marriage for both partners. . . . The kind of sex literature which merely gives statistics on frequency of sex relationships and reported types of satisfaction, so that a man or woman can compare his or her record with some national norm, is the least fitted to inform such revery. Rather do women—and do men—need to know how infinitely varied the sex capacities of human beings are, how complex the patterns which release emotion, how various and wonderful the ways that lead to ecstasy. As they come to realize the extent and depth of sex feelings—in the feeling of the young child and parent, in the young lover who lives on in the middle aged, and in the vision of old age which makes the kisses given by the young already falter in uncertainty—the place of sex in the world, the importance of understanding sex, should take on a new dimension." (Meade, 1953, Introduction.)

Premarital Counseling

While everything that we have been saying has been primarily focused on marriage counseling, much of what has been said previously in this chapter could also be applied to premarital counseling. There are, however, some special situations in regard to premarital counseling which need some attention.

While professionals from many different disciplines engage in premarital counseling, probably the bulk of premarital counseling is done by physicians or clergy.

The Physician

While some physicians consult with couples regarding the dynamics and interaction of their relationship, the majority of physicians limit their consultation to the premarital physical examination and/or contraception and family planning. Because physicians are trained to be knowledgeable in these areas and because women and/or couples expect physicians to be knowledgeable in these areas, communication about sexual matters is expected and hoped for.

The Clergy

Clergy persons, on the other hand, are in a rather different position. While today many parents and couples anticipate that the minister will want to counsel with them prior to the wedding, some parents and some couples anticipate that the minister's expertise should be limited to surveying the couple's dynamics and interactions, not their sexual relationship. In contrast to the physician where sexual communication is expected by the couple, the clergy operate in a situation where communication regarding sexual material is not always expected or desired by the couple.

Because couples planning a wedding have different expectations regarding the clergy's role, premarital counseling in the parish setting which includes a discussion of sexual attitudes, values, feelings, and behaviors can be problematic. Knowledge of three different dimensions is important in determining when to include sexual information and communication in premarital counseling.

First, the minister needs to have some knowledge of his/her present congregation. That includes both being familiar with whether previous pastors have in fact dealt with sexuality in the context of premarital counseling and some knowledge of the general value system and attitude toward sexuality and sex education in general. While it could be argued that all people could benefit from education in general and sex education in specific, what professionals think is good for people is not necessarily what they want. To run roughshod over the congregation's expectations will only lead to frustration on the part of the pastor.

Second, the minister needs to have some knowledge of the specific couple that is preparing for marriage. While a majority of a given congregation might be favorably disposed to the minister including sexual information and material in premarital counseling, a given couple could be upset or irritated with the inclusion of such material. In some cases a minister will know both partners preparing for marriage because of pastoral contacts with their families. In other situations the pastor may know only one partner of the relationship and in other situations may know neither party well. It is important, therefore, that the pastor spend some time at the beginning of the premarital counseling session outlining his/her expectations for what is going to be accomplished in the sessions and getting some input from the couples regarding their expectations. If the pastor moves into premarital counseling by making a contract with the couples, there will be less chance of running aground of the issue of expectations.

Obviously it is a fine line between deciding how much sexual education and communication to include as part of premarital counseling and when that should be left to other professionals. This issue will be treated more fully in Chap. 23.

Conclusion

All of this is a way of saying that the counselor by how he/she communicates, both verbally and nonverbally, will be a model for the couple. If the counselor has a sense of confidence in him/herself and in his/her ability, the counselor will lend not only an atmosphere of permissiveness and acceptance, but will facilitate communication regarding sexual matters and sexual problems. While no one of the many suggestions given in this chapter is to be regarded as an axiom in itself, they may be helpful in helping the counselor to rethink his/her own skill in communicating with couples about sexual material and sexual problems.

REFERENCES

Blood, R. O.: *Marriage.* Free Press, Glencoe, New York, 1962.

Butler, R. N., and Lewis, M. I.: *Sex After Sixty.* Harper and Row, New York, 1976.

Gadpaille, W. J.: *Cycles of Sex* (Freeman, L., ed.) Charles Scribner, New York, 1975.

Goldstein, M. and Haeberle, E. J.: *The Sex Book.* Herder and Herder, New York, 1971.

Hastings, D. W.: *A Doctor Speaks on Sexual Expression in Marriage.* Little, Brown and Co., Boston, 1966.

Kaplan, H. S.: *The Illustrated Manual of Sex Therapy.* Quadrangle/New York Times Book Co., New York, 1975.

Kinsey, A. C., Pomeroy, W. B., and Martin, C. E.: *Sexual Behavior in the Human Male.* W. B. Saunders, Philadelphia, 1948.

Kogan, B. A.: *Human Sexual Expression.* Harcourt Brace Jovanovich, Inc., New York, 1973.

Lang, R. C. (Chairman/Editor): *Human Sexuality.* American Medical Association, Chicago, 1972.

Masters, W. H., and Johnson, V. E.: *Human Sexual Inadequacy.* Little, Brown and Co., Boston, 1970.

Masters, W. H., and Johnson, V. E.: *The Pleasure Bond.* Little, Brown and Co., Boston, 1974.

McCary, J. L.: *Human Sexuality.* Van Nostrand, New York, 1973.

Meade, M.: *Women, the Variety of Meaning of Their Sexual Experience.* Dell, Inc., New York, 1953.

BILL H. ARBES, Ph.D.

17

Counseling the Sexually Dysfunctioning Couple

It is quite easy in our current society to obtain information regarding the "correct way" or "best way" to feel about sex, talk about sex, and perform sex. Practically every popular magazine has printed an article on some aspect of human sexuality, ranging in emphasis from "how to be married to a bisexual" to "sexual self-fulfillment." The commercial success of these articles and the abundant popular books on sex indicate the level of curiosity, if not the feelings of self-doubt and uncertainty, that surrounds this recently liberated topic. Sex is definitely "in," not only for the public but also for the helping professionals who serve this public. There is no doubt our society is in the midst of a complex process of change in relationship to sexual attitudes. Sexual needs, concerns, and problems are discussed more freely and with greater knowledge than in the past. It is perfectly fashionable, and indeed expected, that clergy, counselors, and physicians present permissive attitudes in their work with people, people who seem to be eager for information and tolerant of a variety of attitudes and values.

Unfortunately, a change in the public's attitude toward human sexuality does not assure a change in an individual's fears, doubts and inhibitions. Being knowledgeable about human sexuality and techniques of lovemaking does not guarantee that the individual will feel more adequate or feel more capable of giving and receiving love. Nor will merely reading extensively in the area of human sexuality enable the helping professional to feel comfortable in talking to a client about sex.

This increased awareness and knowledge regarding human sexuality has resulted in more people questioning their sexual attitudes, feelings, and behaviors. Also, there is increasing public awareness of the existence and availability of effective short-term therapies for sexual problems. As a result, most women will not live contentedly with nonorgasmic sexuality, knowing that help is available for this problem. Likewise, men with inadequate or infrequent erections or rapid ejaculations are less willing to tolerate the dysfunction. As a result, most helping professionals are being asked and even expected to spend increasing time in helping persons with sexual concerns and problems and the associated feelings of frustration, depression, inadequacy, and failure.

Conceptualizing Sexual Dysfunctions

Sexual problems are often less the cause of marital discord than they are expressions of other underlying dynamics in the relationship of two people. Sexual incompatibility frequently is the secondary result of problems in other aspects of the couple's relationship. It is, therefore, imperative that the counselor conceptualizes the problem in terms of systems theory (Ackerman, 1967; Bowen, 1961; Jackson, 1959; Minuchin, 1974; Satir, 1964), where the presenting symptom is viewed as an expression of an interpersonal problem within the framework of the couple's relationship. The behavior of one partner directly influences and in turn is influenced by that of the other. For example, in working with a female "identified patient" who complains of "frigidity," the counselor should consider how the male partner contributes to her frigidity in the marriage. Is her problem helping him protect his feelings of sexual doubts and insecurities? The problem is, therefore, not viewed strictly as frigidity, but rather that stress is present in the relationship and this stress is being expressed by her problem. A sexual problem is never just his or her fault. It is their problem, and as such they need to be willing to participate equally in the treatment program. As Masters and Johnson (1970) have repeatedly observed, there is no uninvolved partner in sexual dysfunction. The counselor's task is to bring both partners together and create a more constructive communications experience which can then be carried over to their sexual relationship.

Frequently, the etiology of sexual dysfunctions can be traced to inadequate sex information or to socially conditioned negative or ambivalent attitudes toward sex (see Chap. 10 and 11). Misinformation about human sexuality can create anxiety incompatible with fulfilling sexual functioning. For example, a middle-aged man or older male who literally frightens himself into impotence comes to the counselor because he doesn't get an erection as quickly as during his youth. The recently married young couple comes to the physician because the woman does not achieve orgasm when the couple uses the "missionary" position. In these situations, information regarding human sexuality and the aging process in the former and pleasuring techniques in the latter may suffice. Couples and individuals who maintain misconceptions about sexual behavior or who are ignorant about sexual techniques can often be helped by simple sex education and supportive counseling.

Couples with a sexual dysfunction frequently adhere to attitudes and beliefs that are self-defeating and inhibiting to their sexual response. These result in stereotypic role behaviors that are inherently destructive to the enjoyment of one's own or one's partner's sexuality. A man's sense of masculinity is contingent on his ability to bring his partner to orgasm. The woman is expected to achieve orgasm and arouse her partner. Inability to achieve these criteria results in feelings of sexual failure. The partners with a sexual problem frequently have lowered self-esteem which is reinforced by society's emphasis on orgasm as the indicator of sexual competence and health. The expectation is not only to deliver the best of sexual skills during an encounter but also to abandon oneself to the heights of erotic pleasure. Many women still feel men should initiate sex, no matter how intense their sexual needs. Likewise, some men feel rejected by their partner's passive attitude and perceive them as poor, inadequate sex partners. Both men and women tend to believe the myth that the male knows what the female wants sexually, and that he is essentially responsible for the sexual relationship. The end result is frequently a couple lying silently in bed wondering what to think, feel, or do. The woman doesn't know what to ask a man to do which will be pleasurable for her because she usually doesn't know herself. If she does know, she is fearful of asking for what she wants because she thinks her husband may be insulted. The man doesn't ask his partner what she wants because he has been told somewhere in his life that he's supposed to know what to do. The result is usually the man going through a silent, blind, groping search for a means of pleasing both himself and his partner. In addition, both partners believe that sex is primarily having orgasms and ejaculations, simultaneously of course, and feel increasingly inadequate and anxious as this ideal is not achieved. As Masters and Johnson (1970) state:

> . . . fear of inadequacy is the greatest known deterrent to effective sexual functioning, simply because it so completely distracts the fearful individual from his or her natural responsivity by blocking the reception of sexual stimuli (pp. 12–13).

As a result of this trial and error learning and the fear of inadequacy, many couples develop a highly structured set of sexual behaviors in order to achieve orgasm. This structuring of sexual intimacy negates most pleasurable behaviors other than intercourse and orgasm, easily breaks down if one thing goes wrong, and the repetition frequently leads to boredom.

As their sexual relationship becomes increasingly less fulfilling, a couple may develop a shroud of secretiveness regarding their feelings. This frequently leads to feelings of hostility, self-doubt, and emotional withdrawal. They tend to be fearful of discussing their feelings because it might "rock the boat" and believe that if their partner "really loved them," he or she would know what they want.

Provided that couples do not hold deeper feelings of guilt and personal inadequacy or manifest their concerns by overt hostility, they are usually highly amenable to brief sex therapy. Their inability to abandon themselves to the erotic experience is a result of fear of sexual failure and the fear of rejection should they fail to please their partner. They frequently adopt a "spectator" role (Masters and Johnson, 1970) where they maintain conscious control of their feelings and responses during the sexual act. Because of the breakdown in their communicative patterns, their ability to cooperate and resolve their conflict is seriously impaired and needs outside intervention. In working with these couples, the counselor should remember that the sexual problem is an indication of negative or ambivalent attitudes, lack of sexual information, a communication breakdown, and relationship conflict.

These couples must be differentiated from those who also exhibit performance anxiety and fears of rejection, but whose fears and anxieties are related to deeper or unconscious feelings of insecurity and intense marital conflicts. The prognosis for sexual counseling in these instances is not as good, but is possible providing the counselor is willing to work with the basic relationship disturbance. In this situation, the counselor must be prepared for frequent resistance, feel comfortable in dealing with unconscious motivation, and be able to decide when to bypass, confront, interpret, or resolve the conflicts presented. These relationship problems are discussed in more detail in Chap. 5 and 6.

Some couples identify their problems as sexual when in reality there is a high degree of psychopathology either in the relationship or on the part of one of the partners. These couples are not amenable to a brief sexual counseling program as outlined in this chapter.

Counselor Characteristics and Treatment Considerations

Just as the public is being inundated with "how to" guides to better sex, helping professionals are on the receiving end of an array of articles, books, and workshops related to sexual counseling. Although most of these offerings are excellent professional works with appropriate attention given to counselor characteristics, some present sexual counseling as a simplistic process with minimal emphasis on the personal dynamics of the counselor or the couple's relationship. Perhaps the most difficult couple to help is the one who has previously been "counseled" by a helping professional who merely applied a technique described in a book or journal article.

The one counselor characteristic that all agree upon is that no one should do sex counseling unless he feels comfortable about it and can do it without imposing his own sexual attitudes upon the client. This does not imply the counselor must be value-free, but that he must be aware of his own attitudes, feelings, and beliefs, and that he understands how they add to or detract from the counseling process. Such awareness is particularly important when the counselor is working alone and does not have the advantage of modeling and same sex identification as is available in the male-female team approach.

As discussed in Chap. 10 and 11, attitudes about sexuality are derived from psychosexual conditioning experiences. These attitudes come from two primary sources: relationships to significant others in childhood and adolescence and sexual role definitions derived from one's personal value system. A clear understanding of one's personal attitudes and beliefs can be achieved by actively participating in an intensive training experience in sexual counseling where one is not only asked to look at his personal feelings and beliefs about his own sexuality, but is also presented with a variety of procedures and techniques used in sexual counseling. Frequently, participation in a same sex consciousness raising group confronts a person with his psychosexual conditioning and his current attitudes, feelings, and beliefs. Reading extensively in the areas of male and female role conditioning, human sexuality, and developmental psychology is valuable in helping the counselor understand the couple, but does not in itself assure the counselor's personal self-awareness and self-acceptance necessary for effective counseling intervention.

The counselor doing sexual counseling should have a clear understanding of the physiology of the human sexual response. A sexual concern does not necessarily imply a "psychological problem" with sex that can be resolved through support, better lovemaking behaviors, and the squeeze technique. Although the majority of sexual problems are functional, the counselor must be aware of symptoms representing physical problems which require medical diagnosis. Increasingly, counselors are being called upon to work with sexual problems resulting from physical disabilities, medical treatment procedures, and surgical procedures. To respond to these problems, the counselor should be particularly knowledgeable in the following areas: (1) sexual concomitants of various major diseases (e.g., venereal disease, renal disease, cancer, diabetes, coronary disease, and pulmonary disease); (2) sexual implications and/or effects on sexual functioning of common treatment and surgical procedures (e.g., abortion, mastectomy, enterostomy, hysterectomy, prostectomy, vasectomy, and amputation); (3) sexual implications and/or effects on sexual functioning of common medications (*e.g.*, antidepressants, tranquilizers, antibiotics, steroids, hormones, analgesics, psychedelics, marijuana, and alcohol); (4) awareness of myths about the relationship of sex and drugs; and (5) impact of congenital or acquired disabilities on sexual functioning and activity and considerations in rehabilitation (*e.g.*, spinal cord injury, brain injury or impairment, cerebral palsy, or blindness). Knowledge in such areas increases the counselor's level of comfort in working with these clients, provides necessary data in defining the sexual problem, enables the counselor to provide accurate information during the counseling process, and to plan an effective counseling intervention.

The sexual counseling program as presented here is oriented toward those couple and family counselors who are involved in a variety of counseling interventions, not just the treatment of sexual dysfunctions. As such, there are certain treatment considerations to be appraised. Although the male-female counseling team is currently the ideal and most advocated method for treating sexual dysfunctions, this program does not require co-counselors. Nor is the ongoing participation of a physician necessary as advocated by Masters and Johnson (1970). The program also provides greater treatment flexibility in that it can be spread over a greater period of time, thus making it amenable to general office practice, *i.e.*, once or twice a week contact.

The counseling program is related specifically to the treatment of sexual symptoms and relies on techniques from a variety of approaches. As such, the approach is not primarily marriage counseling or psychotherapy, although the systems approach is necessary to understand fully the nature of the dysfunction and to plan an appropriate intervention. In general office practice, sexual counseling is frequently one aspect of an ongoing couple or family counseling contract and should be seen as a treatment procedure separate from the ongoing counseling. The focus and direction of sex counseling are easily sabotaged by frequent reference to general relationship problems.

Since a primary goal is to enable the couple to relax and focus attention on incoming erotic stimuli, this program, like most brief procedures for the treatment of sexual dysfunctions, relies heavily on the assignment of sexual tasks. These tasks are used to emphasize the mutuality of the couple's problem, to open and assess communication patterns, and to elicit and assess reactions to the tasks. Sager (1974) emphasizes tha the accomplishment of this requires a relatively non-hostile level of cooperation that is not required for marital therapy in general. He states that the couple must meet certain requirements before sex counseling can be attempted:

> . . . first, to put aside their fights and hostility for a period of a few weeks so that these negative components do not determine significant actions;

second, to accept one another as sexual partners; . . . third, to have a genuine desire to help one another and themselves . . . the fourth condition requires that one or the other spouse often put his own gratification aside for several weeks and the fifth that he participate in maintaining a sexually nondemanding ambience (p. 503).

Although it is extremely uncommon to find no relational problems in patients with sexual dysfunction, sexual counseling can often facilitate the communication skills necessary to clarify and work on marital problems. Since the program presented here has the primary goal of overcoming a sexual dysfunction, assessment of relationship problems, especially hostility, is mandatory to determine whether sexual counseling will be productive.

It is important to differentiate between primary and secondary sexual dysfunction since the program is oriented primarily to the treatment of secondary sexual problems. Primary refers to a condition that has existed throughout adult life or has been chronic, and secondary describes a dysfunction of relatively recent onset. A man with a secondary impotence is usually able to have an erection through masturbation or while asleep, but is unable to respond effectively to his partner during intercourse. A woman with secondary sexual unresponsiveness is typically able to respond to her partner through caressing or self-stimulation. A man who has never achieved an erection or a woman who has never achieved an orgasm is unlikely to respond to the short-term counseling outlined in this chapter. Treatment of primary sexual dysfunctioning usually requires more in-depth counseling of both the individual and the relationship. This is a crucial point of differentiation for the counselor who applies this program.

Initial Contact

Generally, the contract of sex counseling evolves out of the context of an ongoing marital or individual counseling relationship or a couple or individual presents with a specific sexual problem. It is a rare treat to have a couple referred who report no major psychological or relationship problems so that the counselor can move directly into treating the specific dysfunction. In terms of the individual, the first barrier can be the partner's refusal to participate. The client may hesitate to ask for her spouse's participation, or even to mention that counseling has been sought, let alone invite him to participate. More husbands than wives tend to refuse participation or feel ambivalent. However, a call to the husband asking for his assistance usually gets him to your office, and the use of judicious interviewing skills usually gets him involved.

The primary goal in the initial meeting is to assess the nature of the presenting problem, the time, and conditions when the dysfunction was first experienced, and the conditions in which the dysfunction now occurs. The counselor's sense of comfort in talking directly and explicitly about sex often reduces the feelings of embarrassment generated by sexual anxieties. Soliciting how the couple feels in the interview situation frequently enables them to relax. Focusing on specifics enables the couple to discharge some anxiety while providing important information.

> Please tell me how you make love. When do you initiate intercourse? Who initiates? What other means, besides intercourse, do you use to satisfy each other sexually? Oral-genital? Anally? How did you feel about this? Describe the feelings you have with orgasm. What do you expect from each other sexually?

The interview continues until the counselor has a clear understanding of how their sexual relationship exists now, how it has evolved during their relationship, and their understanding of and reactions toward the dysfunction.

Throughout the first session, the counselor takes special note of the differences in perception of each spouse toward the dysfunction and their sharing of previous feelings and behaviors, the verbal and nonverbal interaction between each partner and the counselor, the individual strengths and weaknesses of each partner, and the strengths and weaknesses of the relationship. Based upon these initial observations, the counselor decides whether the sexual problem can be separated from the rest of the marital relationship and dealt with directly, or whether the relationship has to be treated first before dealing more specifically with the sexual problem.

If the counselor decides to proceed with the treatment program, the remainder of this meeting is utilized to describe the individual history-taking sessions and the roundtable session. The spouses are told not to discuss the history-taking sessions with each other until the roundtable discussion. Each partner is directed to have a physical examination and the woman a gynecological examination. It is particularly important that the counselor have a close liaison with the examining physician and that the physician is informed of the counselor's impressions following the initial contact. The physician should know how to perform a sexual problem-oriented examination. Hartman and Fithian (1973) and the Zussman's (1974) present a model for a foursome sexological examination and demonstrate how they use this procedure as a learning experience.

Individual History Taking

The primary goal of these sessions is to explore feelings and behaviors, current and past, that the individual is hesitant to share in front of his partner. It is best to accomplish this in one session with each partner, although frequently the session lasts longer than an hour. Although Masters and Johnson (1970) and Hartman and Fithian (1973) describe detailed history-taking outlines, it is usually more comfortable for the counselor and client to individualize each session. The client is asked to tell the counselor those things not to be shared with the partner. Some "secrets" are detrimental to counseling success and usually have to be shared for counseling to proceed, for example, sham orgasms, extrarelationship sexual encounters, and lack of sexual attractiveness to partner. Unless shared, these issues often block future communication and sexual relearning.

The individual is again asked "Why are you here?" The individual's and couple's motivation for seeking treatment are appraised throughout—was either partner forced to come? What are the partners' expectations of treatment? What does each partner expect from the other?

The history includes relevant details of the client's childhood (family relationships, friends, first sexual feelings, masturbation, fantasies and dreams, watching anyone else having sex, etc.), adolescence (school, parental and sibling relationships, menstruation or nocturnal emissions, social and sexual activity, sexual activity with same sex, first sexual experience, etc.), and adult life prior to marriage (engagements, why terminated, friends, social, and sexual behaviors).

In terms of the client's marriage or marriages, the nature of the original attraction, duration of the courtship, premarital and extramarital sexual activity, difficulties on honeymoon, and sexual expectations are discussed. Various aspects of their current relationship are discussed—do they share confidences with each other? What are some sexually displeasing habits or behaviors of their partner? What is the frequency of intercourse? Is it too much, too little? What are the circumstances influencing lovemaking? Who chooses the time? What is missing in their partner's sexual behavior or attitudes? What is positive?

Finally, the client's feelings about self are explored—does he feel attractive? What is his best attribute? Would he like to change something about himself? How would he describe his sexual identity, attitudes, and feelings toward touch, sight, hearing, and smell? Each individual is then asked similar questions about his partner.

Throughout the individual history taking, careful note should be made of sexual misconceptions and misinformation, clients' attitudes toward their own and their partner's sexuality, and the dynamics of their relationship. Regardless of the counselor's skill, only a tentative hypothesis regarding the nature and dynamics of the couple's sexual problem can be made. However, enough information must be obtained to determine whether their sexual problem is amenable to change given their current relationship.

The Roundtable Session

Both partners are present as the counselor reviews the medical and laboratory reports and discusses the significant findings from the sessions conducted. The clients are instructed to interrupt whenever the counselor presents an error or misrepresents one of their staements, to disagree, or to ask a question. During this session, a probable explanation of the causes for the couple's problem is presented. Special attention is given to myths held by one or both partners that contributes to their sexual problem, misinformation regarding human sexual functioning, unrealistic expectations, communication breakdowns, and destructive behavior patterns. The counselor shares his perception of their sexual problems, of how they are hurting each other and how they fail to communicate with each other. This requires the counselor to assume a teaching, more authoritarian role.

The counselor re-emphasizes that neither partner is to blame but that the relationship between them is the focus of treatment. He explains how their values and attitudes influence their sexual functioning. Further discussion centers around attempts to abolish goal-oriented performance and fear of failure. Timmers et al. (1976) have developed an effective technique for re-educating couples about goal-directed sexual experiences. The technique discourages an hierarchical framework of sexual beaviors and substitutes a circular view of sexual interaction. They emphasize use of the word "sexplay" instead of "foreplay" in working with couples to help them remove goal-oriented behaviors. Emphasis is placed on mutual participation in a spontaneous and natural process as opposed to concern with achievement of a result.

Up to this point, communication has primarily been between the clients and the counselor. The counselor's goal during this part of the counseling program is to facilitate the communication between the dysfunctional partners. Continually checking and counterchecking reactions and feelings facilitates the communication between the dysfunctional partners. Continually checking and counterchecking reactions and feelings facilitates this process. For this reason, the roundtable may last anywhere from two to five sessions. The use of various audiovisual materials not only is educational but also enhances the communication between the couple.

The counselor and the couple must decide at this point whether to continue the counseling program. If there is no major disagreement with the material presented and if the sexual dysfunction is amenable to change, the discussion is directed toward a description of the pleasuring experiences.

Pleasuring

The teaching of pleasuring involves teaching the couple to touch each other and to communicate what is pleasurable and what is not pleasurable. Sexual intercourse is forbidden during this phase of the program, and emphasis is placed on learning how to give and receive pleasure from each other. The fear of failure is removed for neither has to produce an adequate response in themselves or their partner. The man does not "have to get" an erection in order to satisfy his partner, nor does the woman "have to lubricate" or "have to have an orgasm" in order to please herself or her partner. In fact, they are discouraged from "having" to do anything except caress and hold each other and to share their experiences with each other.

The couple is given clear instructions regarding the pleasuring exercise. These instructions can be given at the end of, or shortly following, the roundtable session. They are to find a minimum of $1^1/_2$ h each day during which they will explore sensory experiences with each other. Complete privacy is necessary. They are told to take a shower together and then to lie close to each other in bed. They are discouraged from doing this in total darkness, even a candle will suffice. One partner is then instructed to begin giving the other the experience of pleasurable touching. However, neither may touch the genitals or the woman's breasts. The "giving" partner is instructed to caress, fondle, kiss, and lick the other using verbal and nonverbal clues from his partner about the location and intensity of touching desired. The "receiving" partner is to communicate verbally and nonverbally what is pleasurable and unpleasurable. Whenever the partners feel inclined, they can switch roles. The use of massage oils usually enhances this experience. The use of films and/or slides is sometimes helpful in explaining pleasuring to couples. Most couples express feelings of awkwardness and artificiality at first, but this usually changes as they begin to give themselves permission to enjoy the experience.

The couple is then encouraged to give the counselor a detailed description of their pleasuring experience. Many couples respond very positively to these pleasuring experiences. Learning that it is possible to give and receive pleasure without "having to get an erection" or "having to reach orgasm" is often felt as relief and excitement. In such situations, the counseling can proceed to the genital-oriented pleasuring experience.

The pleasuring experience also generates negative reactions, especially in those couples where the relationship itself is destructive or where one or both partners have some degree of psychopathology. Thus, these pleasuring experiences serve as an additional diagnostic check point for the counselor and, therefore, should be included in the treatment of all sexual dysfunctions. These negative reactions can be expressed in a variety of ways—"It's too mechanical," "He's too clumsy," "It was boring," "I couldn't wait." They can be a result of feelings of hostility toward the spouse, guilt about receiving or giving pleasure, fear of rejection, or fear of intimacy (Kaplan, 1975).

Before therapy can proceed, the counselor must help the couple resolve these negative feelings. Sometimes, merely repeating the experience will suffice. At other times, it may be necessary to terminate the sexual counseling contract and either refer the couple or institute a separate contract for marital counseling. If the anxiety is primarily experienced by one spouse, optional relaxation training with guided imagery can be tried (Wish, 1975).

The second part of the pleasuring experience is oriented toward genital pleasuring. The partners are again instructed not to strive for orgasm or ejaculation, but to learn what is pleasurable in regard to their genitals and to communicate this to each other. The man is instructed to sit comfortably, with the woman leaning back against his chest with her feet on the outside of his legs. The woman is instructed to participate actively by putting her hand over the hand of the man and directing his hands and fingers where and how she wants to be touched and verbally instructing him. The partners then switch with the man "receiving" and the woman "giving." This is best accomplished with the may lying on his back with the woman sitting between his legs.

Again, a detailed description of their reactions and feelings is solicited. By removing the pressure to perform or reciprocate, many couples experience intensive erotic feelings. The man may find himself getting numerous erections or the woman discovering herself lubricating frequently. Couples with positive reactions then proceed to a specific treatment program.

Negative reactions to genital pleasuring usually revolve around specific sexual anxieties. Feelings of guilt or anxiety about touching the opposite sex's genitals or about having one's genitals touched often have to be resolved before counseling can proceed. Sometimes feelings of shame or disgust arise; these are frequently associated with early childhood sexual experiences or teachings. The counselor must decide whether to repeat the experience, to terminate the sexual counseling contract, or attempt to proceed with the program. Generally, only after a couple has learned to give and receive pleasure from each other and to communicate their feelings about these experiences can the counseling program progress to the specific treatment programs with confidence and assurance.

Specific Treatment Program

The general program outlined above is followed for all couples with sexual dysfunction. However, the program is individualized for each couple. Perhaps additional time is needed in helping the couple to develop intimate, sexual communication skills. Some partners need help in increasing their feelings of self-esteem, especially their body image. Others need additional training in anxiety reduction. Sometimes, certain techniques have to be modified, or the entire program slowed considerably, so the couple can progress comfortably through the various tasks and experiences.

Space does not permit a description of the specific counseling procedures utilized in treating the various dysfunctions. Although some theoretical and procedural differences exist between those most prominent in the field, the basic techniques utilized in treating the specific dysfunction are quite similar. These techniques are clearly outlined by Kaplan (1974, 1975), Hartman and Fithian (1973), Masters and Johnson (1970), and McCarthy et al. (1975).

Throughout the program, couples are taught that the healthy and fulfilling aspect of sexuality is flexibility and variability in functioning and satisfaction of both husband and wife. The length, timing, or frequency of sexual pleasure is irrelevant compared to the importance of the couple's discovering their own kind of satisfactions and dissatisfactions. Do the partners live up to their own standards and hopes? If a couple feels satisfied or fulfilled having sexual pleasure three times a day or every 3 weeks, it shouldn't matter that other couples their age are averaging 1.8 times per week. As in all counseling, the couple provides the framework within which the counselor works. The goals of helping sexually incompatible couples are those which the partners choose, and the counselor's job is to assist the couple in achieving those goals utilizing all of the suitable skills and techniques.

Summary

Enjoying healthy sexual involvement between two people implies a generally healthy interpersonal relationship. Conversely, when a couple complains of a sexual problem, the counselor must evaluate the functioning of each of the partners and the relationship. To work effectively with a couple, the counselor needs to understand the underlying attitudes, beliefs, and feelings of each partner and their unfulfilled and unexpressed needs. The meaning of their sexual problem must be understood in terms of their relationship. In some situations, a sexual counseling contract can be established quickly. In others, where the interpersonal relationship between the partners is pervaded by feelings of guilt and hostility, the counselor must first modify the relationship before sexual counseling is undertaken.

The program presented in this chapter enables the counselor to undertake a sexual counseling contract as part of his ongoing counseling with a couple. Spreading the counseling over a longer period of time allows the counselor more flexibility in his approach and allows the couple to proceed at their own pace. It also offers the advantage of helping the couple integrate their sexual relationship into their life style as opposed to an intensive counseling program where the couple is placed in a somewhat artificial situation.

Sexual counseling cannot by itself create a close interpersonal relationship between two people nor eliminate individual psychopathology. However, it frequently uncovers interpersonal problems within the relationship and personal problems on the part of one or both partners. At these times, the counselor is faced with the decision whether to revise, repeat, or terminate the sexual counseling contract. It is important that the counselor not perceive these situations as failures, but as part of the counseling process in helping the couple achieve sexual health.

REFERENCES

Hartman, W. E., and Fithian, M. A.: *Treatment of Sexual Dysfunction.* Center for Marital and Sexual Studies, Long Beach, California, 1973.

Kaplan, H. A.: *The Illustrated Manual of Sex Therapy.* New York Times Book Co., New York, 1975.

Masters, W. H., and Johnson, V. E.: *Human Sexual Inadequacy.* Little, Brown & Co., Boston, 1970.

McCarthy, B. W., Ryan, M. A., and Johnson, E. A.: *Sexual Awareness and Enhancement: A Practical Approach.* Scrimshaw Press, San Francisco, 1975.

Timmers, R. L., Sinclair, L. G., and James, J.: Performance anxiety and goal-directed intimacy. *Social Work,* in press.

Wish, P. A.: The use of imagery — biased techniques in the treatment of sexual dysfunction. The Counseling Psychologist, 5: 52–55, 1975.

Zussman, L., and Zussman, S.: The Foursome Physical Examination. Mimeographed paper. Long Island Jewish-Hillside Medical Center, New York, 1974.

CLARK E. VINCENT, Ph.D.

18

Counseling Involving Premarital and Extramarital Pregnancies

Statistical Perspective

In the late 1960's it was assumed by many that the availability of contraceptive pills and the legalization of abortion would result in a sharp decrease in the annual numbers of births out of wedlock. However, data on illegitimate births reported by the National Center for Health Statistics indicate 339,000 such births in 1968 and 418,100 in 1974. (There is a delay of approximately 2 years in the availability of complete data on the number, ratio, and rate of illegitimate births by age and race of the mother.)

The following figures on illegitimate births to various age groups of women provide some perspective on the potential number of women who might seek counseling regarding their illegitimate pregnancies. These figures would appear to indicate that it is primarily women 35 and older who have taken advantage of the increased availability of contraceptives and abortions as means to avoid illegitimate births.

A more accurate measure of increases and decreases, however, is the *rate of illegitimacy*. This measure (which controls for the changing population of married women in various age groups by indicating the *number of illegitimate births per 1,000 unmarried females*) shows that the illegitimacy rate has decreased for every age group except the 15 to 19-year-old during the 7-year period of 1968 to 1974. Thus, it would appear that contraceptives and abortions are lowering the illegitimacy rate among all age groups of unmarried females except teen-agers who, however, still had a lower illegitimacy *rate* in 1974 than did women 20 to 29 years of age.

Data on illegitimacy available from the National Center for Health Statistics do not specify whether the mothers are single, married, or divorced. Therefore, we have no way of knowing how many of the more than 400,000 illicit births occurring annually in the United States at the present time involve single women, divorced women, or married women impregnated by men other than their husbands. Nor do we have any way of ascertaining how many of the approximately 3,000,000 live births occurring in this country annually result from postmarital and extramarital coition, but are not reported as illicit.

Only a very few studies have differentiated among premarital, extra-marital, and postmarital pregnancies. One study (Vincent, 1961, 1969) conducted 20 years ago in a metropolitan county in California found that of 736 illegitimate births attended during 1 year in county, di-vorced women accounted for 19% of these births and married women for 4%. To project the results from one study conducted 20 years ago in California onto the national scene today may represent little more than a wild guess, but such a projection would mean that of the 400,000 current annual illegitimate births, 76,000 are to divorced women and 16,000 are to married women.

With the foregoing statistical perspective as background the remain-der of this chapter is based on information, impressions, and sugges-

TABLE 18.1
Number of illegitimate births*

Year	Total	Age of mother						
		Under 15	15–19	20–24	25–29	30–34	35–39	40+
1968	(339,100)	7,700	158,000	107,900	35,300	17,200	9,700	3,300
1974	(418,100)	10,600	210,800	122,700	44,900	18,600	8,200	2,300

* The figures presented have been compiled from: Table 11, Page 11 of *Monthly Vital Statistics Report*, Vol. 23, No. 3 Supplement (3) (June 7, 1974), National Center for Health Statistics, U.S., Department of Health, Education, and Welfare; Table 11, p. 11 of *Monthly Vital Statistics Report*, Vol. 23, No. 8 Supplement (Oct. 31, 1974), National Center for Health Statistics, U.S., Department of Health, Education, and Welfare; Table 11, p. 11, *Monthly Vital Statistics Report*, Vol. 24, No. 11 Supplement (Feb. 13, 1976), National Center for Health Statistics, U.S., Department of Health, Education, and Welfare.

TABLE 18.2
Rate of illegitimacy

Year	Age of mother						
	Under 15	15–19	20–24	25–29	30–34	35–39	40+
1968		19.8	37.3	38.6	28.9	14.9	3.8
1974		23.2	30.9	28.9	18.6	10.0	2.6

tions derived from (1) an earlier questionnaire study (Vincent, 1961, 1969) of more than 2,000 women impregnated out of wedlock, (2) individual interviews and counseling sessions with more than 600 such women and at least 200 of their sexual partners during the past 20 years, and (3) lawyers, ministers, nurses, physicians, and social workers from whom I have learned a great deal during consultation sessions, workshops, and referrals.

The material (Klemer, 1965; Vincent, 1973) that follows is divided into four categories representing four types of pregnancies: (1) *nonmarital* (women who have never been married and do not plan to marry the man involved), (2) *premarital* (pregnant brides), (3) *postmarital* (divorced women), and (4) *extramarital* (women impregnated by men other than their legal husbands). Some of the points presented in regard to any one of these groups of women will have applicability to one or more of the other groups, while some points will be uniquely relevant to the particular group under discussion. One universal point is that whether the woman with an out of wedlock pregnancy becomes his private patient or never returns her initial visit to a physician to ascertain her pregnancy is a highly memorable experience—either positive or negative. The words and very manner in which the physician confirms or negates that she is pregnant are etched indelibly upon her mind and emotions.

The members of the various professions have some contributions in common and some unique to their individual professions for counseling women impregnated out of wedlock. My comments in the following discussion of the four categories of pregnancies are directed toward physicians and counselors. In some categories, however, my comments are more directed to physicians because of their initial contact with the woman in ascertaining pregnancy and because the physician's performance in that initial contact has implications for subsequent counseling by those in our professions. In addition, my comments are focused on consulting and counseling services rather than psychotherapy.

Very Young Unwed Mothers: Nonmarital Pregnancies

Establishing Who is the Patient

To be helpful in a consulting relationship with the unmarried mother-to-be, particularly if she is a very young one, the physician will need to communicate clearly to her that *she* is the patient, not the parent(s) who may have accompanied her to his office or the couple who might be waiting to adopt the child. This distinction is undoubtedly not an easy one to make when the girl is a minor (particularly if she is a juvenile and the parents are paying the bill); but it is crucial if the physician is to establish a meaningful relationship with unmarried girls.

The very young unmarried girl who is brought to the physician by her parent(s) because pregnancy is suspected probably is already feeling both guilty and rebellious toward her parents. If the physician permits the mother to be present during the interview with the daughter or confirms the pregnancy first to the mother, the daughter will see the physician only as an extension or tool of her parents; the doctor's subsequent efforts to help her, even medically, will be impeded.

Failure of physicians to establish clearly that she herself is the primary patient is one of the criticisms expressed most frequently by young unwed mothers. Many of them—particularly those of juvenile age to whom the physician fails to point out the technicalities of the law—feel that he is simply "under the thumb" of their parents. Many unwed mothers report that this is the major reason they did not return to the physician who diagnosed their pregnancy. The physician will have been very successful in the initial visit if, in addition to medical management, there is established the kind of relationship that leaves her feeling this is the kind of physician she can talk to. There is a very viable grapevine among single females who become pregnant and who pass the word very quickly concerning the kind of treatment received by given physicians, thus accounting, in part at least, for the fact that over a period of time certain physicians build up quite a clientele of unmarried mothers.

When She Comes Alone

When the young single girl comes alone for her initial visit to ascertain pregnancy, the physician has not only a unique opportunity, but also a responsibility, to make sure that she does not become "lost" until the onset of labor pains. For the health and welfare of both the unmarried mother and the child to be, it is important that the physician be able to communicate the importance of regular medical checkups and proper care during the pregnancy. Too frequently, young females of inadequate means disappear after the visit to ascertain pregnancy and reappear only when the baby is about to be born. If proper care is to be provided for those females who do not become private patients, the physician will need to have and to impart accurate and up-to-date information about other resources in the community and to follow through on referrals to such other resources.

The Impressionable Moment

The impressionability of unmarried females at the moment their pregnancies are confirmed is reflected in their varied interpretations of perhaps a single comment made by the physician. Some unwed mothers report that the physician completely condemned them and their sexual behavior; others interpret a few words to mean that the physician completely accepts them and condones their behavior. These two opposite interpretations are frequently derived from almost identical statements made by the physician; the females' selective listening accounts for the difference in interpretation. For clarification, one physician of my acquaintance deliberately asks the patient what she thinks he, her physician, thinks about her pregnancy.

Because of this selective hearing and interpretation on the part of the patient, the physician who confirms to an unmarried female the truth of her pregnancy has no choice as to whether or not to serve her as a consultant. Should the doctor refuse to say anything except that she is pregnant, the very absence of any comment will be interpreted as either supportive approval or as condemnation and rejection. The tone, the words, and the timing used in conveying the information, therefore, need to be carefully considered. An offhand remark, a facial expression, or the most casual of comments is usually given far more weight than the physician intended.

Learning from the Experience

Some very young unmarried mothers manifest all too clearly the failure of parents, physicians, and professional counselors to distinguish between the doer and the deed. Some parents reject both in so devastating a manner as to preclude ever being of future help to their daughters. Other parents are so accepting and "understanding" that they encourage their daughters to "con" themselves into believing that no mistake was made, thereby precluding the learning experience and dignity that can accrue from admitting one's mistakes and accepting responsibility for them.

Some of these girls do not perceive the pregnancy as a mistake because it was desired, but this is different from the denial of any self-responsibility, or being convinced that the pregnancy was entirely the fault of their male partner, or their parents who were either too rigid or too permissive. Others, who did assume some responsibility for their pregnancies, did not perceive them as mistakes but as inconveniences — inconveniences which were viewed as worthwhile by some girls because they received a parent-financed sojourn to another state during the later months of pregnancy and were able to provide a childless couple with an adopted baby. They were explicit in their belief that they would not have come by such a trip had they not become pregnant. They also reported that their younger sisters thought their parents would provide them a similar "fun" trip when they were older.

The Importance of Timing

The physician who has confirmed to hundreds of women that they are indeed pregnant is likely to underestimate the impact of such confirmation on one who is unmarried. Although every sign may be to the contrary, she harbors hope until the last moment that she may *not* be pregnant. Many unwed mothers have reported that, although the physician may have talked to them for approximately 15 min, they "heard" nothing after receiving the news that they were indeed pregnant.

The physician's overcrowded schedule makes it difficult for him to take the time necessary for an unmarried patient to assimilate the confirmation of her pregnancy. Some physicians wisely allow for such assimilation time by providing the patient with a Coke or a cup of coffee and arranging for the nurse or receptionist to sit with her in private for 10 to 15 min while he sees another patient before returning to have a further talk with her.

In giving information and in listening, timing is all important. Few physicians would seriously consider discussing the relative merits of bottle and breast feeding during the initial interview with a pregnant patient. Yet some physicians feel compelled to discuss contraceptive measures with an unwed mother-to-be during the initial session, even though such information is even less relevant at that time than advice on infant care. Immediately after pregnancy is confirmed, supportive listening is crucial.

The Danger of Rushing Decisions

A second major complaint of young unwed mothers is frequently voiced in the form of a plea: "Please tell them (professional people) for the sake of other girls like me not to ask us immediately who the boy is and whether we plan to marry him." Although the question of marriage must inevitably be decided, it unfortunately is asked much to early by ministers, parents, physicians, and social workers. In retrospect, the girls point out how they become identified with a decision that they had not really made. When a young, pregnant teen-ager is asked what her plans are, she tries to demonstrate adult status by stating almost off the cuff either that she does or that she does not plan to marry the male involved—hoping perhaps that she will have much more time to think about it. In their haste to make plans however, the parents and the professional people involved tend to react one way or another to her "decision." Their reaction—although it may be either negative or positive or may not even be expressed in words—will then influence her to crystallize a decision she was not at all ready to make. They physician, parent, or counselor can be of considerable help by taking the initiative and indicating quite explicitly that there is "no hurry" about reaching decisions in a number of areas. (At this stage, 2 weeks will seem an eternity to the young girl.)

Maintaining the Context

In a wide variety of cases involving nonmarital and premarital coition, it is difficult for both the male and the female to maintain an historical and contextual view of their sexual experience. In a minimum amount of time the counselor can give them considerable help in maintaining the context in which a given sexual union occurred. The single female, for example, who has had coition with a male during the time she thought they were in love and were going to be married, will need to be reminded that *at the time of their sex union* the context for her was one of love and of planning for marriage. Too often, in cases where the couple later decide not to marry, the girl subsequently takes the sexual experience out of the context in which it occurred and condemns herself too harshly, even feeling that she is unworthy of any man who may want to marry her in the future.

By emphasizing the need to maintain the context in which the conception occurred, the counselor can also, in many cases, counter the girl's tendency to believe that she has to proceed with marriage in order to preserve her self-image as a "nice girl" — thus trying to rectify one mistake with what may be an even greater one.

The results of the failure to maintain the context are seen all too often in counseling and therapy sessions years later when, for example, the 35-year-old woman is judging what she did at 16 as if she had at age 16 the wisdom, experience, and values she now has at age 35.

Helping Parents Ventilate

Receiving confirmation of an unmarried daughter's pregnancy is also a highly traumatic experience for most parents. Their reaction is likely to be one of anger and disappointment, which they may express with destructive hostility and bitterness. The physician can help both the daughter and her parents by encouraging the latter to vent some of their anger with the physician or with a professional counselor before talking with their daughter. During a brief session with the parents, either in the office or over the phone (after the daughter has told them of her pregnancy or given the doctor permission to tell them), the physician can help them realize that their anger toward their daughter represents, to some extent, a projection or displacement of their own feelings of failure as parents. They can be encouraged to listen and to try to be constructive rather than destructive in their discussions with her. They need also to be aware of their daughter's need to act temporarily as if she had thought and planned for everything and not to press her too early for answers to questions such as whether she plans to marry the boy. The parents also need to understand the probability that if they verbally attack the boy, their daughter will feel she must defend him because their criticism of him is a reflection of her judgment in developing an intimate relationship with him.

Laws Concerning Teen-Agers and Sexual Behavior

The legal statutes and practices regarding teen-agers vary so greatly among the different states and among different regions within a given state that the physician consulted by an unmarried girl who is pregnant will need to seek good legal advice in the locality of his practice. Generally, a distinction is made between *juveniles* (children up to 15 years of age) and *minors* (young people 16 through 18 or 21 years of age). If the pregnant girl is a juvenile, the physician may have very little choice but to inform the parents that their daughter is pregnant. It is to be hoped that the physician obtains the girl's "consent" to tell them or persuades the girl herself to tell them. In the case of a minor, however, the issue of informing the parents is not so clear-cut.

Statutes concerning minors are frequently ambiguous, and application of the statutes varies considerably. This confusing situation, which reflects society's ambiguity in awarding adult status to young people, is familiar to the physicians in other areas of his practice. For example, parents are generally regarded as the guardians of their children until the latter are married, at which time guardianship of a minor female usually passes to the husband. In the case of a 17-year-old girl married to a 19-year-old boy, however, who signs the authorization for surgery for the 17-year-old wife or other type of medical treatment requiring consent in a state where majority age is 20 or 21? In actual practice, most physicians are undoubtedly guided more by common sense or by probabilities than by a literal interpretation of the relevant legal statues.

A literal interpretation of many of the laws dealing with sexual behavior is almost impossible. In the majority of states, for example, there are statutes making *voluntary* coition between unmarried adults a criminal act. Yet many of those same states license and support a variety of agencies, hospitals, and maternity homes to care for unwed mothers, who present undeniable evidence that they have violated the statutes on fornication. These females are rarely prosecuted—and although the personnel of maternity homes and social agencies aid the unwed mother and seek to cloak her identity from the public, they are neither condemned nor punished as "accessories after the fact" of fornication. The existence of unenforced laws against fornication, together with the ambiguity concerning the legal status of minors, makes it very difficult for the physician to know exactly where he stands legally when confronted by the young unmarried pregnant teen-ager desiring medical services.

Another example of ambiguity in the laws and practices regarding teen-agers and sexual behavior confronts the teacher-counselor when (1) school administrators are not prosecuted for expelling 14- or 15-year-old girls who are illegitimately pregnant, and (2) the law stipulates that children *must* attend until they are at least 16 years old. The most persistent ambiguity, or outright contradiction, is to be found in the social practices and attitudes by which our society *inadvertently encourages, if not implicitly condones, the cause (illicit coition) and explicitly censures and condemns the result* (illicit pregnancy). I have illustrated this contradiction at length elsewhere (Vincent, 1961, 1969) and will only note here in passing that the physician is confronted directly by it in such cases as that of the mother who confidently brings her teen-age daughter in for contraceptives, but who subsequently and angrily brings that same daughter in with a premarital pregnancy.

Pregnant Brides: Premarital Pregnancies

Many young women who become pregnant before marriage are already engaged to the father of the child, and many others marry the boy before the baby is born. The number of pregnant brides in this country has been variously estimated to be between 200,000 and 300,000 annually. While some of the points made in the foregoing section are relevant to this group of females who marry during pregnancy, the following points are uniquely relevant.

Helping the Couples Make a Wise Decision about Marriage

When marriage is being considered, it is highly important for the counselor to see the male partner as well as the female. The experienced counselor can often obtain more helpful information and impressions in 5 min with the couple together than in ¹/₂ h with the female alone. One of the important reasons for talking with the male is to form some impressions regarding his motivation for marriage. Some men express definite interest in marriage and may even be pushing the female in this direction, but the counselor needs to help the male make sure that he is not motivated solely by guilt or by a desire to protect the female and his own image of masculinity. It is my strong impression that few males feel guilty about having coital experience with a female, since in our society such experience has historically been associated with masculinity. Men are much more likely to feel guilty if they fail to carry out their learned masculine role of protecting and looking out for the female; but sympathy, protectiveness, and perhaps some pity are insufficient ingredients for a lasting, durable marriage.

In cases where the counselor has strong doubts about the sources of the couple's motivation for marriage, it would be well to make explicit to both of them this aspect of the male's dilemma and to describe in detail the several alternatives involved, including the one of waiting until the baby is born and perhaps even released for adoption before deciding if they still want to get married. In such cases, the counselor needs to emphasize that this does not represent advising and certainly not *prescribing* what they should do; rather, it is providing more complete information, so that their decision can be based on a realistic understanding of themselves and the possible consequences of alternative solutions.

Because people are accustomed to having a physician *prescribe* treatment for them, it is particularly necessary for the physician to provide explicit examples to illustrate his role as *consultant*. Very young couples need quite explicit examples to counter their reaction to other people making decisions for them and need to differentiate between (1) prescriptions and (2) information about options consistent with their values, goals, and means.

A number of counselors have indicated their belief that the young couples who have definitely decided to proceed with marriage are sometimes helped by the suggestion to carry out their wedding plans with as much publicity, dignity, and pride as would have been the case if the bride had not been pregnant. These counselors have found that sometimes a hurried, covert wedding is subsequently more conducive to feelings of guilt than is the illicit conception. In years to come, friends and relatives will no longer be counting months on their fingers, but the couple's periodic attendance at other weddings may still remind them of their own very hurried and not very satisfying wedding arrangements.

The Unanswerable Question

Inevitably, the female who is pregnant at the time of marriage is plagued at various times throughout her married life by the recurring question, "Would he have married me had I not been pregnant?" The counselor can go a long way toward preventing future marital strife by helping the young couple (1) face this question and accept the fact that it can never be answered; (2) recognize and accept the inevitability that each of them during heated discussions and marital exchanges in future years will throw the fact of the premarital conception in the other's face; and (3) realize that such questions and arguments are fairly universal, rather than peculiar to their situation. It can be illustrated that almost every married woman and man at different times in their life will need and want their partner's reaffirmation that if the partner had it all to do over again, the marriage would still have taken place. The counselor can also point out that almost all married couples, in moments of anger, are likely to resurrect events of 10 years ago, to rehash dislikes during the dating period, and even to call upon negative features in the parents and siblings of the spouse. The tendency to bring up issues and behavior that occurred during courting days, either with each other or with other persons, is not peculiar to couples married in the context of pregnancy.

Without an awareness of the universality of her unanswerable question, "Would he . . . ," the pregnant bride will begin all too early to overemotionalize and overpersonalize many of the normal frictions of married life and to assume erroneously that all would have been rosy had she not been pregnant at the time of marriage.

Divorced Women: Postmarital Pregnancies

Physicians, more than any other professional group, have long been aware of the problems posed by *postmarital* pregnancies occurring in divorced women. Although the incidence of such pregnancies is impossible to ascertain, the limited and highly selective information which is available suggests that during the past 3 decades such pregnancies in this country either increased in number or were more openly admitted.

Understanding the Factors Involved

For at least two reasons, the physician who is consulted by a pregnant divorcee needs to be aware of some of the social and psychological factors contributing to postmarital pregnancies. (1) Such an awareness will increase the doctor's own understanding of the problem, and (2) the patient needs to know that her physician understands some of these contributing factors. In most cases, the patient does not seek the physician's approval so much as she seeks and needs one person's understanding of how an out of wedlock pregnancy could happen to a woman who regards herself as normal and moral. The physician who has read some of the case history excerpts in William Goode's book, *After Divorce* (Goode, 1956), will have greater empathy with the pregnant divorcee and hence will be better able to help her gain perspective concerning the circumstances and factors involved in her illicit conception.

Reduced Sexual Caution

One of the factors contributing to postmarital pregnancies is the reduction in the sexual caution of divorced women. This is due in part to a desire to remarry and thereby to escape the socially stigmatized category of the divorcee as soon as possible and, in part to habits of heterosexual interaction acquired during marriage. Most divorcees and some widows discover very quickly that readjustments have to be made in their relationships with other men after the loss of a husband. Many men perceive the divorcee as easy sex prey, since they assume that she is accustomed to sexual intercourse, misses it, and therefore will welcome their advances as a favor. The divorcee herself may inadvertently foster such a view. While married and accompanied by her husband, she may have become accustomed to fairly open and frank discussions of sex in mixed groups; now, however, she has to relearn some of the coyness and subtleties that traditionally accompany courtship. Without such coyness, and under the implicit pressure of society to prove, by means of a successful marriage, that it was not *she* who failed in the first marriage, she may permit her involvement with men after divorce to progress much more rapidly than she means to — until she finds that she is pregnant and the man has lost interest.

Sporadic Postmarital Coition

A second contributing factor is that an unknown proportion of divorces involve a period of continued, sporadic coition between the ex-partners. In cases of "friendly" divorce, many couples report that the continuation of coition, with no love or family obligations expected, is mutually enjoyable. If pregnancy occurs, it is terminated by abortion in an unknown number of cases. When abortion is unacceptable to the woman, however, she is very reluctant to name her former husband as the father. Understandably, she feels that others would think her foolish for having continued to have coition with her husband after divorcing him.

In cases where the divorce was not mutually desired, the wife may view intercourse, and even pregnancy, as a potential means of reclaiming her husband. Pregnancy may also be desired by divorcees who, as one stated, "want a memory of him . . . I hope it's a boy that looks just like him . . . that way a part of him will always be with me." There are also ex-husbands who desire a reconciliation and who finally suceed in persuading their ex-wives to engage in intercourse "for old times' sake" — only to find that the resulting pregnancy makes a reconciliation even less acceptable to her.

Perceiving Divorce as a Treatment Method

The counselor's emphasis on *divorce as a treatment method,* not a disease or failure, can provide needed perspective for the pregnant divorcee who may feel as much guilt and anxiety about her divorce as about her postmarital pregnancy. That the traditional values concerning marriage in our society still predominate becomes obvious when researchers as well as the general public continue to ask "What causes divorce?" Such a question is as meaningless as "What causes surgery?" As surgery is but one of many treatment methods for a serious medical problem. Other treatments for serious marital distress include murder, suicide, alcoholism, workaholism, development of neuroticism, prolonged hostility and personality deterioration, and constructive restructuring of the marital relationship.

The perspective of divorce as a treatment method for a critically disabled marriage may help the pregnant divorcee to gain self-dignity and respect as she reconsiders the prices associated with methods used by others for treating a destructive marital union.

This perspective also opens the door for her to examine, with the counselor's help, the more fruitful question "Was divorce the best, most effective or appropriate treatment method in my case?" If so, this realization increases her self-confidence. If divorce is seen upon examination not to have been the best or wisest treatment, then the awareness that other methods with worse results could have been employed, by choice or default, also provides some degree of self-confidence that far surpasses the negative feelings associated with implicitly or explicitly viewing divorce as a disease or a failure.

Married Women: Extramarital Pregnancies

Why Does She Tell?

Perhaps the most puzzling question concerning the extramarital pregnancy is why a married woman ever reveals that it was not her husband who impregnated her. The answers provided by counselors and physicians fall into three categories. The first includes those cases in which the wife seeks help from the counselor because the husband knows he is not the father and the marriage is threatened. The second category includes cases in which the wife seeks the counselor's help in resolving her own feelings and planning her course of action without telling her husband of the problem. The third category pertains to those women who feel they need at least one, but only one, confidant and who tell their physician in order to minimize the risk of revealing the information to others inadvertently while under the influence of anesthesia during delivery.

Whether there is any subsequent discussion of thoughts, attitudes, and wishes which the mother may express under the stress or anesthesia of delivery will depend on the physician's view of the professional ethics involved. Some physicians report that they ignore, or compartmentalize such information, considering it to be unrelated and irrelevant to their medical role. Others state that they may discuss with the patient any "confidences" revealed during delivery if (1) the patient subsequently requires such a discussion, and (2) it seems likely that the "confidences" revealed are relevant to the patient's physical, emotional, and marital health. The ethical requirement that the physician not divulge any confidential information given him by a patient is of long standing; but the ethics involved in holding subsequent discussions with the patient about "confidences" uttered during periods of extreme stress of partial anesthesia are ambiguous. The procedure followed will obviously depend upon a number of factors peculiar to each case and to each physician—the most important consideration being the present and future welfare of the patient. More open discussion of the professional ethics involved and of the results that might be expected from each method of handling such problems is needed to provide guidelines for medical students and young physicians.

Extramarital Affairs

Since extramarital pregnancies are the result of extramarital liaisons, it seems appropriate to discuss at this point some of the factors both inside and outside marriage that are responsible for the development of such liaisons and to consider ways the physician can help married couples who feel this marriage has been endangered by the involvement of either partner in an extramarital affair.

Arthur Miller's play, *The Seven-Year Itch*, contains many insights concerning the almost imperceptible manner in which the marital relationship becomes sufficiently dull, boring, and unrewarding to set the stage for an affair. The "itch" for a more vital, romantic, and meaningful relationship is not limited, however, to the 7th year of marriage. It can as easily come in the 4th, 14th, 20th, or 30th year. More on how extramarital affairs develop and evolve can be found in Chap. 4 by Williamson.

What Kind of Adultery?

The counselor confronted by the client who is castigating his or her spouse for committing adultery may provide the client with perspective by asking, "What kind of adultery?" In response to the client's look of puzzlement, it can be noted that it is possible to commit "religious adultery," "recreational adultery," "ideological adultery," and so forth. This statement will require the further explanation that many individuals who never commit sexual adultery have far more religious, recreational, or ideological intercourse with another person of the opposite sex than with their own spouse. The total exclusion of the wife from some of these areas is sometimes associated with more hurt and humiliation for her than is sexual adultery, since the latter is usually less public and does not exclude her entirely. One 33-year-old wife bitterly stated, "I wish to hell he *would* sleep with her, that would be private. But what does he do? Two or more times a week, he plays tennis with her where everybody watches. That hurts! He refuses to play (tennis) with me." Curiously enough, those who appear to be most traumatized by sexual adultery are frequently the ones who avow that sex is of minor importance; yet, they are far more upset by sharing their mate in this area than by sharing their spouse in what they regard as other more "important" areas.

By asking "What kind of adultery?" the counselor can stimulate the client to re-examine his or her hierarchy of values and the degree of consistency between belief and practice. Some individuals regain confidence when they perceive how many marital areas are still shared and unadulterated. Others may acknowledge for the first time that sex is a far more important aspect of marriage than they had previously admitted; these individuals then begin to develop a more meaningful sexual relationship with their spouse in order to preclude outside competition. Still others discover that few, if any, areas of their marriage involve any meaningful intercourse and that the sexual adultery is symptomatic of lack of development in several areas; they may then resolve to enrich the total marital relationship.

Closure of an Affair

If it is the husband who is involved in the affair and the wife has sought help or supportive understanding from the counselor, she may need help in understanding that there is a need for dignity and finesse in the closure of an affair. If the relationship with the other woman has developed gradually and has been a meaningful one, the husband will find it difficult to terminate the affair abruptly—and in many cases, too abrupt termination will exact a price from the marriage. If the husband is to maintain his respect and dignity, as well as his image as a male, he will not wish to hurt the other woman unduly. This reluctance is particularly strong if the period leading up to actual sexual involvement included the sharing of ideas, problems, values, and so forth. If he terminates the relationship too rapidly and hates himself for doing so, he may subsequently redirect this hostility toward his wife. The counselor can sometimes help the wife to appreciate that one of the reasons she loves her husband is his compassion and dislike of hurting other people; she may then have more patience during the closure period and not misinterpret the time taken to bring the affair to an end as meaning that her husband loves the other woman more than he loves her.

Time Scabs or Heals

Whichever partner is involved in an extramarital liaison, the counselor can reassure both husband and wife who desire to strengthen their marriage that extramarital involvement *can* provide the motivation and stimulus for developing a marital relationship much deeper than the one which existed previously. This statement is not to be interpreted as encouraging extramarital affairs; it is analogous to reassuring the businessman who has already suffered bankruptcy that others in similar circumstances have benefitted from the lessons learned and have subsequently established highly successful businesses. Such a businessman is well aware that there are other ways to learn. For more discussion on the uses and abuses of extramarital affairs and their management in counseling see Chap. 4.

Much reassurance will be needed often during the ensuing months, which seem to be years for the married couple trying to resolve the aftermath of an affair in which at least one of them has been deeply hurt. The counselor can help them to accept as inevitable, but nondefeating, the recurrent flare-ups when a word, a look, or a memory will evoke fresh pain from a wound that has crusted over but not healed. They will need reiterated reassurance that healing takes time, that flare-ups will become less frequent, and that other couples in their situation have eventually found the wound no longer tender to the touch.

A Postscript and Partial Summary

The current fashionableness of sexual permissiveness of a variety of alternate life styles and of young couples as well as senior citizen couples living together, sans marriage, may lead the reader to dismiss some of my comments, concerns, and observations as too traditional or conservative for applicability to woman who find themselves pregnant out of wedlock in the late 1970's. Thus, it may be worthwhile to note that it is precisely those women with traditional and conservative value orientations who are most likely to seek couseling help with their pre- or extramarital pregnancies. Those whose basic values (not just lip service) support a sexual permissiveness for themselves are far less likely to seek out the professional counselor or to need the consultant role of the physician when experiencing conception outside of a marital union.

Also, at an historical time when sexual permissiveness is fashionable there is a tendency to forget that, by definition, a fashion is fashionable only so long as it has not yet been adopted by the majority—at which time it is no longer "fashionable." The popular notion in the late 1960's and early 1970's that most, if not all, teen-age females were engaging in coition was not supported by the detailed findings and projections which Kantner and Zelnick (1972) reported in a series of publications and which were based on interviews of a national probability sample of the 15- to 19-year-old female population. Approximately 28% of the never married young women in the United States aged 15 to 19 were estimated to have had some coital experience as of 1971. Moreover, one-half of these women with some special experience had their coital experience only with one man—the one they intended to marry. The figures for only the 19 year olds indicated that 40% of the white and 81% of the black unmarried females had experienced some coital experience by the time of their final year as a teen-ager.

Thus, the very young unmarried female who is white, who has coition in her teen-age years, and who becomes pregnant, and who decides to complete her pregnancy is one of a very small minority of girls her age. In the initial professional contact with such a female, the physician and/or counselor can make a significant contribution to her as a worthwhile person and an awareness of her feelings, needs, and unspoken dilemmas. At that time she is desperately in need of a significant relationship with at least one adult with whom she can openly discuss not just the fact of being pregnant out of wedlock, but her thoughts and feelings about the relationship from which the pregnancy derived.

The changes and pendulum swings and in the fashionableness (and even legality) of given trends in sexual behavior and practices (sterilizations in the late 1930's, abortions in the early 1970's) should alert the counselor to the need for an historical perspective for understanding quite different "residual guilt feelings" of different age groups. Thus, as was noted earlier, one of the needs common to a wide variety of women involved in illicit pregnancies, whether before, during, or after marriage, is that of maintaining an historical and contextual perspective concerning their sexual experiences. Adult women may condemn themselves too harshly by imposing adult judgments upon their adolescent sexual experiences. Married women may judge too harshly in retrospect their earlier "love" affairs involving coition with other men. Knowing at 35, for example, the depth and quality of love she now has for her husband, a woman may continually reinforce guilt feelings about an earlier sex union she had with another man before marriage. Certainly it is not easy to always maintain the context within which a given event or experience took place 10, 20, or 30 years previously; but it is important to try to do so. A mature woman of 45 should not judge an extramarital experience she had at 28 as if she had had at that time her present wisdom, judgment, and values. The couple who have resolved some of their marital difficulties a year after one of them was involved in an affair should try to remember the situation as it was when the affair developed. The married woman impregnated during an affair will need considerable help in maintaining the total context within which her affair took place. Otherwise, her guilt and condemnation of herself or her husband may greatly reduce the chances for subsequent strengthening of the marriage.

Sexual Permissiveness and Fear

A sizeable number of counselors and physicians have experienced an increasing polarization (anger or enthusiasm) of patients' attitudes and feelings about the current liberalization of sexual attitudes (Klemer, 1973). The anger may reflect to a considerable degree the patients' underlying fear of sex generally or doubts about their own sexual competence specifically. This underlying fear, for which anger is frequently a symptom, also comprises a much broader thread in contemporary society. Certainly some, if not much, of youth's anger with the establishment, with parents, and with older people in authority positions during the past decade was symptomatic of their fear of a sense of inadequacy in coping with and participating in the system. Reared in a permissive and affluent era, many were not sufficiently prepared to be self-reliant, and the fear of the unknown in becoming financially and occupationally independent was accompanied by "dropping out," while masking their fear and sense of inadequacy by faulting the established system and by angry acts of violence against those in authority. In many such cases, it was not simply a refusal to follow the rules, but an anger symptomatic of the fear of failure combined with a bona fide anger at parents and society for not better preparing them to be self-reliant.

Their parents' anger also is partially symptomatic of fear—fear of the unknowns of co-ed dormitory life, of hippie life, of drugs, or of communal living.

Even youths' delay in getting married and their even greater delay in having children can be viewed, in some, as a concomitant of the fear and doubts they feel about being successful spouses and parents.

Fear is healthy in moderate amounts; in fact, it is needed for survival—only in death or when we abandon hope are we without fear. However, the physician needs to consider whether the patient's extreme anger against liberalized sexual attitudes may be symptomatic of the fear that arises from the unknown (for which the antidote may be straightforward information) or from a sense of sexual inadequacy (which can then be discussed in an open and supportive context).

In the case of the "true believer" proselyte, excessive enthusiasm for liberalization of sexual attitudes may reflect the patient's efforts to convince oneself that what he or she is doing or would like to is really all right. In cases of "methinks thee proselytes too much," the physician may want to help the patient examine whether he or she is really comfortable with the new attitude which may have been adopted to pave the way for new sexual behavior they are not very sure about and also to help them examine whether their degree of proselyting is consistent with their own value system. For example, if the patient favors a pluralistic society with many different life styles, then presumably there should be as much respect for the old as for the new, as much dignity accorded traditional sex attitudes as is granted very liberal sex attitudes.

REFERENCES

Goode, W. J.: *After Divorce.* Free Press, New York, 1956.

Klemer, R. H. (Ed): Counseling in cases involving premarital and extramarital pregnancies, in *Counseling in Marital and Sexual Problems: A Physician's Handbook,* Williams and Wilkins Co., Baltimore, 1965; and from subsequent revision of Vincent, C. E.: Illicit pregnancies and extramarital affairs, Chap. 9 in *Sexual and Marital Health: The Physician as a Consultant:* McGraw-Hill, New York, 1973.

Klemer, R. H.: Side effects on the family from liberalized sexual attitudes. *Medical Aspects of Human Sexuality,* **7**:80–96 (June), 1973.

282   Counseling in Marital and Sexual Problems

Vincent C. E.: *Unmarried Mothers*. Free Press, New York, 1961; Paperbook Ed, 1969.

Vincent, C. E.: *Unmarried Mothers*, Chap. 1, Free Press, New York, 1961; Paperbook Ed, 1969.

Vincent C. E.: Ego-involvement in sexual relations. Implications for research on illegitimacy. Am. J. Sociology, 65:287–295 (November), 1959.

Zelnick, M., and Kantner, J. F.: Sexuality, contraception and pregnancy among young unwed females in the United States, in *Demographic and Social Aspects of Population Growth*. Westoff, C. F., and Parke, R., (eds), U. S. Government Printing Office, Washington, D. C., 1972; Zelnick, M., and Kantner, J. F.: The probability of premarital intercourse. Social Science Research 1:335, 1972; and Kantner, J. F., and Zelnick, M.: Sexual experience of young unmarried women in the United States. Family Planning Perspectives, 4:9–18 (Oct.), 1972.

ROBERT N. RUTHERFORD, M.D., AND
JEAN J. RUTHERFORD

19

The Climacteric Years in the Woman, Man, and Family

The 40's are a time when men and women seem to be thrust into preformed molds which few desire. There are certain physical facts of aging which must be accepted, albeit reluctantly. The physician-counselor can occupy a vitally important role, if he will but accept it, in helping a mid-life couple to seek positive attitudes rather than to look at their "liver spots," to worry over their failure as parents, or to contemplate upon which barren shore their old carcasses, with spirits dwindling, will be left to wither and die. The "empty nest" syndrome may present itself as a distressing new projection for the future.

These days there is much for the physician and the patient to be positive about. Away back at the turn of the century — some 70 odd years ago — the life-span of the typical woman ended in her mid-40's. Often she died of overwork and overbabies as if she were a spent skyrocket. Today she has an average life expectancy lasting into her 70's, because of the many things which can help her mentally, emotionally, and physically.

Not so dramatic, but equally encouraging, has been the increased longevity for men.

Just living longer, though, is not enough. Unless mid-life patients can be helped to make creative adjustments to the menopausal and postmenopausal years, they may not have really gained anything. Fortunately, both hormone therapy and counseling skills are now available to help the physician help his patients. Both are important and both will be discussed herewith, in their relationship to women, to men, and to family living.

The Physician's Role

Increasing awareness has come regarding the new role of the physician in the family constellation. No longer does he occupy the traditional position as a physician only—patients now identify the physician "as a primary source of sexual information and counseling—but physicians often are not prepared to meet this responsibility"—so declared the American Medical Association House of Delegates in 1973. Dr. William H. Masters has pointed out "physicians probably know no more and no les about the subject than do other college graduates." Masters has coined the term "sexual dis-ease," both for physician and patient.

As an example of this profound lack of formal training in past medical school curricula, the following table may illustrate this deficit in a most significant area.

Fortunately, in answer to the many requests from all levels—most frequently from physicians in practice who had found their inadequacies for this type of counseling most upsetting—medical school programs plus postgraduate programs now are functioning with increasing value for the medical student as well as the practicing physician. Comment often is made by those completing these courses that their own personal lives have been bettered considerably as well as in the quality of their professional advices to their patients. One of the pioneers in this program has been Dr. Harold I. Lief of the University of Pennsylvania.

Appended is a list of books recommended by sexologists for the physician's library.

TABLE 19.1
Some sexual misconceptions of medical students*

Sample questions	% of incorrect answers	
	Male	Female
There are two kinds of physiological orgasmic responses in women, one clitoral and one vaginal (false)	38	43
Impotence is almost always a psychogenic disorder (true)	37	35
An immediate result of castration in the adult male is impotence (false)	35	51
Only a small minority of married couples ever experience mouth-genital sex play (false)	25	35
25% of men over the age of 70 have an active sex life (true)	36	31
Certain conditions of mental and emotional instability are demonstrably caused by masturbation (false)	15	15
Direct stimulation of the clitoris is essential to achieving orgasm in women (false)	22	33
Menopause in a woman is accompanied by a sharp and lasting reduction in sexual drive and interest (false)	21	13

* *Medical World News* March 24, 1975.

The Female Climacteric (Menopause)

Our earlier concepts of the menopause often made it a wastebasket into which could be consigned many female "megrims and miasms" of difficult classification. The writers have seen this diagnosis pinned upon patients as early as age 17 and as late as age 73. It has been as useful and as acceptable as the diagnosis of "hypochondriasis" or "functional illness" or "problems of unknown etiology," or even "psychiatric problems."

What goes on within the female body and psyche at this time? These changes can be ascribed to many causative factors other than estrogen deficit alone: less activity, poor diet, obesity, hypertension, as well as the inevitable catabolism of aging. The large majority of these factors are amenable to treatment programs and any deficits, including estrogenic deficits, should be corrected. A number of things can be documented:

1. Osteoporosis—a loss of protein and calcium from the bones resulting in a thinning and weakening of the bones. Even if this fails to progress to the point of causing loss of height, "dowager's hump," backache, or collapse fracture of the vertebrae, it can never be considered a "normal" or "good" change. The 80-year-old woman who suffers a fractured hip in a minor fall may blame it on the fact that her ovaries ceased functioning 30 years before and substitution treatment was never given—plus a "tea and toast diet" with no exercise except maintenance household duties.

2. A loss of the normal female protection against atherosclerosis.

3. A tendency to gain weight and to develop diabetes in those who have the hereditary potential.

4. A withdrawal of protein from the skin, thinning it, and giving the fine wrinkles usually blamed on aging.

5. An increased irritability and vasomotor instability leading to such symptoms as hot flashes.

6. The atrophy and drying of mucous membranes. This includes drying of the lining of the nose and throat, eyes and tear ducts, and of the neck of the urinary bladder and vagina. Individuals vary widely as to the degree of symptoms that result, but many times the local irritation or itching is a cause of serious discomfort.

7. An increased tendency of the kidneys to waste salt in the urine, leading to a decreased volume of blood which may cause weakness and dizziness.

8. An increased incidence of cancer of the breast and uterus.

What are the subjective, emotional, difficult to measure things which may be far more important than changes in lipid metabolism?

Beginning with marriage the first major strain the family unit will have is the advent of the first baby. This requires mutuality in every sense of the word. Interestingly enough, the second major strain is the last child's leaving the parental home.

Then, the middle-aged couple turn toward each other for strength and reassurance, comfort, and inspiration for further living. But, what if this partnership has foundered long since—foundered by reason of the wife who has given herself completely to "her" children at the expense of a husband's love. The husband now has compensated for his wife's inattention toward him with his job, his hobbies, and his community responsibilities. She turns to him only to find that he has little more than a basic simple courtesy toward her. Often he wants no other woman, he is just busy with other things.

It is unfortunate that events are timed so that in the mid-40's a series of family-shaking changes converge on the family unit all at once:

1. The children physically leaving home for the great wide wonderful world, whether to jobs, higher education, the armed forces, marriage, or what you will. No longer is the mother in her erstwhile role of past great significance.

2. Even though the mother may have called her menstruation "the curse" for many years, when it suddenly stops she may realize that this means she cannot have another baby to make her of paramount importance again to some dependent person. Of course, there is the sorry substitute of grandmotherhood, but this usually is of little consolation.

Some women equate the cessation of menstruation with loss of femininity. Fortunately this is not true.

3. Father is just reaching his stride, even though he may be balding. His importance is still on the upgrade, his community efforts and increasing recognition keep him busy, almost too busy, and too importantly happy.

The mother looks about at a wasteland which can be most heartbreaking. She may be troubled by easy emotional upsets which even a Phi Beta Kappa mind cannot seem to control. The body she has lived in and controlled over the last 45 years is changing and shifting in its responses. Her feelings of attractiveness may falter, and consequently her sex urge may be disrupted, even though she consciously wishes no basic change in her relationship with her husband.

Treatment in Women

In this day and age, a great deal can be done for the menopausal woman, probably more for her than for her husband.

In the realm of medications which can be prescribed we have the estrogens. Excellent work emerging from geriatricians has shown that many women may need positive medication at this time. Prior to the last 2 decades, an occasional lonely medical prophet such as Dr. Fuller

Albright advised routine use of estrogens whether the patient was having menopausal symptoms or not. The bulk of medical thinking then felt that menopause was a normal and natural physiological phase completed within a few months or a few years by every normal female and should not be interfered with. But, evidence has continued to pile up that certain basic benefits can be given to all aging women by judicious use of estrogens.

In the majority of women, the ovarian source of estrogens withers in the late 40's. However, the adrenal sources of estrogens continue until roughly age 60. From this age, on it was noted that women now shared the same incidence of vascular problems as men, *i.e.*, coronary occlusions, cerebral vascular accidents, and the like.

In any event, increasing support was given to the concept that women who show estrogen deficiency by Papanicolaou smear may be benefitted by supplementary administration of estrogens. These benefits are as follows.

1. There is less loss of elasticity of the skin (*i.e.*, "wrinkling," to our patients).

2. There is less atherosclerosis.

3. There is less osteoporosis.

4. There is less shrinking and drying of the vagina, less cervical stenosis, less shrinking of the bladder capacity and urethral problems, and less anal stenosis.

5. Lipid and lipoprotein metabolism remains unchanged, with less of the "dowager's hump" and thickening of the midriff.

New retrospective studies are suggesting that there may be an increased incidence of endometrial carcinoma associated with the use of estrogens. Continuing studies are indicated for this and other possible harmful side reactions in the use of estrogens. Additional research is being done before this care concept is either valid or important. There is a wise middle ground between the "estrogens for all" school of thought and the "never estrogens at all" concept. Certainly any potent medication should be given under supervision and not as a routine treatment program.

If there is loss of libido (this is reported in some 10% of menopausal women), androgen can be added with benefit, should estrogen alone not be an adequate stimulus. If androgens are combined with estrogen, side effects of masculinization are minimal, particularly if treatment is interrupted from time to time. Usually, explanation of the slowing cycle of sex interest in the wife and reassurance that this often is shared by the husband will help a great deal, with or without hormone aid.

In the realm of psychological treatment, the promotion of positive attitudes is tremendously important. It is a matter of simple arithmetic to show the menopausal woman that the children have been her concern for only 20 years, and that now she faces what can be a promising vista of 30 years with her husband. Usually income is less encumbered as is leisure time. This can be made to sound like an insurance brochure hailing the delights of retirement insurance. The suggestion from the physician that there is no loss of femininity — courtesy of estrogens — is of great value to every female patient.

Reassurance that life still can hold a great deal of rich, creative living is an important therapeutic procedure in helping middle-aged people. But it might be well to point out that in order to make his reassurance convincing, the physician must really believe it himself. The physician-counselor needs to have genuinely positive attitudes about the aging process.

The Male Climacteric (Menopause)

The male climacteric is a sly, subtle change which makes no such dramatic announcement as the stopping of menstruation in women. There are no sudden physical changes which can be noted. No night sweats or hot flashes occur, neither does impotence or premature ejaculation or lack of sex interest (those dramatic evidences that "something is wrong" with the male machinery).

The male menopause is a term that should never have been coined, yet it is with us for some time to come. It has no physical basis. It does not mark the stopping of sperm formation or of male hormone production. Instead, it is an emotional-attitudinal change.

The man in his late 40's may suddenly realize that his physical powers are limited somewhat. He does not bounce quite so well the next morning. He may be confronted with the realization that he has gone about as far as he will go, or can go, in his job. Younger men seem suddenly to loom as challengers. Also, his children seem to doubt many of his ideas and values and to seek his advice less often. But then, so does his wife, who seems to be emotionally upset most of the time. His behavior toward her has not changed, he thinks, yet all he gets is into trouble.

In other words, his entire world seems to focus upon him as if he were at fault, or as if his values were not as good as he had always thought they were, or as if whatever he has accomplished is not really worthwhile. These things bring many uncertainties at a time when he suddenly realizes that there *is* only one real certainty — he is on the downhill slide.

He realizes that he is mortal, is aging, and will someday die. True, he has left children as evidence of his immortality and possibly a number of fine works. This is the time when the professional fund raisers hit him for stained glass windows for the church, for alumni gifts, or for endowment of any of many monuments to show that he once was here and important.

It can be a very unsettling moment of truth for the strong and for the weak, for the religious and the irreligious, for the happy man, and the unhappy man. This is a spiritual menopause which often has been precipitated by certain physical realizations.

If this man can turn to his wife — as we hope she can turn to him for support and understanding — their marriage may go on for another very happy 30 years (remembering our current life expectancy).

On the other hand, if he has no support from his life partner, from his job situation, from his financial planning for the future, from a progressively devaluated dollar, or from his physician-counselor, what may he do?

He may check his sexual prowess with another partner.

He may say "To hell with it!" and chuck the whole thing and go over the hill.

He may look his situation over and decide that it is better to stay where he is, unhappy though he may be, rather than to change his familiar road for unknown new responsibilities.

None of these alternatives offers any real solution to his problem.

This man at this juncture needs understanding, help, sympathy, and reinspiration for what could be productive years ahead.

Treatment for Men

For the man, medical treatment is largely that of counseling and not of endocrine therapy. If we note that the male has a higher incidence of cardiovascular problems than the female up until the age of 60, it would seem that that the use of androgens for "supportive" reasons has little value. Their use improving libido is thought to be largely a placebo effect.

It is possible to measure the levels of androgen in the male. If there is the problem of lessened potency, psychological factors should be explored but also those of androgen levels. If indicated, androgens can be of great value both in sexual performance but also in mood elevation derived from increasingly able sexual performance as well as a possible anabolic effect.

A sympathetic discussion and hearing on the part of the interested physician is a treatment "must" for the middle-aged male. Simply helping a man of this age group to understand the physiology involved, both in himself and in his wife, can be reassuring. While he may be on the "downhill metabolic slide," it can be presented in such a fashion that it represents a happy challenge for the next 30 years. The man mentioned above who thought only of stepping out, going over the hill, or resigning himself to unhappiness really has another possibility which, perhaps with a little counseling help from the physician, he can come to see. He can, if he will, pull himself up by his own bootstraps. He can take the initiative and say to his wife, "These are our green years. Our children are launched. Our responsibilities now are only for you and me. Let's start these new fruitful years, not fruitful from our loins but from our minds."

The Family Climacteric

The "family climacteric" is not often discussed as such. But in its own way it may be most dramatic. It occurs when the family has a "change of life" and the children are suddenly gone.

One parent pair may have trained their children for maturity and for leaving the nest. They will be delighted by the children's adulthood and independence. After this graduation from the family, the children may take on the status of good friends to their parents because of mutual enjoyment and respect.

But another parent pair may despair at the departure of their children, at the loneliness of life with only themselves, the overwhelming boredom of facing the future with only the other sterile partner. Put this way, these are melancholy prospects.

In middle age, we find only too many couples who no longer "are in love with each other." On the other hand, the old familiar resentments have become chronic and there is not enough motivation to cause either to want a divorce.

The physician is in an ideal position not only to counsel but to suggest avenues of a new enriched life, to go back to school, to return to a job, whether paid or volunteer, part-time or full-time, to exploit a latent talent. Whatever the doctor's prescription, it should emphasize the need for the couple to become interesting to themselves as individuals and then to each other as individuals and partners.

This is not just sentimental talk. As we live with our patients and watch the human patterns form again and again, certain patterns for helping emerge. The basic problems are the same. Just the individuals change. Often the physician-counselor is able to make a larger contribution to his patient's mental health than any other helper, because of the intimate association with all the family members over the years. The counseling provided in the latter years of the family life cycle may be as important as the prescriptions and treatment given when the family was just beginning to grow.

Fallacies and Myths as We Age

Man has reached the moon. Our life-span is increasing due to many factors but still the Wheel of Life with aging and ultimate death is inevitable. However, there has been an appreciable change in many attitudes regarding aging. Previously, according to deBeauvoir (1972), the aging individual was "To live as your conscience should tell you, you must conform to social image and dress, be deprived of privacy, show inactivity and retirement from work. One must not seek pleasure in sex nor upset the incest taboo of the young. One must be afraid of scandal or ridicule as 'a lecherous old man' or a 'shameless old woman' and believe in the myth of lost sexuality with age." (Glover, 1975, p. 165.)

These social restraints upon the elderly have been lifted. It may be because of financial necessity wherein two individual Social Security checks are better than the single check to which they would be reduced were they to marry. The sexual restraints have been lifted as well, if only by the permissive sexual activities of their grandchildren. The social unit of marriage with its past imponderable responsibilities is under fire at all levels—not the least of which is in the twilight zone of from 50 years on. It is interesting that one of the most distressed patients of recent years was a young man who had turned 30—he now was an old man and would be ostracized by his younger friends!

Exact stress information has been developed for the "maturing" individuals. Sex after a heart attack may be selected as a case in point. The "death in the saddle syndrome" is the figment of coroners' imaginations. The actual burst of energy in an orgasmic relationship is equivalent to 150 calories or two slices of buttered bread. With these reassurances, starting 3 months after a "coronary," the usual couple can begin a rewarding sexual contact. Until then, the benefits of touch, stroking, and even of manual release may be prescribed.

As the years go by, the reassurance can be given to patients that sexual expression is many-sided. Simply living together in a mutually sharing and giving relationship is one aspect of adult sexuality. However, if both partners are physically able, consistency of sexual expression (less of quantity but with no diminution of quality) is most important in maintaining sexual potency. This reassurance is vital.

It is well for the conscientious physician to heed the admonition of the American Medical Association Committee mentioned earlier in this presentation. No longer is the physician a dispenser of nostrums for megrims and miasms—"his patients identify him as a primary source of sexual information and counseling." And so it is—so we are charged as physicians ministering to the multiple needs of our patients.

REFERENCES

deBeauvoir, S.: The Coming of Age. G. P. Putnam's Sons, New York, 1972.
Glover, B. H.: Family practice and problems of aging. Postgraduate Medicine, 57 (8): 165, 1975.

Part IV

Premarital Counseling

ROBERT F. STAHMANN, Ph. D., AND
ANNE BARCLAY-COPE, M.S.

20

Premarital Counseling: An Overview

Premarital counseling is a widely accepted idea and practice. Most professionals recognize that premarital counseling in some form is valuable, yet there has been little written as to what is really involved. The purpose of this chapter is to review some of the major writing that has appeared related to premarital counseling and synthesize it into an overview of current practice. The chapter does not deal with specific techniques for premarital education and counseling. Techniques and specific topical considerations are treated in the referenced readings and in chapters following which consider: the religious dimension of premarital counseling, psychosocial factors in premarital counseling, sex education and family planning, the premarital physical examination; and contraception and family planning.

What have marriage counselors said about premarital counseling? Butterfield, some 20 years ago (1956), stated that if one were to judge by the current divorce rates in the United States, it would be easy to conclude that many marriages take place with little, if any, serious planning for marriage and family life. Those comments are being validated and reiterated by marital counselors even today.

Mace (1972) concluded that people drift into marital relationships with all their "maddening complexity on pink clouds of sentiment." He said that people are prepared to spend considerable effort and money on the wedding and ceremonies which are over in a few hours, yet leave to chance the outcome of the marriage, which is supposed to last a lifetime. He proposed that one of the main reasons for trouble in marriage was that young couples do not get the help they need and the information they need about marriage either before or after they get started in marriage.

Rutledge (1968) postulated that although marriage itself can be a maturing process for an individual, persons must have attained a resonable amount of adult growth and responsibility if they are to carry their share of the multifaceted responsibilities of modern marriage. Rugledge identified discovery of selfhood, continued growth as a person, and communication and problem solving skills as basic factors in preparing for marriage. He further stated that much of the process of preparation for marriage was opening up these crucial areas of life and projecting the young couple into the future, enabling them to foresee the kinds of problems and challenges awaiting them.

Ellis (1961) stated that still another cause of failure in marriage was ignorance about the nature of the marriage relationship itself. Many people do not have even the most elementary preparation for the demands that marriage will make of them, and it is assumed that they will automatically know how to adapt themselves into this, the most important partnership of their lives. He indicated that this lack of preparation was really quite amazing since a person is not expected to know how to "drive a car, to dance well, to strum a guitar, or hit a golf ball without definite instructions! Surely there is no reason to consider modern marriage less filled with dangers and pitfalls than far less stressful occupations and pastimes as these."

Butterfield (1956) agreed that just as there are skills in social life, so there are skills in family life and in every detail of the marital relationship. One needs to acquire these skills if he/she expects to make a success of marriage. Many young people are disappointed in marriage because they bring to it so little in either useful skills or helpful attitudes.

Mace (1972) postulated that marital failures stem from ignorance about marriage and suggested that counselors move out of the remedial routine and go into marriage preparation and enrichment. (See Chap. 12.) Rutledge (1968) has concluded that if all clinicians would devote one-fourth of their time to premarital counseling they could make a greater impact upon the health of this country than through all of their remaining activities combined. Such comments make good sense and are usually embraced by marriage counselors. However, it has been our observation that many marriage counselors are so set in the therapeutic approaches to dealing with marital pathology that they find it difficult to make the transition into premarital counseling which is most appropriately an educational function. That is to say, that most premarital counseling does not deal with persons and relationships with serious dysfunction. Premarital counseling is done with relatively healthy persons and is a counseling experience to enhance and enrich growing relationships, rather than to treat pathological ones.

Who Does Premarital Counseling?

There are three major professional groups that provide most premarital counseling. They are: (1) clergy, (2) physicians, and (3) professionals in clinics and agencies.

Of these three groups of providers of marital counseling, the clergy and physicians tend to see people who are preparing for marriage and are doing so with positive anticipation and planning. These professionals work with clients in an educational preventive format rather than a remedial or pathological focus. On the other hand, the third group, professionals in mental health clinics and agencies, probably see as the majority of their premarital clientele people who are uncomfortable about their wedding plans, or couples who are having difficulty deciding whether they should get married, or couples in which one or both have been married and are concerned that their second marriage might not work out. This chapter, and the section on premarital counseling in this book, is directed to the providers who deal with the majority of premarital people, in other words, the clergy and physicians. Premarital counseling with problematic relationships parallels the treatment of couples discussed in the other sections of the book.

Historically, the clergy have probably been in the premarital counseling business for a longer time than others. From early beginnings in the church, in the first century until the twentieth century, the premarital sessions were primarily didactic in nature and related to the following types of issues: permission from the pastor/bishop to get married, instruction on the nature of the Church marriage, instruction on the nature of the wedding service, and instruction on Christian life. In the twentieth century, with the advent for the pastoral counseling movement, the emphasis in the premarital session by pastors changed from advice giving to a counseling orientation. The clergy began to focus on the relationship and began to see their work with couples to be an opportunity to prepare the couples for greater interpersonal skills (see Clinebell's discussion in Chap. 22).

Schonick (1975) provided some data that lend credence to the idea that the clergy provide most of the premarital counseling. She reported that in 1972 in California of 4000 couples who applied for a marriage license, 2745 used the clergy for premarital counseling. She pointed out that this was probably the case because the clergy typical required only one couseling session and the couples frequently found out about a premarriage counseling requirement when they applied for the marriage license! California had instituted (required) premarital counseling for couples when one of the partners was a minor. The California law passed in 1970 required that minors (persons under 18 years of age) applying for a marriage license may be required to participate in premarital counseling concerning social, economic, and personal responsibilities incident to the marriage.

Physicians are also in a role to provide counseling. In relationship to the legally required physical examination, the physician is in a natural and logical position to provide some counsel. Since the premarital physical examination in many places is required within 30 days before the application for a marriage license, there is though, really little time for long-term premarital counseling.

What Are the Purposes of Premarital Counseling?

From discussions with clinicians, a survey of the literature, and presentations at professional meetings, the following conclusions can be drawn about the practice of premarital counseling today.

1. The focus on premarital counseling is educational and preventative rather than therapeutic and does not focus on pathology.

2. The typical premarital counseling is done seeing the couple conjointly rather than individually.

3. Most counselors prefer to work with the premarita' couple when they seek counseling voluntarily and early, approximately 3 months or so prior to the marriage.

4. In contrast to the typical marital counseling session, premarital counseling often is in 2-h sessions, for a set (four to five) number of sessions, and in small groups.

5. Many counselors are using various inventories and questionnaires in an attempt to provide specific assessment and feedback to the clients. The majority of these inventories are developed specifically by counselors for their own clinical use and not published or standardized.

6. Counselors are more and more using audio tape and video tape to serve as an adjunct to the counseling process and to give clients the advantages of immediate and accurate analysis of their interaction.

7. Premarital counseling has long involved the use of bibliotherapy and it appears that with the current availability of appropriate materials that bibliotherapy is still widely used as an adjunct to the counseling process.

8. Many persons who have been divorced or widowed are seeking "remarital" counseling, a form of premarital counseling.

What Are Approaches to Premarital Counseling?

The teaching and development of *communication skills* for the premarital couple is a common goal for premarital counseling. Some counselors approach communication and the development of communication skills very directly as a primary identified purpose in the counseling. When this is the case, communication exercises are usually practiced with the couple and "homework" assignments to develop and practice the skills outside the counseling session are frequently prescribed. One such program, the Minnesota Couples Communication Program (Miller *et al.*, 1976), has been widely used as a program itself and as a model for similar programs. Among the dimensions underlying the Minnesota Couples Communication Program model are:

— an educational and developmental orientation
— a focus on the system
  . . . dyad versus individual or group
  . . . focus on *how* rather than *why*
— a skill orientation

Others approach communication as a desired outcome but less directly. In this case the focus might be upon developing listening skills, empathy, or self-disclosure with the indirect outcome being the articulation of communication skills for the couple.

The teaching of *constructive conflict* or "fighting fair" (Bach and Wyden, 1969) has become a popular focus in premarital counseling. Of course, the focus here is preventative and developmental, assuming that conflict will be a part of a marital relationship and the desired outcome is to teach the couple adequate ways to cope with the conflict (Vanzoost, 1973).

Horejsi (1974) described a small group *sex education* program for engaged couples. Here the focus was upon the sexual relationship and sexual information with the secondary outcome being a focus upon communication between the premarital couples. Small groups of three engaged couples were presented case situations as a focus for discussion about sexual relationship and interpersonal difficulties. Such a focus was helpful in generating interaction and questions among the participants, which had as a side-light improved communication between the future spouses, plus gaining specific sexual information which was of particular interest or need to the couple.

In the churches, numerous denominations have curriculum and materials available for group study in sex education. Such materials, which have primarily appeared in the past few years, are of great use and significance to premarital couples as they integrate their religious values and sex education and planning.

The authors have been involved in premarital counseling using material focusing upon *values clarification* (Simon, 1974). Our primary focus has been interactional in working with premarital couples conjointly, either as an individual couple or in a small group of three couples. By using dyadic exercises focusing upon values and the clarification of values the couple moves from an examination of their own individual values (the "I" dimension) into the position of generating and articulating their new value system for their particular relationship (the "we" dimension). This is seen as a beginning of the lifelong process which is the key to the marital relationship. Thus, a related part of the values clarification is the teaching and practicing of effective communication for the couple.

What is the Format for Premarital Counseling?

Premarital counseling is preferably done in *conjoint sessions,* either with the single couple or with a group of couples. In this respect it is similar to marital counseling. However, because of the educational nature of premarital counseling, there are a number of different formats and techniques that are appropriately used.

The *lecture* is commonly used in many large group settings where the content is informational. Thus, authorities on topical areas such as communication, sex education, parenting, money management, religious dimensions, etc., present information by lecturing. The lecture is typically followed by a discussion and/or *question and answer period.*

Small group interaction is often an important part of the premarital counseling workshop or program. The stimulus and content for such discussion can be the topical lecture, but may be from a study guide, reading, films, etc. In such small group discussions, *professional counselors* or *paraprofessionals* are used to facilitate the group interaction and format.

With today's high quality of media materials and presentations, *films* and *slide-tape presentations* on specific topics are used frequently and effectively in presenting material. The preference for the use of such materials is in conjunction with discussion, question and answer sessions, small group interaction, or some other format to allow the participants to clarify and integrate the information rather than to assume that they have adequately understood it from the media presentation.

What are Topical Areas in Premarital Counseling?

The topical areas which are typically covered in premarital counseling are discussed in the other chapters in this section, particularly in Chap. 21, "Premarital Counseling: Process and Content."

What is the Future of Premarital Counseling?

Our overview of premarital counseling has yielded several observations. First, the practice of premarital counseling is now emphasizing the premarital dyad and couple interaction. That is to say, the primary focus in premarital counseling is not unlike that in marital counseling, the relationship.

Second, premarital counseling programs and practices appear to center very much upon communication. This is undoubtedly related to the recent literature in marriage counseling which has identified communication problems and deficits as being a major cause of marital disharmony and divorce.

Third, and related to the focus on communication, there has been a move away from specific problem solving approaches in premarital counseling. Thus, skills are taught in a general, preventive, positive, and developmental way rather than a problem-oriented focus. This appears to be in keeping with the preventive approaches to mental health and mental health education.

Fourth, there is, and probably always will need to be, some content information presented in premarital counseling. It is true that one of the reasons for couples seeking premarital counseling is to gain specific information and advice. However, the practice has shifted from a "standard" set of information imparted to clients to the current practice of the counselor "listening harder" to the clients and attempting to meet specific needs.

The practice of premarital counseling is based upon the idea that it can be beneficial to the couple and assist them in establishing a lasting marriage relationship. Research studies appear to support this goal. We also believe that conscientious premarital counseling can facilitate this objective. Similarly, divorced persons frequently talk about the lack of adequate preparation and premarital counseling in their previous marriages. They tend to seek out and value "remarital" counseling which is really premarital counseling.

Furthermore, we believe that competent premarital counseling has the outcome of introducing the couple to a process of professional assistance that they can turn to in time of need later in the marriage. Thus, when and if crisis situations occur in a marriage, the couple who has been involved in premarital counseling which they felt was of value will perhaps more likely turn to marriage counseling assistance. Certainly, we believe that the premarriage counselor should extend such an invitation and make such a suggestion in the final session of premarital counseling.

REFERENCES

Bach, G., and Wyden, P.: *The Intimate Enemy.* William Morrow and Co., New York, 1969.
Butterfield, O. M.: *Planning for Marriage.* Van Nostrand Co., Inc., Princeton, New Jersey, 1956.
Ellis, A.: *Creative Marriage.* The Institute for Rational Living, New York, 1961.
Horejsi, C. R.: Small-group sex education for engaged couples. *J. Family Counsel.,* **2 (2):** 23–27, 1974.
Mace, D. R.: *Getting Ready for Marriage.* Abingdon Press, Nashville, Tennessee, 1972.
Miller, S., Nunnally, E. W., and Wackman, D. B.: Minnesota couples communication

program (CCP): premarital and marital groups. In *Treating Relationships*. (Olson, D.H.L., ed), Graphic Publishing Co., Lake Mills, Iowa, 1976.

Rutledge, A.: *Premarital Counseling*. Schenkman Publishing Co., Inc., Cambridge, Massachusetts, 1968.

Schonick, H.: Premarital counseling: three years' experience of a unique service. The Family Coordinator, **24 (3):** 321–324, 1975.

Simmon, S. B.: *Meeting Yourself Halfway*. Argus Communications, Niles, Illinois, 1974.

Vanzoost, B.: Pre-marital communication skills education with university students. The Family Coordinator, **22 (2):** 187–191, 1973.

ROBERT F. STAHMANN, Ph.D., AND
WILLIAM J. HIEBERT, S. T. M.

21

Premarital Counseling: Process and Content

This chapter is designed to focus on the premarital counseling process and the social-psychological factors related to premarital counseling. Other chapters have dealt with the review of the field of premarital counseling, the introduction of sex education material and family planning, and the religious dimension of premarital counseling. This chapter focuses on the process, goals, and nature of premarital counseling.

Motivating Factors in Marriage

Professional people see themselves in many different ways. Sometimes they see themselves as healers. But professioals are not the only healers; people attempt to heal themselves as well. Marriage has been called many things, but sometimes we wonder if it isn't an amateur attempt at psychotherapy. That is, a way of saying that people marry for some purpose, that they expect marriage to do something to them or for them, that marriage in some way makes sense.

Before moving into an examination of the counseling process, we want to examine briefly some of the factors that impel individuals into a marital relationship. Let us look at some of them.

Emotional Maturity

Some couples move into the marital relationship because they are ready to deal with each other as individuals and are ready to establish a relationship in which each maintains their own identity and yet fulfills the need of being with someone.

Emotional Immaturity

As discussed in Chap. 20 and pointed out by various authors (Mace, Rutledge, and others), many individuals are inadequately prepared for marriage. Their family of origin and society in general has not provided them with an adequate resolution of their childhood dependency needs. Their parents did not get the job done in terms of helping them to mature. They want to be children and are looking for the "good parent" who will take care of them. These relationships are often characterized by rigidity or incapabilities for new ideas and immature jealousy concerning their future spouse's behavior manifesting itself in temper tantrums.

"I Will be Different after Marriage"

There are a number of myths or false ideas that people often accept as valid and attempt to live their life by them. These myths are perpetuated by society and frequently couples are not aware of their influence on their relationship. For example, some people believe that "I will be different after marriage." These are people who enter marriage having had previous unsatisfactory interpersonal relationships and experiences. They move into the marital relationship in an attempt to try and find some satisfaction in a new relationship to solve the pain and bruising that came from their own parent-child relationships or that came came out of their own peer relationships at an earlier age. The marriage relationship, however, will not likely be a completely different relationship utilizing or creating different interpersonal behavior than has existed already in the individual's parent-child relationships or in the individual's peer relationships.

"Everybody Ought to be Married"

Another cultural myth is the idea that it is necessary to be married, particularly by a specific point in time. It is often helpful for couples to examine carefully their ideas about why they are getting married. The social construction and expectation in our society moves people along the path toward marriage. Some people get married because it is the thing to do, everybody is doing it, their friends are getting married, their parents want it, their parents were married, etc. Probably today more than ever, couples have the alternative of postponing marriage or perhaps not even marrying at all. While society may be raising questions with this myth, it is important that the individual couple look at their own circumstances.

"Marriage is for Adults"

Another myth that influences people in our society is the idea that when they get married they automatically reach the status of adulthood. This seems to be related to the fact that in some families and in some subcultures marriage is looked at as a rite of passage from childhood into adulthood. This frequently occurs in families where there is a tremendous battle between parents and children, parents attempting to keep their children in a childish status. The children, attempting to get out from under the influence and control of the parents, will get married as a way of making a bid for adulthood. Marriage becomes a way of saying to parents, you can't tell met what to do now, I'm married. Marriage becomes an attempt, therefore, to change their relationship with their parents and peers.

"We Will Be One"

Another idea which is perpetuated by society and parents regarding marriage is the false idea that marriage is a state of togetherness that is absolute, forever, the same. Individuals experiencing themselves as incomplete, as less than whole, as being a half person search for another person to make themselves complete, a whole. It is as though they view marriage as being a relationship in which two halves make one whole person. More can be read about the difficulties this myth causes later in marriage in Chap. 8.

Sexual Urge

The sexual urge is an important factor compelling people into marital relationships and is a natural and normal process. As children grow up in families, they begin to experience a growing attraction toward members of the family. When sexual feelings begin to appear in early adolescence, it becomes difficult for children to reconcile their sexual feelings with the closeness that exists in relationship to family members. In an attempt to resolve the conflict, the adolescent's sexual needs push him/her out of the family to eventually find a closeness with sexuality in marriage.

All of these factors, and many more, are important, vital, and dynamic forces propelling people into marital relationships. In addition, each of these tremendously powerful forces is an attempt, each in its own way, at coping, healing, and reaching for personal growth and health. As such, these powerful forces are difficult to break or change. Indeed, it is questionable whether it is possible to break or change them, or, whether it ought to be done at all. Many marriages, in spite of the fact that they are beginning with potential problems or a less than desirable motivating base, do well, at least initially. Perhaps the time to intervene comes when the crisis occurs later.

Nature of Marriage

Many people believe that a "marriage beings with a wedding." We would contend, however, that this is a myth. Marriage does not begin with a wedding; a marriage begins when the commitment takes place between the couple. Psychologically speaking, a marriage begins when each says to the other, "You're for me." As we see it, the marriage has already taken place by the time the couple comes for premarital counseling. What we are doing as counselors is *not* premarital counseling. It is prewedding counseling. The marriage, psychologically speaking, has already taken place.

Nature of Counseling

We have already established in this chapter that there are many factors which propel people into marital relationships; that people do not get married by accident. We have also established the fact that usually the commitment is made prior to the wedding; that couples coming for premarital counseling are already "married."

What do we mean, then, by *premarital counseling*? Simply this: premarital counseling is not usually and primarily either counseling or psychotherapy. We do not see premarital counseling as a process dominated by the medical model, with its orientation toward pathology. Nor do we see premarital counseling as an examination of the emotional maturity and the readiness for marriage of a couple. Rather, we see premarital counseling as a more generalized process, focused on enhancing the couple's skills in their interpersonal relationship.

In our experience we have discovered that counselors who attempt to construct the prewedding sessions into therapy meet with frustration. Most couples involved in prewedding counseling are not anticipating problems, do not want to focus on them, or for that matter, may not need such a focus.

For us, then, *premarital counseling* could be viewed as *pretherapy* or *education for marriage* or *prewedding counseling*. A further explanation of this orientation can also be found in Chap. 24.

If *premarital counseling* is really all of the various things we have suggested in the above paragraph, then, you might be wondering, why don't we call premarital counseling something else? Why do you use the words *premarital counseling* to mean *education for marriage*? Our answer is two-fold: (1) it is easier to say *premarital counseling*, phonetically speaking; and (2) Alice in Wonderland: " 'The question is, said Alice, whether you can make words mean so many different things.' 'The question is, said Humpty Dumpty, which is to be the master—that's all.' "

Focus of Chapter

In Chap. 20 the authors suggested that the primary providers of premarital counseling are the clergy. And, that the majority of people seeking premarital counseling are couples preparing for the wedding. This chapter, thus, focuses on the premarital counseling that is done in the process of prewedding counseling. To be sure, there are numerous couples who seek premarital counseling because of special circumstances or specific problems. For example, they may be couples who have been previously married and are concerned that their new marriage not duplicate the dynamics of their previous marriages. Or, they may be couples who are struggling with whether to get married, one or both parties resisting the wedding; or they may be couples who are struggling over the issue of a premarital pregnancy. These special circumstances call for a more specialized kind of counseling that is more therapeutic in nature and more typical of, and similar to, marriage counseling. This chapter will not address itself to those specific circumstances and situations. Rather, this chapter focuses on those professionals who are engaged in prewedding counseling.

Not only is this chapter focused on the major providers of prewedding counseling, but the content can be used with either an individual couple or a small group in mind.

The Counseling Process

There are a number of decisions that the counselor must make regarding the structure of the prewedding sessions.

First, the counselor will need to decide whether the premarital couple counseling will be offered in a small group setting with one to three couples or whether the counselor is going to work with each couple individually.

Second, the counselor will need to make some decision in regard to the amount of time that will be spent with each couple or small group, both in terms of the number of sessions and the amount of time or length of each session. Since the process of premarital and/or prewedding counseling is a process that could be described more as educational rather than therapeutic, the situation lends itself to structuring in terms of a set number of sessions. Many counselors working with prewedding couples do so in 2-h blocks of time rather than the standard 50-min h.

Third, the counselor needs to make some decision as to whether the couple will be seen individually and concurrently, or together (conjointly) in the session, or some combination of the two.

Fourth, the counselor will need to make some decision regarding fees. Most usually, clergy working with couples in prewedding sessions are not accustomed to charging fees, especially when one of the individuals is from that congregation.

Fifth, the counselor will need to make some decision regarding literature. Is the counselor going to make use of a resource packet with inventories, reading marterials, and questionnaires? If so, who is going to pay for it?

Sixth, since prewedding counseling lends itself to structure, the counselor will need to choose the focus for each of the sessions and have some outline regarding the implentation of the process.

Goals of Premarital Counseling

We have now defined the premarital counseling as prewedding counseling. In order to clarify and distinguish it from counseling and/ or psychotherapy, we provide a list of the following goals of prewedding counseling as we conceive it.

Discovery of the Basic "Selfhood" of Each Partner

Prewedding counseling is a process of establishing the "I" position of each person, sketching out their thoughts, feelings, and fantasies.

Discovering the Other's Selfhood

Premarital counseling is a process of filling in the partner's "I" position by sketching out and filling in the other's thoughts, feelings, and fantasies.

Making Sense Out of Behavior

During the prewedding counseling, many opportunities are given for looking at and understanding each other's behaviors. Prewedding counseling can enhance not only the understanding of each other's behaviors and meaning behind them, but can facilitate new behaviors and the expanding of one's repertoire of behaviors.

Development of Communication Skills

Premarital counseling can be a process of helping the couple to improve their interpersonal skills by learning how to send clearer messages, how to check out the meanings of messages sent and received, and becoming more ware of their own thoughts, feelings, and behaviors.

Opening up Vital Areas for Communication

One of the goals of premarital/prewedding counseling is to facilitate the couple's talking about areas that they could not previously talk about. In some ways the most significant work between a couple happens after they leave the office and are away from the sessions. Something said in the sessions may spark a conversation between them on something they had not thought about or been able to discuss. For this reason, counselors might attempt to prescribe and set up areas of discussion in the counseling sessions that are purposely not resolved during the sessions. Following up on these areas during subsequent sessions will allow the couple to experience carry-over beyond the sessions.

Premarital Counseling Process

We are going to discuss the premarital/prewedding counseling process in two parts: the *content* and the *relationship*. By content we mean the subject matter, the focus of the session, what the couple(s) and counselor talk about. By relationship we mean what happens between the couple(s) and the counselor while they are relating together. First, we will examine *content*.

There are many topical areas which are appropriate for examination in premarital/prewedding counseling. All of the areas we list below are valuable for exploration during the premarital/prewedding sessions, whether it be by a couple themselves or in a group procedure. The primary idea is that the counselor should raise these areas as considerations for the couple(s). The couple may have already discussed and worked through some of the areas and have no concerns about them. On the other hand, couples frequently overlook some of the areas and/or are ready for new ways to resolve other situations or improve their relating skills.

The writers suggest that the counselor include a consideration of the following areas during the premarital/prewedding counseling sessions. These areas can well be considered throughout the entire process and do not necessarily need to be covered in any particular order or sequence. We have suggested the topical areas with related questions. The topical areas and questions are only suggestive and other areas and questions should be generated by the counselor based on his or her own approach and upon the needs and the context of the particular counseling setting.

Content Focus

Parental Modeling—Parental modeling is extremely important. The first person that an individual learns to know is his or her parents. Mother is the first female a child learns to know; father is the first male a child learns to know. In addition, many people feel that their parents did a good job of bringing them up to this particular point in their lives. Parents have a way of doing things and usually these are accepted as right or mostly right. Parental models often assume a correctness for couples, and frequently they get locked into a right/wrong dichotomy. Our goal is premarital/prewedding counseling would be to help the couple grow beyond this dichotomous way of looking at their families, to teach the couple that there are many ways of doing things. We suggest the following six areas as worthy of exploration.

1. What about the demonstration of affection as modeled by parents? Where, when, and what was "proper" in terms of the demonstration of affection by the parents? For example, walking hand in hand in the street is inappropriate to some couples and very commonplace to other couples. Problems may arise in a marriage where there are differences in the expectations and needs in regard to the demonstration of affection. For example, an undemonstrative husband may result in a wife feeling unloved, or an undemonstrative woman may result in a husband feeling rejected or unloved.

2. What about the use of alcohol and drugs? How parents make use of these substances will depend upon their own value system and their religious background, as well as social-economic or cultural situations. It is commonplace, for example, for a male in some settings to stop for beer on the way home from work each day. If that behavior is uncommon in the background of a wife, it certainly could be an area for misunderstanding and contention.

3. What about the area of companionship? Did the parents socialize as individuals or primarily as couples? In some areas male companionship excludes the wife and takes the form of "male only" activities such as hunting, fishing, and racing, etc. In rural areas, for example, it is common that the sexes tend to socialize individually. In urban areas, the sexes more frequently socialize together.

4. What about money and its use by parents? Sometimes couples come from very different standards of living. In addition, while couples may come from similar living standards, there can be great differences in the spending habits of parents. It is valuable to explore how each set of parents handled their money, how they valued it, and how they went about making decisions regarding its spending.

5. How did parents handle the children? Often young couples have ideas about raising children based upon the experiences they had as being children and being raised according to certain guidelines and assumptions (Satir, 1974). There can be significant differences in parental homes between permissiveness and strictness. It is valuable to explore the issues of who will discipline the children and what methods will be used in discipline.

6. What part did religion play in the parents' lives? When examining the area of parental modeling, it is important to note how parents dealt with the religious dimensions of their lives. The issue here is religious practice rather than theology. What are the expectations and practices relating to religious customs and habits and how are they similar? Chap. 22 explores this dimension in greater detail.

Individual Personality Differences—Whether the counselor uses formal assessment techniques or simply observation, differences between the partners in personality will become apparent. These differences and assessment of them are useful content areas for focus by the counselor. Sometimes couples are not aware of the psychological differences between themselves which manifest themselves in the form of personality. The educational function of premarital/prewedding counseling is to assist the couple in identifying and understanding such personality differences. We suggest the following dimensions would be useful for consideration by the counselor.

1. Extraversion and introversion are dimensions for identifying and discussing the socialization needs for each of the partners.

2. The use of the Jungian model of thinking versus feeling and sensing versus intuiting can be a useful tool in exploring this conceptualization of personality.

3. Differences in peace-keeping dimensions of the two partners are important. In other words, who tends to have difficulty with negative feelings and anger?

4. What about dependence versus independence? Does one partner appear to need the other more?

5. How do the two compare and contrast in regard to the thinking of conventional versus unconventional thoughts? Who tends to be more "different" in relationship to cultural values?

6. The dimension of low energy versus high energy is often fruitful to explore. Are there differences in the typical energy level between the two of them? Can on individual be identified as always needing to be on the move while the other prefers to be left sitting?

7. Self-esteem is an area of great importance in individual and interpersonal functioning. The counselor can help the couple investigate their individual and joint conception of self-worth and acceptance and look at their relationship and other personality dimensions as well as considering this as an important dimension by itself.

8. How do the individuals deal with depression and anxiety? While depression and anxiety are not necessarily considered to be positive aspects of the personality, their prevalence is significant in the everyday functioning of many people and would be of particular importance when this is the case. Even when persons tend to be nondepressed and of low anxiety this area is valuable to explore.

Communication — As has been pointed out in several chapters, communication is a very important content area in both marital and premarital counseling. Anger has been labeled as the "great American hang-up." Anger can be viewed as a love message, although it is usually seen as bad. In arguments, who apologizes? Who has the worst temper? Who submits or leads the argument and attempts to please? Who wins arguments? Similarly, in verbal communication, who talks the most? Can one partner outtalk the other? What about the areas of nonverbal communication and its effects and power in the relationship?

Interpersonal Dimensions — We suggest the following areas as fruitful for exploration in regard to how the couple deals with each other and what is going on in the interaction.

1. Friends-Social
   a. To what extent are your friends primarily "his/hers" or mutual friends?
   b. Do you seem to be making new friends as your relationship has developed or are you carrying over your old friends from days prior to your relationship?
   c. Do you seek a few "close" friends or "casual" friendships?
2. Geography
   a. What has been your geographical environment when growing up? How have your geographical upbringings been similar and different?
   b. What are your geographical preferences after marriage?
   c. What about your relationship geography? How do you project that you will deal with physical separation?
3. Religion-Values
   a. What is the meaning of marriage to you? Consider the psychological and emotional aspects as well as the legal aspects of marriage.
   b. What has been the influence of organized religion upon you?
   c. What is the importance of religious activity and involvement to you and your marriage?
4. Activities
   a. What kinds of avocational and recreational activities do you enjoy alone and together? How do you anticipate working out your personal goals with your mutual goals?
   b. What are your vocational plans? How does your future mate fit in?
   c. How do you feel about your partner's vocatonal activities and plans now and after marriage? How will you maintain a balance between your personal goals and mutual goals in your relationship?
5. Budget
   a. How do the two of you plan to handle the money that you have? How did you decide this?
   b. What are the responsibilities for decision making about budgeting and money matters in your relationship?
   c. How will you apportionalize the "I" and "we" money in your budget?
6. Affectional-Sexual
   a. To what extent is your upbringing and experience about affection likely to influence your marital relationship? Is the "courtship attitude" important to maintain?

    b. Do you have adequate sex information and have you discussed male and female physiology and contraception?

    c. What are your expectations about giving and receiving affection after marriage?

7. In-Laws/Parents

    a. What are the expectations that your parents have for you individually and as a couple?

    b. What has been the effect of your interaction with your future in-laws (parents, brothers and sisters, aunts and uncles, etc.) during your premarital relationship and what are the implications for your marriage?

    c. In what ways do you see the influences of in-laws and parents as being positive and growth producing for your relationship?

8. Children

    a. Do you have adequate information and have you together discussed family planning?

    b. What do you believe would be the optimal number of children for your marriage?

    c. What kinds of goals do you have for your children?

9. Roles

    a. What does it mean to you to be your partner's wife/husband?

    b. What roles are your expected/willing to fill as husband/wife?

    c. How will you create and negotiate roles in your relationship?

10. Physical Health

    a. What kinds of activities do you plan to pursue to maintain your physical health?

    b. Are there any major illnesses in your medical history which might have an impact on your marriage?

    c. How do you see yourself coping with illness when your spouse is ill?

Relationship Focus

The second part of the counseling process is the *relationship*. By relationship we mean what happens between the couple(s) and the counselor while the content is being discussed. This is a significant part of the interaction between the counselees and the counselor (Benjamin, 1974). The following dimensions characterize the significance of the counselor-couple(s) relationship.

First, the counselor will be seen as a resource by clients. That is one of the reasons why couples seek out voluntary premarital/prewedding counseling. Thus, prewedding counseling is an important opportunity for the counselor to act as a resource of the latest and perhaps most appropriate knowledge and information in the field of marital and human relationships. While many counselors prefer to play down this role of the "knower," few counselors deny the fact that they are a resource. The counselor needs to be very sensitive to the client expectation regarding him/her as a resource and to be very sensitive as to how he/she is influencing the couple.

Second, the counselor serves as a model and creates an environment in which understanding the communication can take place. The counselor is a model of communication by speaking clearly and directly. Similarly, the counselor is a model by assisting the couples in clarifying misunderstandings and articulating various aspects of their verbal and nonverbal communication during the counseling sessions. By serving as a model for communication, the counselor facilitates new behavior and interaction for the couple.

Third, it is important to remember that the counselor above all is a person. While couples will perceive the counselor in a variety of ways, he/she will facilitate couples' growth when he/she is perceived as a person who clarifies, understands, and enables couples to change in positive ways. Thus, the counselor sets the tone in premarital/prewedding counseling for future help in marital crises.

Summary

This is what premarital/prewedding counseling is all about—letting the counselees know who you are, that you care, that you can help. Premarital/prewedding counseling is exposure to a process and to content that has short-term and long-term effects.

REFERENCES

Benjamin, A.: *The Helping Interview*. 2nd Ed, Houghton Mifflin Co., Boston, 1974.
Satir, V.: *Peoplemaking*. Science and Behavior Books, Palo Alto, California, 1974.

22

Premarital Counseling: Religious Dimensions

"In the fullest expression of intimacy there is a vertical dimension, a sense of relatedness to the universe which both strengthens the marital relationship and is strengthened by it. Quite apart from any churchy or churchly considerations, the spiritual dimension of marriage is a practical source of food for marital growth and health. No single factor does more to give marriage joy or to keep it both a venture and an adventure in mutual fulfillment than shared commitment to spiritual discovery. The life of the spirit is deeply personal, so that moments of sharing on the spiritual level are tender, precious moments in a relationship." (Howard and Charlotte Clinebell, 1970.)

The spiritual or vertical dimension of a marriage often is a crucial variable in determining the strength, creativity, and growth of that relationship. This may be as true of couples who do not perceive themselves as "religious" as of those who do. It is important, therefore, for a counselor to do everything possible during the process of preparation for marriage to encourage couples to discuss, clarify, and enhance this dimension of their relationship — the dimension of meanings, values, beliefs, and what Abraham Maslow called "peak experiences."

We do our work with people in the context of turbulent changes in values, faith systems, and religious institutions caused by a planet-wide weakening of old authority-centered ethical and religious systems. Old certainties no longer seem plausible, let alone certain, to countless millions of people. Traditional values are being challenged and often rejected by young adults. The global crisis in meanings, values, and faith systems has a profound, although often subtle, impact on inti-

315

mate relationships such as marriage. It is, therefore, particularly important, in our times, for the counselor to help couples deal with this dimension of their relationship in open, growth-enabling ways.

It's obvious that ministers, priests, and rabbis have a special interest in and training for facilitating growth in the religious dimension. But clergy have no corner on the opportunity to help couples deal with this area in creative ways. Everyone who does counseling—before, during, and after marriage—encounters implicit spiritual issues and needs, inextricably intertwined with all other aspects of relationships. Every counselor, of whatever professional discipline, has opportunities to encourage couples to deal with the religious issues in their relationship constructively.

Prewedding Counseling or Enrichment

Let me first review the overall model of prewedding sessions of which the methods of spiritual growth facilitation are a significant part. What is ordinarily described as "premarital counseling" actually is not counseling (in the sense of dealing mainly with problems) in most cases. Rather it is *personalized training* the aim of which is to enhance the couple's relationship-building insights and communication skills. It is the most common form of what I have described elsewhere (Clinebell, 1966) as "educative counseling." This is an integration of cognitive input and counseling methods which offers a couple both functional concepts and coaching in those relationship-developing skills which are relevant to their particular needs and growth goals.

Within this educative enrichment process there should be ample opportunities for dealing with conflicts and problems if the couple chooses to do so. However, my experience in doing prewedding sessions with some 100 couples suggests that focusing mainly on problems, present or anticipated, is emphatically *not* what most couples want or, for that matter, need. The primary focus of prewedding sessions should be on positive, growth-oriented prevention. It should be on a couple's strengths, assets, and potentialities for continuing growth together. Prewedding sessions should help couples learn the love-nurturing communication and conflict resolution tools to develop their rich individual and relational potentialities through their time together. Learning to enrich the vertical dimension of their lives together is an important aspect of a couple's growth work.

Most couples are open and receptive to such a *growth counseling* approach because it offers them assistance in doing what *they* really want to do, *i.e.,* develop the most mutually fulfilling marriage of which they are capable. The growth counseling philosophy offers a conceptual framework for premarriage sessions which is far more enabling than the pathology-medical model which has dominated much counseling theory and practice. Using terms like "Premarriage Enrichment" or "Preparation for Creative Marriage" in publicizing such events expresses the affirming, human potentials orientation better than "premarital counseling."

Institutions as Growth Centers

There is both research evidence (Compaan, 1973) and clinical evidence that a new style of marriage has emerged among young adults. In this "mutually potentializing" marriage, the relationship is central and is valued as a place for communication, mutual growth, and egalitarian sharing. This new marital style is both more difficult and more fulfilling than traditional styles. To respond to the needs of couples who are struggling to develop such relationships our churches (when I use this word I also mean temples), schools, and social agencies need new, innovative programs. By setting up a network of growth groups they can help couples continue to "growth" their marriages throughout the life cycle. Churches have a key role and responsibility in this since the majority of couples are married in churches and many continue to have continuing contact with a church after the wedding. Schools and counseling agencies should also offer preparation for marriage and marriage enrichment opportunities for couples who prefer these settings. All three kinds of institutions also should offer *divorce (and remarriage) growth groups* and *creative singlehood groups.*

Prewedding sessions should be described to couples as an important phase of a continuing marriage enrichment process in which they are encouraged to participate. Ideally, prewedding enrichment should be a bridge linking *remote preparation for marriage* (e.g., relationship skills groups and classes for adolescents) and *early marriage enrichment* during the first 5 crucial years. An important goal of prewedding sessions is to attract couples into an ongoing enrichment program. This involves helping them realize that couples who are still friends and lovers after 5, 10, or 50 years almost always are those who have worked at nurturing and enriching their relationship, with the help of others.

A number of churches are setting up programs for young couples with three parts: first, participation in a "Getting a Head Start in Marriage" group of three to six couples, offered two or three times each year; second, attending one or two prewedding training sessions as a couple with the clergyperson; third, having a marital enrichment "checkup" with the minister after 6 months and after a year of marriage or participating in a marriage enrichment group during the 1st year. One west coast church has a highly effective premarrieds/newly marrieds group composed of five premarried and five newly married couples. If a minister sets up the appointment for postwedding enrichment meetings during the prewedding sessions, most couples keep their appointments and use the growth opportunity well.

To maximize participation, a church's program and expectations should be publicized widely so that couples will be likely to know what is available and plan to participate before the hectic prewedding days. The program should be approved by the governing board or education committee of a church and publicized as the expectation of the congregation for couples planning to be married there.

To free couples to use church-sponsored prewedding interviews and/or growth groups to enrich their relationship, it is crucial to create an atmosphere of openness in the relationship with them. To do this, it is important to move beyond the *screening function* as quickly as this can be done responsibly. Until this is done, a couple's defensiveness usually remains high because they sense that they are on trial. As soon as a minister can give a positive answer to the question, "Can I with professional integrity participate in the marriage of this couple?" it is important to say, in effect, "I'm pleased to have a part in this important milestone in your relationship!" Defensiveness can also be reduced by a clear statement of the goals of the sessions in positive, growth-oriented terms.

Growth in the various facets of a relationship, including the religious dimension, will be more likely to occur if a couple participates in a preparation for marriage group, workshop, or retreat. Such groups have many advantages. Although they take time to set up, in the long run they save the leaders' time. In such growth groups, couples discover each other, learn from each other, and have their relationships enriched by the trust and sharing which is experienced among group members. One couple, after a premarriage group, reported, "For the first time we really experience what the church is all about!"

A small group is an ideal setting in which to use communication exercises such as those described in this chapter. Couples who have had a preparation for marriage group experience plus one or two prewedding couple sessions with their minister generally are substantially better prepared for marriage than are couples who have had only the sessions with the minister.

In setting up premarriage groups it is wise to invite one or two couples married less than 5 years to serve as catalysts and resource persons by sharing their struggles and satisfactions in marriage with the group. It is important to have male-female co-leaders of all marriage and premarriage enrichment events and to choose leaders who themselves have liberated, egalitarian marriages.

One premarriage group approach which has proved effective is a series of four to six weekly, 2-h sessions involving short didactic segments and longer experiential segments using structured communication relationship-strengthening exercises. Chap. 4 to 6 of *Growth Counseling for Marriage Enrichment, Pre-Marriage and the Early Years* (Clinebell, 1975) describe a variety of such exercises, gives other formats, and suggests schedules for marriage workshops and groups.

The Goal of Premarriage/Early Marriage Enrichment

The overall goal of the process is to provide continuing opportunities, coaching, and reinforcement for each couple as they create their own unique, mutually actualizing relationship. Relationships which liberate couples to use their full gifts in mutually enhancing ways are open, intimate, equal relationships with intentional commitment to each other's growth. Such a liberating or potentializing marriage is one in which both persons grow toward what in biblical language is called, "life in all its fullness." (John 10:10, New English Bible) A firm commitment to one's own and the other's growth nurtures love in a relationship and gives strength for handling the inevitable pain and crises of the marital journey.

What is the Religious Dimension?

Growth occurs in a marriage as *mutual need satisfaction* occurs in the give and take of that relationship. A couple will experience their marriage as an environment for growth, to the degree that their basic needs—physical, emotional, psychological, sexual, and spiritual—are satisfied in their interaction. The religious dimension in the life of a person consists of the ways in which she/he satisfies seven interrelated spiritual or existential needs. It is noteworthy that psychoanalyst Erich Fromm, a nontheist, recognizes that all persons need a "frame of orientation and an object of devotion" shared by a group. (Fromm, 1950.) These needs are existential needs in the sense that they are inherent in human existence. Their presence is a part of what defines human existence as human. As existential needs, they are present in all persons including those most secularized in their thinking and those most alienated from institutionalized religions. The adequate satisfaction of these spiritual needs is essential for mental wholeness or health. What constitutes adequate satisfaction varies tremendously within and among cultures; in fat, it is unique for each individual. In most cultures, including our own, the majority of people seek to satisfy these needs through organized religions. However, in secularized Western cultures, such as ours, more and more people search for answers outside religious institutions.

The basic spiritual-existential needs include: (1) the need for a viable philosophy of life, a belief system that will give one's existence meaning and purpose; (2) the need for clear values and priorities to serve as inner guidelines to behavior that is personally and socially constructive; (3) the need for an integrating relationship with and commitment to that which is seen as ultimately real and significant—called "God" in conventional religious language; (4) the need for an ecological consciousness, a sense of trustful, organic belonging to humanity and to the biosphere; (5) the need for the renewal which comes from regular moments of transcendence or "peak experiences"; (6) the need to develop one's uniquely human or spiritual potentialities—i.e., one's capacities for self-transcendence, creativity, awareness, altruism, responsible freedom, and communion with the highest; and (7) the need for a community of caring which undergirds one's world view and values by means of shared rituals, beliefs, and religious practices.

These seven spiritual needs can be satisfied in growth-producing ways that enrich and expand one's life and relationships. Or they can be satisfied in inadequate ways that retard personal growth and impoverish or disrupt relationships. One's religion can be creative or crippling; it can enhance or diminish growth toward fuller personhood. *Salugenic (health producing) religion* results when people satisfy their spiritual needs in open, life-affirming reality-respecting, inclusive ways. *Pathogenic (sickness producing) religion* results from attempting to satisfy these needs in immature, authoritarian, exclusivistic, reality-avoiding, rigid ways.

A person's religion tends to be salugenic and growth-producing in his/her relationships to the extent that it: (1) builds bridges rather than barriers between people; (2) stimulates the growth of inner freedom, mature consciences, and personal responsibility; (3) provides clear and significant ethical guidelines; (4) handles the vital energies of sex and hostility in responsible and affirming rather than repressive ways; (5) encourages intellectual honesty and acceptance of reality; (6) emphasizes love and acceptance rather than fear and guilt; (7) provides effective means of moving from the alienation of guilt to the reconciliation of forgiveness; (8) strengthens self-esteem; (9) provides for the regular renewal of basic trust through meaningful rituals of belonging; (10) encourages the maturation of one's belief and value systems; (11) enhances the appreciation and celebration of life; (12) provides pathways for relating to the resources of one's unconscious through meaningful symbols, rituals, and myths; (13) nurtures inner security by a sense of belonging to a group sharing common commitments; (14) provides an uplifting object of devotion or integrating commitment; and (15) allows one to respond creatively to the awareness of one's finitude (existential anxiety) through a trust-giving philosophy of life or belief system. These criteria for salugenic religion can serve as guidelines for ministers and other counselors as they seek to facilitate spiritual growth. (For a further discussion of these criteria see H. Clinebell, 1972.)

It is axiomatic in pastoral counseling that the religious dimension of a person's life is inextricably interrelated with all other aspects of his/her personality and relationships. The goal of counseling and enrichment is to maximize growth in all the interdependent dimensions of the couples lives and relationship.

In the development of a new relationship, the differing ways in which the two persons have satisfied their spiritual needs encounter each other. In open, growing relationships there is respect for each person's autonomy but also the desire to increase areas of creative interdependency, spiritually and otherwise. In the shared life style which two people are creating, each person's values and meanings will be modified and enriched. There is inevitable conflict in this process of co-creation. The counselor should encourage couples to move toward increasingly salugenic and shared ways of satisfying their basic spiritual needs.

The Spiritual Search of Young Adults

During late adolescence and early young adulthood — the time when the majority of couples enter into marriage — many people are still engaged in identity-formation struggles. An essential part of this movement toward autonomy is deciding on their own values and beliefs, as distinct from those of their parents. Their need is to deparentify their ways of satisfying their basic spiritual needs and to form their own unique faith and values. The minister or other counselor should affirm them in their search and provide psychological space within which they are free to struggle and find their own answers to questions of meaning. If young people have grown up in families in which religion was constricting and repressive, they often need to reject formal religion for a while in order to move to more freeing, growth-enabling ways of satisfying their needs. Such persons should sense in the counselor an accepting ally who values their liberated responses to their spiritual needs.

The breakdown of traditional, authority-centered sources of ethical guidelines and beliefs has produced both heightened anxieties and an unprecedented opportunity to develop one's own adult values and intellectually acceptable beliefs. There probably has never been a time when spiritual searching by young adults was more intense. It is obvious that in the sessions that are available with a couple before and after the wedding, it is unrealistic to expect to make more than a modest contribution to their total growth, including their spiritual growth. But a significant contribution *can* be made in some cases. The goal is to do everything possible to help a couple learn to satisfy their spiritual needs in ways that will strengthen their love, deepen their communication, increase their capacity to cope with crises, and enjoy life together.

The marriage counselor-enricher can facilitate exploration of issues related to spiritual needs in two ways—by recognizing and responding to these issues when they are raised in an interview or group discussion and by creating opportunities for communicating about such issues by using approaches such as will be described below. In recognizing spiritual issues when they arise, it is well to remember that in our secular society, spiritual issues are often described in nonreligious language. For example, covert spiritual and value issues often are present when someone mentions topics such as loss, death, life styles, attitudes toward the future, and the use of time (which usually reflects implicit values). Let me now suggest some practical methods for helping couples enrich the spiritual dimension of their relationship. These methods can be used in both premarriage and marriage enrichment groups, and in interviews with individual couples.

Communicating about the Spiritual Issues

This communication exercise may be used during an enrichment group or given to a couple as a "self-enrichment assignment" to do between sessions and report back. Or, questions can be selected from the list by a counselor and used to help a couple open up dialogue in the area of their spiritual needs. *Instructions*: the incomplete sentences in the list below are designed to help you talk about your religious attitudes and beliefs. Look over the list and decide together which sentence you will discuss first. Take turns completing the sentence; discuss similarities and differences in your responses. As soon as you both feel finished with your discussion of the issues raised by completing that sentence, select another sentence and do the same.

 —The times when I feel most alive (most hopeful) are. . . .
 —The things that are the most worth living for now are. . . .
 —Life has the most meaning (the least meaning) for me when. . . .
 —I feel closest to you spiritually (most distant) when. . . .
 —What I really believe about God is. . . .
 —I feel closest to God when. . . .
 —I feel most inspired (feel spiritually high) when. . . .
 —My religion increases (diminishes) my enjoyment of life because. . . .
 —The beliefs from my childhood that still have meaning (no longer have meaning) are. . . .
 —The religious beliefs that mean the most to me are. . . .
 —The strengths (and limitations) of my parents' religion are. . . .

—My faith and values are similar to (different from) my parents in these ways. . . .

—The way I feel about the church (my church, your church) is. . . .

—The things I see as strengths (limitations) in your religion are. . . .

—Participating in a church is (is not) important in our marriage because. . . .

—The things I'd like to do or to share more in the spiritual area are. . . .

—I get help from my religion in these ways when things go badly. . . .

—If or when we have children, I would like them raised in the following way religiously. . . .

—Other issues in this area I'd like to discuss are. . . .

—The way I feel about discussing issues raised by these statements is. . . .

The counselor should encourage couples to build on their discussion of these issues by making concrete plans for improving this aspect of their relationship.

A less structured way of facilitating communication about religious issues is for the counselor to inquire, "What part did religion play in your parents' marriage?" (This often helps increase a couple's awareness of the significance and differences of their religious backgrounds.) After they have responded, the counselor can ask, "In comparison with your parents' religion, what role would you like religion to play in your marriage?"

A simple way by which a minister can help a couple explore the significance of spiritual issues is to inquire, "Why did you choose to be married in a church?" This query often leads to a productive discussion of whatever meaning religion has in their lives. Or a minister can open up discussion of the religious dimension during that part of the prewedding training in which the wedding ceremony is discussed step by step. If a couple chooses to use a traditional wedding ceremony, there are many opportunities, as they discuss its various stages, to explore the meaning to them of the religious words and the symbolic acts. One pastor I know points out that the ceremony is a celebration and asks, "What are you celebrating?" The discussion which ensues can heighten a couple's awareness of the dimension of wonder and mystery in their creating a new relationship. It may help them experience their wedding as a peak experience shared by their caring community of friends and relatives. A minister aims at helping a couple experience the meaning of "holy matrimony" on a very personal level. Couples who choose to write their own ceremony can be encouraged to include words which express an awareness of the vertical dimension of their growing relationship.

Values Clarification and Reformulation

Value clarification exercises are useful in both group and individual couple sessions to heighten awareness of the guiding values and priorities which are implicit in a person's life style. As young couples seek to create a shared life style, value conflicts need to be faced openly and every effort made to negotiate a workable synthesis of their values and priorities. A variety of value clarification exercises are available. (See Sidney Simon, 1972.)

Here, for example, is a simple values-priorities exercise. *Counselor:* "To help you get a clear picture of the things that matter most to each of you, write down the 10 things (relationships or activities) which are of the most value to you." "Now, number these in order of importance from 1 to 10." "Now, share your lists with each other, discussing the implications for your marriage of similarities and differences in the values and priorities you have listed." "What changes do you each need to make in your values or priorities to make your life together more fulfilling?"

The following exercise can help a couple clarify their goals and values. It also helps their sense of *intentionality, i.e.,* of their control over the direction of their own development. *Counselor:* "To help get a clear picture of the direction in which you'd like to see your relationship develop, write a brief description of the ways you'd like to have your marriage be a year from now." "Compare your lists of growth goals for your marriage." "Make a joint list of goals for your marriage on which you both agree." "Now, plan the things you each will do to move toward your joint goals; include a schedule for implementing your plan." Either of the above exercises can be given as homework for the couple to do between sessions and report back on the results.

Value exercises often reveal overcommitment to self-centered values which eventually will contribute to an impoverished marriage. In marriage and premarriage enrichment groups it is appropriate to challenge couples to test their life styles (and the values these reflect) in terms of whether or not they are ecologically sound. Will they contribute to the survival of the human family on a livable planet? One perceptive student of the world situation has observed, "The contemporary global crises of poverty, overpopulation, ecological disaster, and energy exhaustion are the realities which threaten the collapse of the whole historical fabric of civilization. . . . The real crisis is . . . a crisis in meaning and value." (LeFevre, 1976.) In the long run, marriage styles which collectively will impoverish the planet are self-defeating. A viable life style for the future must involve outreach—more commitment of our time and resources to causes that are bigger than ourselves or our marriage.

During a marriage enrichment interview, one young married couple from a Roman Catholic background mentioned what they called "the guiding vision of their marriage." When asked what they meant, they described the dream they shared that they would develop effective ways to reach out, as a family, to help those in need. In the interview they explored plans for implementing their vision.

Marriage Enrichment and Inner Renewal

When one's inner space becomes cramped, cluttered, or impoverished, one's intimate relationships inevitably suffer. Taking time to experience renewal at one's "center," the inner world from which a person relates to others, has a salutory effect on his or her close relationships. In the hectic whirl of modern life, it is important to encourage couples to enrich their inner lives regularly so that they will have more to give and share in their marriages.

Many couples are discovering that twice daily "meditation breaks" pay big dividends in terms of personal-marital enrichment. If a couple shows interest, I may suggest that they try the simple steps described in Herbert Benson's *The Relaxation Response.* (Benson, 1975.) If both partners are into a meaningful form of inner renewal, sharing usually occurs spontaneously.

In discussing "peak experiences," Abraham Maslow (1964) points out that these "little mystical moments" are moments of self-actualization. They are one of the ways we move toward experiencing unity with ourselves and each other. Couples can be encouraged to discuss the kinds of experiences each finds conducive to peak experiences and to plan their schedules to include frequent opportunities for sharing such high moments. Many couples find energizing lifts in sharing music, communing with nature, religious worship, intimate communication, and sex. Peak experiences are precious moments of feeling one's connection with the energy of growth and healing in the universe. In sharing such experiences, a couple can become aware that they are a small but significant part of the larger life!

A Spiritual Maturation Method

One block which prevents many adults from trusting and from being aware of peak experiences is the inner lump of unfaced doubts, obsolete beliefs, and religious fears from their childhood. Clearing out this logjam of childish feelings and magical beliefs opens up the channel within a person for the flow of creative energies. It also increases the person's ability to perceive and enjoy spiritual reality in the present. I find the "empty throne" method, (an adaptation of the empty chair method in Gestalt therapy) an invaluable tool for facilitating spiritual maturation work.

The technique consists of inviting the person to "put God into that empty chair you are facing and talk to him." After the person expresses whatever is on his/her mind, then she/he is invited to sit in the empty chair and say what "God" is speaking back. Repeated rounds of this dialogue often are required to allow obsolete, blocking feelings to be worked through. The person usually discovers that the feelings are vestiges from early experiences with parent figures and with the religion of that person's childhood. Verbalizing these feelings in the presence of a counselor and letting go of them allows the person to reclaim the energy that has been invested in the feelings. Most people respond to a session of such spiritual growth work with feelings of release and of a load lifted.

Using Religious Resources Constructively

Because spiritual growth is one aim of marriage and premarriage enrichment and counseling, it is important to use traditional resources such as prayer and scripture, if they are used, with sensitivity and care. Their misuse can block rather than facilitate spiritual growth. Here are some guidelines for their constructive use. (1) Use such instruments sparingly and only after one is aware of what they mean to a particular person or couple. (2) Use religious resources only with persons for whom they are meaningful and with whom they will deepen the sense of trust. (3) With persons from pathogenic religious backgrounds, spiritual growth often is more likely if one avoids using "religious" language or tools. (4) After the use of prayer or reading scripture with anyone, it is ell to ask the person(s), "What was going through your mind while I was speaking?" (5) Avoid praying in ways that create magical expectations, diminish the sense of responsibility, or block the catharsis of negative feelings. (6) Be aware of the fact that the use of religious practices usually strengthens the authority image of the person using these; deal with this by discussing it openly. (7) Never feel that you *have* to use religious instruments. The issues at the heart of all enrichment and counseling—wholeness, growth, guilt, alienation, anxiety, reconciliation, and rebirth—are essentially spiritual issues. Remember that the Power of which these instruments may be a channel is a reality in all relationships where growth and healing occur, whether or not religious terms or practices are used.

Spiritual Growth and Liberating Marriage

There is substantial evidence that religion has been used to keep women "in their place." (Charlotte H. Clinebell, 1976.) Premarital enrichment (like all sound counseling and enrichment) should aim at liberating people from those sex role stereotypes which keep both women and men from using their full potentialities. Ministers have an opportunity to encourage couples to eliminate archaic elements reflecting obsolete patriarchal practices from the wedding ceremonies e.g., the use of a single ring or the practice of the bride's father "giving her away."

Marriage growth work should provide opportunities for couples to claim and develop their "other side." As Carl Jung made clear, inner wholeness involves developing one's neglected side—the so-called "feminine" side in men (the soft, nurturing, feelingful, vulnerable side) and the so-called "masculine" side in women (the assertive, analytical, rational side). By encouraging couples to claim and develop their full personhood, a counselor can help them enrich what they bring to the relationship. The feminist theologians have shown how the patriarchal orientation of the Hebrew-Christian heritage has impoverished our spiritual lives. Reclaiming the feminine in our experience of divinity can be spiritually liberating and personally enriching. (Mary Daly, 1973.)

Mixed Religious Marriages

Every marriage is a "mixed marriage" in the sense that the two persons grew up in different families with different attitudes, values, communication patterns, and religious orientations. In marriages involving two persons from radically different religious or ethnic backgrounds, a number of issues become crucial in premarriage and marriage enrichment. First, it is essential that they be encouraged to communicate openly and fully regarding their religious beliefs, attitudes, customs, and values. Second, each person should be helped to appreciate the strengths in the other's religious orientation. Third, it is important to help such couples realize that the key to allowing their differences to enrich rather than diminish their relationship (through chronic conflict) is their willingness to respect each other's position and each other's right to differ. Fourth, it is important for the couple to examine how they will respond to the pressures which will probably come from their families of origin, particularly around the rearing of children in one family's, or the other's religious tradition. These issues need to be resolved, as far as possible, before the wedding. Marked disparity between a couple in the intensity of their religious interests may be more of a source of alienation in marriage than differences of denominational or faith groups. However, differences of religious affiliation still represent, for many people, a broad complex of family attitudes, traditions, practices, and status.

Contracting on Religious Issues

As a part of the process of clarifying each person's expectations for a marriage, many couples find it helpful to write out an agreement about what they will expect and give in the relationship. Such an explicit contract or covenant may be particularly helpful for couples from very different backgrounds. One clause in such a covenant should spell out their understanding about the place of religion in their marriage. In the prewedding training, it is important to practice the skill of developing and revising such an explicit covenant.

Preparation for Remarriage

In 1975 more than a million couples divorced in the United States. Approximately two-thirds of these women and three-fourths of these men eventually will remarry. Effective preparation for remarriage or for creative singlehood is an increasingly urgent need in our society. The process of doing this is different than helping people prepare for first marriages. There are at least two essential steps. The first consists of providing ample opportunity for the persons to complete their "grief work" related to the past relationship by expressing and working through feelings such as failure, anger, guilt, relief, and resentment which otherwise will block the healing of the psychological wound. Some of the feelings, especially feelings of guilt and rejection, cluster around religion and the church. Participating in a divorce growth group can help persons do their grief work so that the feeling will not infect their next relationship.

The second aspect of preparation for remarriage consists of using the painful crisis as a growth opportunity. This involves learning what one contributed to the disintegration of the previous marriage and how to nurture future relationships to keep them well and growing. Churches have an exciting opportunity to help set up divorce growth groups to facilitate this process. (See H. Clinebell, 1977.)

The Counselor's Spiritual Growth

All techniques of spiritual growth will be empty and ineffective unless those who use them in counseling and enrichment are congruent in their use. Thus, the crucial variable in facilitating spiritual growth in others is the quality of our own values, commitments, and consciousness. It is essential for those of us who are concerned about strengthening the religious dimension in marriages to prize and nurture our own inner lives and relationships. To be aware of and prize what Roberto Assagioli, the founder of psychosynthesis, called the "higher Self" within another it is necessary to be in touch with that Self within ourselves.

Every person and every marriage has a gold mine of unused possibilities within them, including the rich potential for greater enjoyment of the life of spirit. Couples who are the best prepared for marriage are those who are beginning the process of discovering and releasing these riches within themselves and their relationship. The most difficult part of being a facilitator in this process is to stay alive and growing oneself. This is both the challenge and the reward of growth approaches to counseling.

REFERENCES

Benson, H.: *The Relaxation Response*. William Morrow, New York, 1975.

Clinebell, C. H.: *Counseling for Liberation*. Fortress, Philadelphia, 1976.

Clinebell, H. J., Jr.: *Basic Types of Pastoral Counseling*. pp. 189–205, Abingdon, Nashville, 1966.

Clinebell, H. J., Jr.: *Growth Counseling for Marriage Enrichment, Pre-Marriage and the Early Years*. Fortress, Philadelphia, 1975.

Clinebell, H. J., Jr.: *Growth Counseling for Mid-Years Couples*. Fortress, Philadelphia, 1977.

Clinebell, H. J., Jr.: *The Mental Health Ministry of the Local Church*. Chap. 2, Abingdon, Nashville, 1972.

Clinebell, H., and Clinebell, C.: *The Intimate Marriage*. p. 179, Harper and Row, New York, 1970.

Compaan, A.: *A Study of Contemporary Young Adult Marital Styles*. Th.D. dissertation, School of Theology, Claremont, California, 1973.

Daly, M.: *Beyond God the Father*. Beacon, Boston, 1973.

Fromm, E.: *Psychoanalysis and Religion*. p. 21, Yale University Press, New Haven, 1950.

LeFevre, P.: Lifestyle as a religious and ethical issue in American thought, *The CTS Register*, p. 57, Spring 1976.

Maslow, A.: *Religious, Values, and Peak Experiences*. State University Press, Columbus, Ohio, 1964.

Simon, S.: *et al.: Values/Clarification*. Hart, New York, 1972.

MAX J. SPENCER, M.D.,
ROBERT F. STAHMANN, Ph.D.,
AND WILLIAM J. HIEBERT, S.T.M.

23

Premarital Counseling: Sexuality

Professionals engaged in premarital counseling are expected by clients to discuss and/or facilitate the discussion of human sexuality as a part of the premarital counseling process. Some counselors find the topics related to sexual information to be difficult to discuss because they have not resolved many questions and attitudes themselves. Hiebert in Chap. 16 discussed such counselor-related problems and offers solutions. Clark in Chap. 25 presents a point of view for physicians and counselors on the content and conduct of the premarital physical examination. Josimovich, in Chap. 24, discusses the various methods of contraception for family planning. Male and female sexual conditioning are discussed in Chap. 14 and 15.

Our purpose in this chapter is to supplement those chapters and focus on the related questions for premarital counseling of *when* should information on sexuality be presented and *what* should be presented.

In premarital counseling the counselor is not doing sexual therapy such as discussed in Chap. 17 by Arbes or described by Masters and Johnson (1970). In recent years there has been a phenomenal increase in material and information related to sex counseling and therapy for married couples, but comparatively little material focused on sexual aspects of premarital counseling. That material and information which has focused on premarital counseling has primarily been developed by churches in the form of pamphlets, books, and study guides for workshops or programs. Certainly, the counselor would do well to inquire with the local denominations in the community/area and obtain such materials and information.

In a recent topical issue of a counseling journal devoted to human sexuality, Mary S. Calderone, President of the Sex Information and Education Council of the United States (SIECUS), pointed out that it is useful to articulate differences among education, counseling, and therapy as they apply to human sexuality. "Actually these lie along a continuum, so the boundaries for each cannot be exact. *Education* is the process by which factual information about sexuality is offered and assimilated so that attitudes about the information undergo modification and internalization by individuals to fit their needs. *Counseling* is the art of helping individuals transmute their sexual education into fulfilling and socially responsible sexual behavior. *Therapy* is highly specialized in depth treatment by which impediments to an individual's satisfactory sexual evolution and fulfillment can be brought to consciousness and dealt with. Generally speaking, the sex therapist is dealing with one or another of the specific sexual dysfunctions identified by Masters and Johnson (1970)" (Calderone, 1976, p. 350). Premarital counseling deals with education and counseling.

Sex education and information is a multidisciplinary area of knowledge and field of practice. Physicians, clergy, and counselors are all expected to have the latest information in the area and (from the clients point of view) to be able to deal with most all concerns and problems that are brought to them. The counselor, regardless of setting and discipline, needs to be well-informed, but we believe must also work in conjunction with related professionals and services. Thus, the counselor should know the availability and telephone numbers of such resources as March of Dimes (for genetic information or counseling), Planned Parenthood, local health department, rape crisis centers, street clinics, and pregnancy testing and counseling services (Gordon, 1976).

We believe that pertinent facts of fertility should be understood by all adults. This is not privileged information for the physician. The newly married couple especially needs information concerning the menstrual cycle, the time of ovulation, and life-span (longevity) of ovum and sperm to enable them to conceive or not conceive.

We concur that the marital dyad should know about the usual behavioral changes during the menstrual cycle. For example, a pedometer placed daily on the ankle of a female in the reproductive years demonstrates up to a ten-fold increase in physical activity on days near the time of ovulation. Another is in many women, marked irritability may occur for several days prior to the menstrual period (called premenstrual tension and caused by rapid changes in physiology). This may require medical attention, if effects become severe. Also, the cramping during menses (called dysmenorrhea) may be prevented in many women by vigorous physical exercise for several days prior to the menstrual period. In addition, there are exercises which may relieve the cramping after menses have begun. In some severe cases, medication may be needed.

Myths Concerning Human Sexuality

The counselor is undoubtedly aware of many myths and misunderstandings that premarital couples may have as they enter marriage. An important part of premarital counseling is to shed light on such misinformation and to explode myths. In doing so, the counselor cannot escape the responsibility of keeping abreast of current knowledge in the field of human sexuality and the specific areas which are dealt with in premarital counseling. The specific resources discussed later in the chapter are helpful to the counselor in meeting the responsibility of keeping abreast of the field, as are the materials for distribution to clients. *Human Sexuality* (McCary, 1973), with its section on "Sexual Myths and Falacies" is an excellent resource for counselors.

The following myths are examples of those which the authors believe should be covered in premarital counseling.

There seems to be a myth related to the idea that men need little sexual information, that they "already know it." Most counselors and physicians concern themselves with the needs of the bride and omit information for, or even consultation with, the groom. With conjoint sessions in premarital counseling, including sexual information, this myth can be corrected. Assume that the man knows no more about himself and sexuality than the woman does about herself and sexuality.

If the prospective groom seems threatened or is resistive, the counselor might talk directly to the bride-to-be, but in the presence of the male. He may pretend not to listen, but will probably learn more than she and will usually show a favorable response as the discussion progresses. He needs to know about his wife and to have myths exploded.

There is the myth of the hymen being imperforate, or that it must be broken with first intercourse. The fact is, the hymen is located at least 1½ cm inside the outlet of the vagina, and it is soft, elastic, and ribbon-like. It circumscribes the perimeter of the inside of the vagina. If the hymen were closed or if the hymen closed the vagina, menstrual periods would be impossible. Such a thing as an imperforate hymen does occasionally occur, but this is a result of incomplete development in embryo. Pain and bleeding are not necessary to prove female virginity. If difficulty in intercourse is first experienced, it is usually the result of inadequate arousal, or it is caused by anxiety of the female which produces increased tone of the muscles which surround the vaginal orifice and give the impression of a "tight hymen." The senior author has seen in practice women who have delivered more than five babies and still had an intact hymen.

Another myth which counselors could well explode is the myth of the relative size of sexual organs causing incompatibility. Masters and Johnson (1966) have demonstrated that the small phalus in the resting state increases in size much more than a corresponding large phalus in the resting state. The same is true for the vagina. The point being this: when excitation phase is completed and plateau phase is reached sexual organs are of a relatively equivalent size with a few exceptions.

Another myth is that orgasm is not necessary for the female. When a female has reached the plateau phase such remarkable vasocongestion occurs that changes take place in the pelvis which need to be resolved. If orgasm does not occur, the resolution phase cannot follow. The resolution phase is when intense vasocongestion and dilatation of structures in the pelvis resolve or reverse, which allows them to reduce to their normal size, shape, and configuration. The vasocongestion must be allowed to recede or the female may experience discomfort or even pain for several hours in some cases, until spontaneous resolution does occur after some time.

Another point of myth, the real anatomy of the vagina should be explained. The vagina on cross-section is H-shaped. Most diagrams of the internal part of the pelvis from the side view are taken through the median sagittal section of the body and pelvis and intersect the vagina through the crossbar of the H. This is the birth canal and is much larger internally than most people realize. The passage of a baby through the pelvis as portrayed in most diagrams really would be a miracle!

A popular concept is prevalent that the vagina is an unsanitary, malodorous receptacle, which needs frequent internal cleansing. Normally, nothing could be farther from the truth. Fortunes are being made on the false premise that "to maintain her feminine daintiness and hold her husband's love" a particular douching preparation must be frequently used. The truth is that the normal vagina, in the absence of infection, is very clean, has no disagreeable odor internally, and is not only a temporary receptacle, but also serves as a bidirectional passage. It can receive and convey the substances which contain the masculine haploid chromosomal (components) to the entrance of the inner (female) reproductive system, and it can allow exit of the products of conception. It possesses a self-cleansing mechanism which produces a mucous discharge far more functional than douching, and it operates continuously. This discharge collects on the external genitalia and is rapidly decomposed. This degraded matter gives off an odor, a ready warning that it needs to be cleansed away. It is this odor from the external parts which has given rise to the misconcept that the internal parts also need lavage. Surprisingly, even at the height of a menstrual period, there is no undesirable odor inside the vagina. (Women who use tampons do not usually have an offensive odor.

Removal of the tampon, however, permits rapid decomposition of biological tissue which has outlived its usefulness and an extremely disagreeable odor soon emanates.) This obtains, only in the absence of infection, obviously. Hygiene for the normal external genitalia requires simple cleansing of the outside parts, preferably with water and a *very mild* nondetergent soap or cleansing agent. Careful drying is essential.

Change of the normally clear or white discharge or strong odor signals the need for a competent gynecologist. While the insult of occasional douching is quite easily tolerated by the normal vagina, too frequent douching can remove the normal protective barrier to infection and make it easier for infection to occur. Internal douching is not usually needed by the healthy vagina. Note: In 1954 this principle was first given attention by Dr. S. Leon Israel, recently deceased luminary in gynecology. He labeled douching as "a barbarous anachronism." A number of gynecologists have reiterated his observations since that time.

The myth that the vagina is a stationary receptacle needs correction. Cinematographs of the inside of the vagina during plateau and orgasmic phases, filmed by the team of Masters and Johnson, using special techniques (which movies are available for scientific teaching purposes) show the very remarkable dynamic qualities of the vagina. Certainly, the efficacy of a diaphragm is questionable. Also the effectiveness of vaginal foam, etc., which must remain in contact with the os of the cervix, unless put in place *early* (not at or after the end of excitement phase), should hardly be expected to be found on a cervix which in plateau phase will have been elevated out of its normal location, and the inner one-third of the vagina will have expanded such that an application would reach the cervix only by sheer chance. The vigorous movements of the vaginal walls during orgasmic phase are quite dramatic, probably reflecting the intense activity of the structures which surround the vagina.

The basic sexual cycle as described by Masters and Johnson (1966) can be very helpful to the premarital couple. The knowledge of such information regarding sexuality will not ensure against problems or questions, but it can be helpful. By analogy, an artistically talented person can learn by himself how to mix paints and then to apply them to a canvas. But much difficulty and wasted time and effort can be avoided by an introduction to form, perspective, colors, media, brushes, canvas, lighting, and display. The new knowledge does not make one an artist, but certainly can facilitate the application of one's creative genius. Nor will knowledge of the basics of sexuality ensure good performance, but it may serve to initiate a better and more appropriate learning and communication process.

When Is Sex Education Done?

Professionals doing premarital counseling and education are often very conscious of the timing and appropriateness of information related to sex education and family planning. Of course, the setting and nature of the counseling will be primary factors in answering this question. However, the question does not take care of itself. Rather, we believe that counselors must always be sensitive to it.

The physician, particularly in the one session premarital physical examination and consultation, will naturally, from his/her and the patient's point of view, provide some information about sex education and sexual relations. However, if the physician is involved in some sort of longer term counseling relationship with the patient(s), such as group meetings with premarital couples, the general information may be deferred for that setting.

Clients typically do not expect the clergy to provide as much or as complete information regarding sex education and family planning as physicians or marriage counselors. It seems to us that this is an inappropriate expectation or assumption, and in fact, the clergy are in an excellent position to provide thorough information in these areas. The clergy in premarital counseling are in an excellent position to assist the premarital couple in the integration of the sexual area of the relationship with the other key areas such as social, economic, religious, vocational, geographical, etc., as discussed in Chap. 21 and 22.

Marriage counselors, psychologists, social workers, and other professionals in agency or clinic settings also confront the question as to when sexual information and content are dealt with in premarital counseling. Again, there is no single answer. Persons in such settings are in the best position to conduct programs, workshops, and seminars, etc., dealing with sex education and family planning. Often such programs serve as an adjunct to the premarital counseling and clients are invited to attend apart from the ongoing counseling. On the other hand, the offerings may be part of a more broadly based program which includes sexual-affection topics and information along with other topics.

Thus, the following conclusions can be drawn about the timing or *when* sex education and family planning information are presented in counseling.

1. Sexual-affectional information can be appropriately presented in all counseling settings. This is not privileged information for any particular discipline of counseling.

2. The role of the counselor and setting for counseling are important in determining the client expectations regarding the presentation of sexual-affectional information.

3. Professionals doing premarital counseling cannot ignore the area of sexual-affectional information for their clients. This does not mean that they must do it all themselves, rather, it means that they see that such information and areas are considered by the clients in their counseling sessions or by collaboration or referral with other professionals. In fact, if the counselor is not comfortable in dealing with sexual information, it is best handled by another counselor who has achieved better resolution of his/her own conflicts. Negative feelings are difficult to mask and are communicated to the clients inadvertently.

4. The overall goals and structure of the premarital counseling will determine the exact sequence and content of sexual-affectional information and considerations. Interdisciplinary communication is needed for assurance that the clients receive the information they should have.

5. As a routine part of the premarital counseling process, we would suggest that the counselor, regardless of setting and discipline, schedule a follow-up session with the couple several weeks after the wedding. Such a session would facilitate the couple's resolution of concerns and/or problems that they have had or are experiencing whether they be emotional or physical adjustment to marriage. The focus would be preventative and positive rather than an attempt to dredge up pathology. The session would set the tone for growth through professional consultation rather than remediation after a problem has developed. Some professionals would disagree with the follow-up session, pointing out that the couple is likely in an ecstatic state and counseling would have no benefit or impact as such a point in time. Our experience has been that such follow-up sessions are of real benefit and apparent significance to the couple.

What is Included in Sexual-Affectional Content?

It is beyond the scope of this chapter to give detailed information as to the content of what the counselor needs to know about sexual-affectional information, values, and attitudes in order to do an acceptable job in premarital counseling. We have identified a number of topical areas that we believe are important for the counselor to have a knowledge in and have included several primary sources for the counselor to consult for complete content. In addition to the specific resources which we have cited, there are other excellent ones available which have not been cited because of lack of space or redundancy of material. Because of the recent growth and mushrooming of material for professionals and the lay public, the counselor has a real responsibility and challenge to keep up in these areas.

First, the topics related to the biology and function of the human sexual system must be included. This includes such areas as sexual anatomy and physiology of the male and female including anatomical structure and function. Books are available which can enrich the knowledge of counselors and the clients who wish such detailed information. Excellent books for the counselor would include Frederick Cohn's *Understanding Human Sexuality* (1974), James Leslie McCary's *Human Sexuality* (1973), and Frank Netter's *Illustrated Atlas of Human Reproductive Systems* (1974), as well as other books. A useful booklet which professionals can make available to clients is Bernard R. Greenbalt's *A Doctor's Marital Sex Guide for Patients* (1973).

We find that couples are surprised and intrigued when they learn that there are remarkable similarities in female and male anatomy and physiology. Frank Netter's *Reproductive System* (1974) graphically indicates anatomical and endocrine considerations. Masters and Johnson's *Human Sexual Response* (1966, Chap. 17) describes numerous similar anatomical and physiological responses during the sexual cycle. Counselors can point out, however, that males will never have the perspective of females, physically, emotionally, spiritually, intellectually, or socially, and vice versa. Relationship in depth of the marital dyad is needed for complete understanding. We feel that the counselor has many opportunities to encourage this concept, and we find that couples respond favorably.

Second, information and discussion of the basic sexual response and sexual act should be included. Cohn's and McCary's books cited above as well as Donald Hasting's *Sexual Expression in Marriage* (1971) are valuable resources for the counselor. Booklets which the counselor may wish to provide to clients would include Greenbalt mentioned above, as well as Lindsay R. Curtis's *Sensible Sex* (1971), Kimberly-Clark Corporation Life Cycle Library's *Getting Married* (1974), and Richard H. and Margaret G. Klemer's *Sexual Adjustment in Marriage* (1966).

To refute the false concept that sexuality is intended for reproduction only, we offer the following observations. (1) Men are attracted to women almost any time, not just when women are near ovulation. (2) Women are receptive most of the time, not only near ovulation. Many women desire sexual relations even during menses, unless under strict cultural taboos. We find no scientific reason to refrain from intercourse during the menstrual period (surprisingly, relief from dysmenorrhea may occur if the woman is able to reach orgasm phase). (3) Both men and women desire and need sexual expression following the reproductive years as well and are active into the 8th decade of life or later if they have had satisfactory sexual experiences earlier, unless strongly preconditioned by cultural environment or debilitated by severe disease.

Third, basic information on family planning and contraception should be discussed with the couple. Counselor information would include Josimovich's presentation in Chap. 24 of this volume, Cohn and McCary, cited previously, and Charles William Hubbard's *Family Planning Education* (1973). Information booklets for the client would include those by Curtis and Greenbalt cited above.

Fourth, the information suggested and cited above needs to be integrated into the values and attitudes of the premarital couple. This is really a primary function and responsibility of premarital/prewedding counseling. Thus, assuming accurate and appropriate presentation of information and content, the counselor's attitudes and relationship with the clients are of primary importance. Clients will likely find a book such as William H. Master's and Virginia E. Johnson's *The Pleasure Bond* (1976) to be helpful and insightful. The counselor may wish to use it as bibliotherapy and part of the counseling process or simply recommend it as an appropriate resource for reading on the honeymoon.

In addition to the books and pamphlets discussed above, the authors have found *The Sex Knowledge Inventory, Form X Revised*, to be a useful tool in premarital sex education counseling. This instrument, developed by Gelolo McHugh (1968), is not a "test" in the diagnostic sense, rather, it is an inventory of items pertaining to knowledge of sexual information, beliefs, and values. The items of the inventory have an interpersonal and relationship focus and can assist the counselor in pinpointing specific areas for clarification and exploration in the counseling session(s) after the clients have taken the paper and pencil instrument. A related instrument, by the same author, is the *Venereal Disease Knowledge Inventory*.

Summary

The presentation of information and the exploration of the premarital couple's attitudes and values concerning sexuality are important aspects of premarital counseling. The chapter discussed *when* and *what* might be presented and attempted to explode some common myths concerning sexuality. Specific resources were presented, both for the counselor's background and knowledge and for bibliotherapeutic use with clients.

REFERENCES

Calderone, M. S.: Introduction: the issues at hand—the counselor and human sexuality. Personnel and Guidance Journal, **54:** 350–351, 1976.

Cohn, F.: *Understanding Human Sexuality.* Prentice-Hall, Englewood Cliffs, New Jersey, 1974.

Curtis, L. R.: *Sensible Sex: A Guide for Newlyweds.* Searle and Co., San Juan, Puerto Rico, 1971.

Gordon, S.: Counselors and changing sexual values. Personnel and Guidance Journal, **54:** 362–364, 1976.

Greenbalt, B. R.: *A Doctor's Marital Sex Guide for Patients.* Budlong Press Co., Chicago, Illinois, 1973.

Hastings, D.: *A Doctor Speaks on Sexual Expression in Marriage,* Little, Brown and Co., Boston, Massachusetts, 1971.

Hubbard, C. W.: *Family Planning Education.* C. V. Mosby Co., St. Louis, Missouri, 1973.

Lief, H. I.: *Medical Aspects of Human Sexuality.* Williams & Wilkins Co., Baltimore, Maryland, 1975.

Life Cycle Center: *Getting Married.* Kimberly Clark Corp., Neenah, Wisconsin, 1974.

Klemer, R. H., and Klemer, M. G.: *Sexual Adjustment in Marriage.* Public Affairs Pamphlets, New York, 1966.

Masters, W. H., and Johnson, V. E.: *Human Sexual Response.* Little, Brown and Co., Boston, Massachusetts, 1966.

Masters, W. H., and Johnson, V. E.: *Human Sexual Inadequacy.* Little, Brown and Co., Boston, Massachusetts, 1970.

Masters, W. H., and Johnson, V. E.: *The Pleasure Bond.* Bantum Books, New York, 1976.

McCary, J. L.: *Human Sexuality.* 2nd Ed., Van Nostrand Reinhold Co., New York, 1973.

McHugh, G.: *Marriage Counselor's Manual: The Sex Knowledge Inventory, Form X Revised.* Family Life Publications, Inc., Saluda, North Carolina, 1968.

Netter, F. H.: *The CIBA Collection of Medical Illustrations; Reproductive System.* CIBA Pharmaceutical Co., Summit, New Jersey, 1974.

Medical Aspects of Contraception and Family Planning

The preceding chapters have considered the enormous increase in demand for contraceptive information in the past 20 years resulting from greater availability of a variety of techniques and earlier age of sexual expression of interpersonal needs. The physician is, therefore, called upon to counsel patients directly or indirectly through his or her nonphysician colleagues on the technical aspects of contraception in general (efficacy, safety, and patient acceptability) and in a variety of special circumstances (variations in age, marital status, or medical conditions). Although most physicians are equipped to counsel with the most up-to-date information on risks and side effects, peculiar sets of social circumstances of individuals continue to present exciting medical and ethical problems in therapy to the physician. The purpose of this chapter, then, is to review the different contraceptive modalities and then to consider specific age and medical condition-related problem situations. An earlier review gave the relative effectiveness of different techniques most commonly accepted in the medical community, even today (Garcia, 1967). This chapter will give updated information in this regard.

Different Modalities of Contraception

Coitus Interruptus and Nonintromission

Although not included in most lists of contraceptive techniques, these approaches are used by a substantial minority of patients in an effort to prevent pregnancy. Their exact efficacy is not known except that many individuals have met with success with them over many years of married life, while others have met with failure after relatively brief experience. The reason for counseling against use of these methods is because we do not know whether they are as effective as other techniques, whose efficacy is better known. The failures are due primarily to passage of some spermatozoa just prior to ejaculation with secretions issuing from the urethra during sexual excitement and because ejaculation on the perineum may still occasionally result in pregnancy.

The Rhythm Method

The efficacy of this method is alleged to be poor in that roughly 10 times as many pregnancies occur with this technique in comparison with the oral contraceptives (OC's) and the intrauterine contraceptive device (IUCD) (Mastroianni, 1974). This technique recognizes the increasing probability of conception if intercourse occurs between the 4 days prior to ovulation as well as the day of ovulation and 3 days thereafter. Each patient must determine the length of this fertile period in which she has no intercourse: a period bounded by subtracting 18 from the shortest cycle length in the past 12 months and 11 days from the longest cycle length. The technique is unsuitable for those women who have marked irregularity in cycle length or if they are anovulatory in more than 1 or 2 months of the year, because of the long periods of abstinence required. Improvements in the efficacy of this technique by pin-pointing the time of probable ovulation through changes in vaginal or cervical secretion pH, chemical, or physical changes, as well as by daily basal body temperature charts, have aided in the predictability of when ovulation occurs. All women ovulate 14 plus or minus a fraction of days prior to the onset of menstruation, except those women who have anovulatory episodes of bleeding or who have premature failure of the corpus luteum ("inadequate luteal phase defect") and a foreshortened postovulatory period prior to menstruation. These latter conditions are associated with a high degree of infertility, however, so that they need not be of concern. Research is going on, however, which may permit those clinics favoring this method for religious or other reasons to shorten the length of the intercourse abstinence period if these techniques of cervical mucus study can distinguish the nonfertile period, particularly after ovulation (Mastroianni, 1974). There is no question of the safety of this technique, except when it results in pregnancy which has health risks of its own. There is one psychological advantage of this method in that it tends to make both sexual partners more responsible toward the possibility of pregnancy in comparison with other techniques which put the burden more on one partner than on the other.

Douches, Foams, and Use of Vaginal Contraceptive Creams and Jellies

Pre- or postintercourse douching for contraception is to be condemned because of its very low efficacy (Garcia, 1967) and because repetitive douching may be irritating to the vagina and perineum of a certain minority of females. There has been renewed interest in the use of vaginal contraceptive foams, creams, and jellies because of their protection against venereal diseases such as gonorrhea. All three are supposed to have an efficacy of approximately one-fourth that of the IUCD and 1% of that of the combined OC's (Garcia, 1967) when used by themselves. The foams may be used in conjunction with condoms, while the creams and jellies are routinely used as an adjunct to the diaphragm (see below).

Condoms

The condom ("prophylactic," "rubber") was the first mechanical contraceptive device used on a large scale in modern times. It was employed (and legally permitted for only such specific use) for prevention of passage of veneral disease from one partner to another. With standardization in quality testing by reputable manufacturers, the chance of rupture had dropped and the increased thinness has permitted more sexual pleasure. There has been a resurgence of use, particularly when combined with vaginal foams, because it is free of side effects, because the use of the two increases psychological responsibility in both partners, and because the varieties in manufacture (color, thinness, texture, degree of prelubrication, thickened areas on some models called "ticklers") are thought to compensate for the artificial "feel" of condoms. Although earlier medical writers have stressed that the erect male organ is the same size, recent studies have suggested that there are variations in erect length and girth, and that degrees of obesity affect "available length." Furthermore, wide variation in the differences between flaccid and erect length makes training in the choice of appropriate condom size and how much to leave free beyond the penis of great importance to the individual male. Thus, it is important that males or male partners of female patients are counseled on the wearing of condoms, and that there is an opportunity for answering the many questions. Tradidtionally, the failure rate of the condom method has been approximately 3 to 100 times that of the IUCD and the OC, respectively (Garcia, 1967). Recent studies, however, suggest that there may be comparable failure rates of the three techniques with the recent improvements in condom design and patient motivation described above (Dumm, *et al.*, 1974).

The Diaphragm Plus Contraceptive Cream or Jelly

Over the past 30 to 40 years, this device has enjoyed immense popularity, especially among married couples. Its use, freeing the patient from fear of harmful side effects, permits her to have control over reproduction in a way that the condom did not, while its effectiveness is moderately good, with a failure rate of 2.5 to 60 times that of the IUCD and the OC, respectively (Garcia 1967). More recent studies have found improved effectiveness (Anonymous 1974a; Wortman, 1976). The use of the diaphragm is usually restricted to married (legally or nonlegally) couples who can expect to have intercourse at a particular time of day. Reasons for these restrictions are two-fold. First, the vagina must have reached a stable set of dimensions for optimal fitting which takes anywhere from one episode of intercourse plus a few days to up to 2 to 3 months in some partner pairs. Second, the contraceptive cream or jelly is only effective for 10 to 16 h and since there is need to leave the diaphragm in place for 3 to 6 h after the last intercourse, the diaphragm can only be used for a limited period of time each day before it is to be removed and reinserted with fresh cream or jelly. Some patients find it unplesant to use because of irritation of the penis or because of dripping of acid-smelling cream or jelly after being in place overnight.

The diaphragm size must be rechecked when a woman gains or loses 10 pounds (because of change in vaginal shape) or after 4 to 6 weeks recovery from each pregnancy.

The Oral Contraceptives ("the Pill")

The oral contraceptives have proven to be the most effective form of birth control so far available as they are greater than 95% effective (Garcia, 1967; Potts et al., 1975). The OC's now available consist of a combination of synthetic estrogen (mestranol or ethinyl estradiol) and a synthetic progesterone-like compound (progestin). Sequential contraceptives (estrogen alone for the majority of a cycle followed by a final 5 days of combined estrogen and progestin) are no longer sold because of their high estrogen dose and because of a suspicion that they might increase the incidence of endometrial carcinoma. Concerning the high effectiveness of the OC's, it should be noted that to test the relative efficacy of different preparations against one another or against other forms of contraception, it requires at least 100,000 woman years of experience (mean number of years use per patient times total number of patients). The effectiveness of the OC's undoubtedly relates to their combined effects on the hypothalamic pituitary axis to prevent gonadotropin release needed for ovulation, plus their effects in making the endometrium inhospitable to the fertilized ovum, in altering tubal motility for sperm and egg transport, and in adversely affecting the hospitality of the cervical mucus to sperm transport. It is clear, however, that OC usage increases the incidence of serious medical disorders and death although to a much less extent than pregnancy itself (Tietze *et al.*, 1976; Anonymous 1974b). The well-known potentially harmful and lethal side effects appear to be almost exclusively related to the estrogen doses and to the enhancement or inhibition of estrogenic effects by the various progestins in each OC. From the original studies, it appears that the majority of serious complaints occurred with the OC's containing higher synthetic estrogen doses (80 to 100 μg per pill) (Vessey and Doll, 1969). It is hoped, but not yet proven, that the OC's containing lower doses, especially 20 to 35 μg per pill, might be virtually free of harmful side effects. The following are the major problems which the physician must consider in prescribing the OC's and about which he should *fully inform* the prospective user (Anonymous 1974b; Potts *et al.*, 1975).

1. Venous thrombophlebitis and pulmonary embolism. The incidence for all users of serious enough pulmonary embolism to result in death has been reported to be approximately 8 times that found in nonpregnant, non-OC users or approximately one-half that seen during or immediately following pregnancy (Vessey and Doll, 1969).

2. Cerebral vascular accidents have occurred with a four-fold greater incidence in pill users than in nonusers (Potts *et al.*, 1975). In the majority, there were premonitory warnings of an increased occurrence of migraine headaches, visual blurring, and/or transient limb paralyses.

3. Induction of arterial hypertension is seen and appears to occur in those already susceptible to development of essential hypertension. The induced hypertension seems to be reversed on withdrawal of the OC medication. The underlying hypertension is approximately threefold higher among OC users than in nonusers (Potts *et al.*, 1975).

4. Myocardial infarctions, according to recent literature, occur fatally with a five-fold greater incidence in women over 40 years of age than in nonusers (Mann and Inman, 1975; Mann *et al.*, 1975).

5. Worsening of glucose tolerance and temporary induction of diabetes mellitus occur with susceptible women just as they occur in pregnancy (Beck, 1973). An increased insulin response to a glucose load, probably caused by some but not other progestins used in OC's, may not compensate for the decreased effectiveness of endogenous insulin caused by the estrogens. The abnormal glucose tolerance or frank diabetes always appears to be reversed on OC withdrawal regardless of length of usage, with some exceptions (in those presumed to be the ones who would have developed diabetes spontaneously).

6. Familial hyperlipemic patients demonstrate a larger rise in the triglycerides and VLD (very low density) lipoprotein fraction of the serum, changes which appear reversible on stopping OC ingestion (Beck, 1973).

7. It is not clear whether or not the incidence of amenorrhea with or without associated galactorrhea is increased by taking the OC's. Women should be warned that there is roughly a 1% chance of having no periods after stopping the pill; while approximately 1% of young women may normally have a cessation of periods without having ever taken the medication. Thus, a cause and effect relationship between taking OC's and "postpill amenorrhea" remains to be established. Nevertheless, a woman taking the pill should perhaps be advised to use alternative types of contraception for a few months prior to beginning a pregnancy, in case she is one of the 1% who might require artificial induction of ovulation with other medications such as clomiphene citrate or menopausal gonadotropins. Those who develop galactorrhea (inappropriate lactation) while taking OC's should have then serum prolactin levels and other endocrine studies performed to see whether they might have a pituitary adenoma (Archer et al., 1974).

8. The incidence of seizures may be increased in epileptics if the estrogen:progestin ratio is excessive for a particular patient.

9. Less concerning but still annoying side effects depend on the relative estrogen:progestin potency and to a lesser extent on the androgenic potency in a particular individual. For excessive estrogen effects, there may be nausea and/or vomiting or psychological agitation; for low estrogen effects, there may be greater androgenic effects such as acne or breakthrough bleeding, while amenorrhea and/or psychological depression results from too low a progestin and estrogen potency. Finally, excessive progestins may cause excessive weight gain in fat or in edema.

Various authors (e.g., Dickey and Dorr, 1969) have suggested particular combinations of estrogen and progestin based on the patient's previous menstrual history and physical examination. Since individuals vary so much in their responses, however, it seems reasonable to begin with a lower estrogen dose pill to avoid serious side effects, e.g., containing 50 μg, or even lower dose OC's in smaller or very young women. If symptoms of progesterone and/or estrogen lack develop, a pill containing more of one or both components may be substituted. Thus, the patient should be counseled that pill dosage may need to be changed after one to three cycles of an initial prescription.

Because of the numerous side effects of OC's, many more details of which are found in the packaging inserts supplied by the pharmaceutical companies and in certain detailed papers (see References), it is essential to see each patient for questioning, pelvic examination to rule out occasional overstimulation of uterine leiomyomata ("fibroids") or cervical polyps, and for checking for excessive increases in weight or blood pressure 1 to 3 months after OC prescription is begun.

The "morning after pill," or the use of large doses of estrogen-containing medication for 1 to 3 days after unprotected exposure to prevent implantation of a fertilized egg, is not advised because of possible risk of the estrogen and possible adverse effects on a developing embryo if the medication fails now that endometrial aspiration (very early abortion) is available.

Intrauterine Contraceptive Devices

The IUCD has been used by a large segment of fertile women because of fears or actual experience of the side effects of oral contraceptives or because certain medical conditions and age have made consumption of OC's too hazardous. All women contemplating use of the device should be counseled that IUCD's may be spontaneously expelled and that they may cause unacceptable degrees of hypermenorrhea or cramping immediately postinsertion. Furthermore, less than 1 in 100 may have more serious complications of endometritis with or without parametritis or perforation of the uterus and passage of the IUCD into the peritoneal cavity requiring laparotomy or colpotomy to remove the device. For those roughly one-half to three-quarters of women who have no immediate problems, the IUCD is the best tolerated and effective of all forms of contraception. Prior to insertion and after making certain that acute or chronic pelvic inflammatory disease is not present, the patient should be further warned that in the event she becomes pregnant, the IUCD should be removed to decrease (but not totally eliminate) the possibility of miscarriage and to prevent the very rare occurrence of mid-trimester chorioamnionitis and septicemia, which has occasionally proven fatal. The latter possibility, although not statistically proven to be related to the presence of an IUCD, is particularly rare now that the Dalkon Shield IUCD has been withdrawn from the market because of its implication in causing septicemia during pregnancy.

In response to questions as to whether the IUCD causes pelvic infection, which may reduce fertility and require major surgery, it should be kept in mind that IUCD's may cause a flare up of mixed anaerobic-aerobic sepsis in the parametrium, tubes, and ovaries in those with postgonococcal pelvic inflammatory disease; and that although not yet proven, there does seem to be a definite increase in unilateral tubo-ovarian abscesses in IUCD users which might be life threatening and require major surgery. The patient should probably be required to sign an informed consent for insertion of an IUCD since it represents an invasion of a body cavity. Recent reviews have shown the relative safety of IUCD's in relationship to OC's, pregnancy, and abortion (Huber et al., 1975; Mishell, 1975; Tietze et al., 1976).

In counseling as to which type of IUCD to use, the patient should be shown a sample. The Lippes Loop and Saf-t-koil, made in different sizes, are the most often employed. For nulligravida, these may be too large, and a Copper-7 device is now most popular.

The patient should be counseled to return for a brief history and pelvic examination after one to three menses have passed to check that the plastic strings are in place and that there has been no excessive hypermenorrhea, cramping, signs of pelvic infection, or IUCD dislocation. The patient should be counseled to manually check the presence of the strings weekly or as often as she wishes, and that additional contraception with condoms, diaphragms, foams, and/or jellies is advisable during the first 3 months after IUCD insertion. If satisified, the patient should return for annual check-ups and may leave the IUCD in place for an indefinite number of years if she desires, except for the Copper-7 which must be removed after 2 years because a part of its effectiveness is dependent on the copper content which declines with time.

Newer devices which probably increase effectiveness by releasing progestins are now becoming available on the market. Whether the benefit of an extra degree of contraceptive effectiveness will outweigh the need to replace these devices annually (because of dissipation of the progestin) remains to be seen in larger series of patients.

Back-up Therapeutic Abortion

In the case of failure of other contraceptive techniques, therapeutic abortion by endometrial aspiration (vacuum suction 1 to 14 days after delay of expected menses), first trimester suction curettage (to 12 weeks after the 1st day of the last menstrual period), or second trimester abortion (intraamniotic injection of hypertonic saline, intraamniotic or vaginal administration of certain prostaglandins, or removal of the fetus via a hysterotomy) may be offered by those institutions and physicians which do not preclude this modality for religious or ethical reasons. The offering of the availability of abortion as the sole form of contraception is not acceptable to the great majority of physicians because it delays psychological development of responsibility in conceptors and because repeated therapeutic abortion, besides their own inherent medical complication possibilities, may increase the incidence of infertility due to damage to the cervix and/or infection.

Sterilization

Female sterilization is usually desired in women after they have had one or more offspring and reached that age where the psychological, financial, and health threats of another pregnancy outweigh the natural desire to retain the possibility of future conception. These patients require extra counseling to make sure that they are not requesting this procedure (be it direct cutting and ligation of the fallopian tubes via laparotomy or colpotomy or a laparoscopic ("bandaid surgery"), tubal cautery, or banding with a Fallope plastic ring) due to pressure from their sexual partner or by another relative. The most difficult cases seen for counseling are young women who have little or no medical contraindications to future pregnancies but who demand sterilization without evident neurotic overlay. In discussing female sterilization, it is important to know the possibility for vasectomy in the male partner, a lesser surgical procedure if this would fulfill the female patients' needs. Needless to say, counseling of males prior to vasectomy should be as thorough as it is before female sterilization.

In the case of proposed sterilization of either sex, an informed consent form should be signed. Besides discussion and summarizing on the form the general surgical and anesthestic risks, the patient should be fully informed that these procedures are essentially irreversible (no more than a few percent can be surgically reversed), but that there would still be a 1 to 3% risk of future fertility due to procedure failure (primarily due to recanalization of the scarred ends of the interrupted fallopian tubes or vasa deferentes).

Choice of Contraceptive in Special Situations

The Adolescent and/or the Woman Without Prior Intercourse Experience

Particular care must be taken not to exaggerate breast swelling with attendant stretch marks, prevent attainment of full stature, or induce sudden, excessive weight gain by excessive estrogen doses in this group of women. It is advised that such patients be started on lower estrogen-containing doses of OC's until they have had intercourse enough times that a diaphragm and cream or jelly or IUCD (Copper-7 for most nulligravida) can be easily fitted.

Anticipating Pregnancy Soon

If pregnancy is desired in the next 3 to 12 months, patients should be counseled to stop OC's and use other forms of contraception to permit correction of rare anovulatory conditions, as noted above.

Postpregnancy

Depending on the ability of the patient and her partner to refrain from having sexual relations, it is essential that intercourse not occur for at least 2 weeks after pregnancy (term or abortion) for fear of causing pelvic infection; and it is recommended that she wait until her first menstrual period (usually 4 to 6 weeks after the end of pregnancy) before insertion of an IUCD (when the uterus has returned to normal size and expulsion of a device is less likely), for resuming OC's (when the chance of abnormal bleeding is reduced), or for refitting of a diaphragm. For those who must use contraceptives before 4 to 6 weeks and when physical methods such as condoms plus foam or the rhyhm method are unacceptable, oral contraceptives or IUCD's may be started earlier with the full realization of an increased risk of diagnostically troublesome, vaginal bleeding, pelvic infection, and expulsion in the case of IUCD's, as well as a variably, but usually moderately reduced milk supply in the case of nursing mothers. In regard to the latter process, nursing, it should be noted that contraceptive efficacy is relatively poor during this physiological event, even though the patient may have no menstrual periods.

Premenopausal Patients

As mentioned above, there is increased risk of myocardial infarction in pill users over age 40, so that these women should be advised to use other forms of contraception. If they decline to stop, they probably should be asked to sign an informed consent prior to continuing OC's at an increased risk to their health.

Physicians no longer advocate the continued use of OC's after menopause, as there is no evidence that indefinitely prolonged administration of estrogen prevents bodily aging or endometrial carcinoma.

Importance of Certain Medical Conditions

As mentioned above, glucose tolerance may worsen on OC's, so that diabetes may have increased insulin requirements although there is no evidence that such a situation leads to earlier vascular complications.

If vascular disease already exists (previous thrombophlebitis, atherosclerosis, diabetic vascular disease, hypertensive vascular disease of any etiology), OC's are generally contraindicated but may be permitted under very special circumstances after thorough consultation with the internist or other physician managing the patient's primary medical problem.

Patients with mental retardation or psychiatric illnesses rendering their legal mental competence questionable continue to be a problem for the physician. Every effort must be made to obtain as informed consent as possible from each patient in addition to that of her legal guardians. Because the rights of the latter to make final decisions have been legally questioned recently, the physician must obtain as much medical and legal consultation as possible before making decisions, especially in the case of irreversible contraception such as sterilization.

Patients at high risk of venereal disease should be discouraged from using IUCD's if an alternative form of contraception is feasible.

Finally, patients with a susceptibility to infertility because of prior history of amenorrhea, oligomenorrhea, pelvic inflammatory disease, pelvic endometriosis, previous unilateral oophorectomy, uterine leiomyomata ("fibroids"), or difficulty in conceiving ought to employ methods other than OC's or IUCD's unless they understand the additional risk of using these two birth control modalities and the pill dose or IUCD model is chosen with special care.

Summary

As the complexity in the modalities and possible adverse side effects and because of the greater sophistication of patients in understanding their rights to control and protect their bodies, the physician and his or her colleagues must spend more time than ever before in serious counseling before a particular method is chosen, while balancing the seriousness of such discussions with a knowledge that all of these techniques provide safety not too different from that of other common medications or devices and which provide security from an undesired pregnancy which has even greater health hazards. The physician must keep abreast of further possible hazards of these methods by reading FDA-approved package inserts.

REFERENCES

Anonymous: Contraception in Britain. Study finds experience and careful instruction lead to low failure rate with diaphragm. Family Planning Digest, 3(3): 8–9, 1974a.

Anonymous: Royal College report on oral contraceptives: 9-year prospective study of 23,000 users finds serious risks few, benefits great. Family Planning Digest 3(5): 1–7, 1974b.

Archer, D. F., Nankin, H. R., Gabos, P. F., Maroon, J., Nosetz, S., Wadhwa, S. R., and Josimovich, J. B.: Serum prolactin in patients with inappropriate lactation. Amer. J. Obstet. Gynecol., 119: 466–472, 1974.

Beck, P.: Contraceptive steroids: modification of carbohydrate and lipid metabolism. Metabolism, 22: 841–855, 1973.

Dickey, R. P., and Dorr, C. H., II: Oral contraceptives: selection of the proper pill. Obstet. Gynecol., 33: 273–287, 1969.

Dumm, J. J., Piotrow, P. T., and Dalsimer, I. A.: The modern condom: a quality product for effective contraception. Pop. Report, H:21–36, 1974.

Garcia, C. -R.: The oral contraceptive: an appraisal and review. Amer. J. Med. Sci., 253: 718–740, 1967.

Huber, S. C., Piotrow, P. T., Orlang, F. B., and Kommer, G.: IUDs reassessed: a decade of experience. Pop. Reports, B: 21–48, 1975.

Mann, J. I., Vessey, M. P., Thorogood, M., and Doll, R.: Myocardial infarction in young women with special reference to oral contraceptive practice. Brit. Med. J., 2: 241, 1975.

Mann, J. I., and Inman, W. H. W.: Oral contraceptives and death from myocardial infarction. Brit. Med. J., 2: 245–245, 1975.

Mastroianni, L., Jr.: Rhythm: systemized chance-taking. Family Planning Perspectives, 6: 209–212, 1974.

Mishell, D. R., Jr.: Assessing the intrauterine device. Family Planning Perspectives 7: 103–111, 1975.

Potts, M., van der Ulugt, T., Piotrow, P. T., Gail, L. J., and Huber, S. C.: Advantages of oral outweigh disadvantages. Pop. Reports, A: 29–51, 1975.

Tietze, C., Bongaaits, J., and Schearer, B.: Mortality associated with the control of fertility. Family Planning Perspectives 8: 6–14, 1976.

Vessey, M. P., and Doll, R.: Investigation of relation between use of oral contraceptives and thromboembolic disease. A further report. Brit. Med. J. 2: 651–657, 1969.

Wortman, J.: The diaphragm and other intravaginal barriers: a review. Pop. Reports, H:57–75, 1976.

LE MON CLARK, M.D.

25

The Premarital Physical Examination: A Physician's Guide

Approximately 20 years ago John F. Oliven in his book, *Sexual Hygiene and Pathology* (1955), gave a very brief outline of a premarital examination. He said, "A complete premarital examination of a couple consists of a general health examination including history, gynecological (and I add, urological) examination, and necessary laboratory work and is followed by an offer of conferences with bride and groom. Individual talks are usually the most feasible approach, but a joint conference is preferred by some couples." (Oliven, 1955, p. 170.)

Dr. Oliven goes on to suggest very wisely that the first examination take place some days before the projected wedding in order to allow time for necessary medical attention if any is indicated. And he also suggests that there should be one follow-up appointment 6 to 8 weeks after the wedding. Given a chance to air some differences very early to a sympathetic yet uninvolved individual may prevent molehills from becoming mountains of misunderstanding.

Blood serology (required in most states), blood pressure, and examination of heart, lungs, and urine is, of course, routine.

Patient Concerns about the Examination

One of the most important things a young person can learn from a premarital examination is that sex, and the part it should play in marriage, is something which can be talked about as easily and naturally as one talks about a toothache to a dentist.

Attitudes are caught. They are not taught. If the examining physician is at ease when discussing any aspect of sex the patient will certainly be much more at ease than if the examining physician himself finds it something to be a bit "up tight" about. What vocabularly should be used? The scientific, medical names for the sexual organs and proc- esses! The colloquial names have an aura of indecency about them, a back alley, behind the barn stigma that makes it difficult for anyone to use them. If necessary the colloquial terms can be used to define the decent terminology, but it is really seldom necessary. Most people know the scientific terminology but have never acquired facility in using it.

A young woman may be fearful that a vaginal-pelvic examination will reveal the fact that she is no longer a virgin. This will give the examiner the opportunity to show that he is not in the least shocked by the finding. The physician may then ask how old she was when she first experienced intercourse. Is it now pleasurable? Does she reach or- gasm fairly regularly and frequently? If not, has she any explanation as to why she does not? Is she somewhat overwhelmed with a sense of guilt? Is there any actual difficulty connected with the experience?

Virginity need not preclude an adequate pelvic examination. The hymen can be stretched almost painlessly after infiltration of a little local anesthetic at 4 and 8 o'clock. If it can be stretched adequately, incision may be unnecessary. Any dilatation or incision of the hymen should be talked over with the young couple and should not be done without their permission.

If all this is done sympathetically yet matter of factly the physician may well be rewarded by having the girl say she is so glad to talk to someone who does not make her feel that she is a "naughty girl" for having had intercourse before marriage.

Anatomical and Medical Considerations

If the clitoris is entirely free is it pleasurable to have it gently stimulated by her sweetheart? If the clitoris is covered with adhesions between it and the prepuce, is stimulation of the clitoris irritating or even downright painful? If so, then the adhesions between the clitoris and the prepuce must be freed. If they are not too extensive this can be done with a blunt probe without an anesthetic. First, of course, warn the patient that it will hurt momentarily, the clitoris being one of the most sensitive spots on the whole body. If extensive, inject a local anesthetic through a weal just above the clitoris, inserting the needle down first one labium minus on one side and then the other. The adhesions are then easily separated without pain. (Dickinson, 1949, Fig. 77a.)

I always show the patient the clitoris having her hold a hand mirror so that she can see the situation both before and after. Then she must be taught the motion with both hands to retract the prepuce after separation of the adhesions and told to apply some unguent morning and night for 10 days so that it will heal that way and not readhere. Vaseline, cold cream, anything which she may have will serve.

While first examining the vulva, separation of the labia minora may reveal a greater or lesser amount of whitish smegma. This should be pointed out to her and she should be told that bathing the vulvar area with the flat of her hand is not good enough. The whitish smegma has a very unpleasant odor. To remove it requires a separation of the labia and washing with one finger. This is especially necessary in this day and age. Kinsey's phrase "good mammalian behavior" for oral genital contacts has made such activity commonplace, a normal part of love-making, which it should be. (Kinsey, 1948 pp. 510 and 574.)

Is there an excessive discharge of mucus? Is it due to infection? A microscopic examination of a smear will answer that question. Is it due to a cervical erosion? Visualization of the cervix with a speculum, virginal if necessary, will answer that. Electric or cryocoagulation will solve that, but it will take 4 to 6 weeks to heal completely, depending upon the size of the area treated. But it will remove the excess discharge and permit a much more pleasurable apposition of the penis and mucous membrane lining of the vagina. The young women who have the excess discharge commonly think it quite normal since they have had it most of their postpubertial lives.

But even more important, an eroded cervix is not a healthy cervix. The excessive discharge invites infection. And it all too easily is "milked" up the urethra by the motion of the penis in the vagina causing frequent bladder infections, the typical honeymoon cystitis.

Is the vaginal opening really free? In a very few cases the hymenal ring may be elastic enough to permit insertion of the penis into the vagina, but it may form a constricting band around the penis which is uncomfortable for both of them. Insertion of 1 cc of a local anesthetic at 4 and 8 o'clock of the hymenal ring and then incision of it with a pair of surgical scissors will end the difficulty. (see chap. 23 for another point of view.)

Is the uterus retroverted? If so, the vagina may be foreshortened and deep penetration be painful. Is it bound down or can it be freely moved? Could it be replaced by bimanual mainpulation and a Smith-Hodge type pessary inserted to hold it in normal position?

If it is not freely movable, why? Is there evidence of pelvic infection? Are there endometriotic nodules palpable in the posterior cul-de-sac? Again, the patient may be shown the retroverted uterus with the hand mirror. Explain the angle of the cervix in the vagina.

Two suggestions may be made to obviate the discomfort of deep penetration if the retroverted uterus is the cause. After insertion of the penis she may bring her legs together somewhat while he puts first one leg and then the other outside of hers. He can then have the satisfaction of pushing almost as hard as he might wish with little fear of causing her discomfort. The other suggestion is that they have intercourse in the "upside-down" position, she above him. She can then ride up to prevent too deep a penetration.

Sexual Counseling

Dr. Oliven (1955), suggests "an offer of conferences." It is far better for the examining physician to take the initiative in suggesting such a conference. Here one has to "feel" his way. Have they had intercourse? If so, there is less reason to see them separately. If not, then possibly one session with each alone would be better. Each could air his or her fears or confusions. Then a session together will show each in the presence of the other that sex can be talked about quite naturally and easily.

Is she fearful of his finding that she is not a virgin? Is he fearful his penis is too small? Too large? Does she know how her mother and father got along sexually? Have negative attitudes been passed on to her from her mother? From her father? She should be told that sexual intercourse should be enjoyed to the fullest extent.

How frequently should a young couple have intercourse? As often as they both want it. Can they have it too ofetn? No, they will finally be so relaxed that they will be quite content.

Sex desire commonly arises much more spontaneously and more frequently in the male than in the female. If the female accepts his attentions, his petting, caressing without rancor or resentment, in a relatively short time she will find that it is much more interesting than she at first thought it might be. I frequently use the illustration of having a starting point and progressing thru time and space from that point to orgasm, some way ahead. If he starts lovemaking and, despite her reluctance, he continues to the point of orgasm he may be partially satisfied. It would be much more satisfactory if she had taken part. But she did not. She backed off from the starting point. The petting, caressing, and the act of intercourse itself cannot help but arouse her. During this period she moves back toward the starting point and even beyond. Now, if he would start all over it would be fun. If she had remained passive, had not reacted negatively to his early advances, she would probably have kept pace with him and gone on to orgasm without difficulty.

A physician must face the fact that getting a sexual history which really gives some information is more difficult than getting a mere physical history. If the girl has had intercourse has she learned to reach orgasm? This can be of vital importance to her health. A smart young orthopedist once told me that many women who came to him for low backache probably needed nothing more than to learn to reach orgasm regularly and frequently in intercourse to relieve the pelvic congestion to cure their backache.

Joseph B. Trainer, M.D., has a trenchant remark in a chapter of Hirsh Lazaar Silverman's (1972) book on *Marital Therapy*. He says, "The same man who inspects with confidence and decision a vulva bearing an infected Bartholin cyst is undone if he has to look at the same structure and tell the patient how to use the components for more sexual fun." (Silverman, 1972, p. 37.)

Can she constrict the vaginal muscles? You can tell her that it is the same sensation as though she were trying to prevent urination. Some 45 years ago Dr. Kegel of Los Angeles and I were working on the same problem quite unknown to each other. I was trying to teach young women to constrict the vaginal muscles thinking it would give their husbands greater pleasure. In almost every case they returned to say that it gave them far more sensation than it did their husbands. Dr. Kegel found the same thing and went on to develop his perineometer to teach women to exercise these muscles more especially for the purpose of increasing bladder control, but also increasing their sexual stimulation. With Dr. Kegel's death the perineometer died also. It is no longer manufactured. (Kegel, 1956, pp. 487–495.) Any woman can achieve the same result without it. To understand the sensation, insert two fingers deeply into the vagina. Then contract the muscles. The feeling is the same as though one was trying to prevent urination. Hold it as long and as hard as you can, repeating it 10 to 12 times each time you think of it, and see that you think of it 10 or 12 times a day. In 4 to 6 weeks you will develop these muscles a very considerable amount.

Many young women do not know how to move their pelvis, to tip it forwards and backwards without pushing up their abdomen. Sometimes it may be necessary to put a hand beneath the buttocks and one on the abdomen and literally teach them to tip the pelvis in the movements of intercourse. Explain to them that this activates the lumbosacral plexus raising the voltage in the pelvic nervous system and thereby increases sensation.

Shocked at the suggestions? You give them exercises for various other difficulties such as low back pain. Why not give them exercises to increase the sexual satisfaction which they and their husbands will attain in the act of sexual intercourse!

Both young men and young women may have doubts as to the effective size of their primary sex organs. Occasionally it is quite worthwhile to have a large test tube, one which is 8 or 10 inches long and at least an inch in diameter. This can be inserted into the vagina until she can feel it impinging upon the posterior cul-de-sac. Mark the depth with the thumb and withdraw it showing just how deep the vagina is.

A young man is usually looking down at his flaccid penis and hence it is foreshortened. The pubic hair covers the base so that it appears even shorter. Point out to him that there is little correspondence between the flaccid and the erect size of the penis. A small penis may increase to 3 times its flaccid size when erect. A relatively large flaccid penis may not increase in size when erect by more than 50% of its flaccid size. Point out to him that the vagina has the power of adapting to almost any size since she can contract the muscles to bring about a satisfactory, snug fit.

I try to impress upon young people that sexual intercourse should be enjoyed. It should be considered play at the adult level. Anything which they want to do to each other which is mutually acceptable is definitely all right. The one with some reservations must be willing to try what the other suggests. It might prove very interesting and enjoyable.

Child-Bearing Considerations

It is undoubtedly worthwhile to inquire about the health of the mother and father of each. A history of diabetes, for instance, in the family of both of the young people would raise grave questions about the danger of juvenile diabetes in their children if they married.

First cousin marriages we know are fraught with possibilities of disaster. A cousin of mine through my mother's side married a cousin of his through his mother's side—no relation of mine—they had two children. The girl was very bright and despite the handicap of severe hearing impairment graduated from college. The boy was a deaf mute. But, there was no evidence of hearing difficulty in either side of the family as far as it could be traced!

Certain types of deafness, serious myopia of both of the young people, and other genetically transmitted diseases known or unknown to the young couple should be found if possible and considered.

Birth Control or Contraception

Does the couple want information on contraception or birth control? They may be hesitant about asking, but will gladly welcome the introduction of the subject by the doctor. See Chap. 24 for a discussion of contraception.

The medication in the birth control pills has been much reduced in the last 5 years. Despite this, adverse reactions do occur. As a result the search for better methods goes on. New IUD's are being developed. But only time will tell what may be the final outcome of their use. The Dalcon shield, which seemed a good idea, proved disasterous.

The increasing problems which seem to be appearing with the use of birth control pills and IUD's and which are discussed in the news media lead many young women to come asking for the diaphragm. I, personally, have always favored the diaphragm. It is absolutely harmless. It does not upset body metabolism. If properly fitted and *always* used it is as effective as any other method.

The one thing that she must understand is that the diaphragm must always beat the penis into the vagina. I tell them to keep it in a bedside table drawer with the tube of spermicidal cream where she can get it "in case of fire." If her husband wants to get his arms around her in the morning and play "for just a minute," without reaching orgasm she must say "uh, uh." "Thirty seconds (which is all it takes) for me to put the diaphragm on."

Fit the diaphragm so that with the fingernail resting against the rim of the diaphragm, the very tip of the gloved finger can be inserted between it and the pubic bone. If, as some directions say, the largest size that will go into the vagina should be fitted, following intercourse she may wake up an hour later with almost unbearable pelvic cramps. Just as the penis shrinks to a smaller than average size almost immediately after the attainment of orgasm returning to the normal flaccid size some minutes later, the vagina does the same. If, upon shrinking, it encounters a foreign body in the vagina it may go into a tonic contraction that is extremely painful.

The diaphragm should be inserted *dome up,* not dome down. The cream should be put on the top of the diaphragm and drawn down through the rim as it is compressed into an elipse for insertion. Do not advocate putting the cream around the edge before inserting it or the vulva becomes a gooey mess. Putting some additional cream into the lower vaginal canal afterwards may also make a gooey mess of the whole procedure and interfere with normal sensation. With the cream above the dome up diaphragm it is rubbed into the cervical os all during intercourse, and any sperm that get around it run into, what is, for them, a perfectly lethal bath.

Above all they must keep open channels of communication. They must be willing to listen and to explain what they would like to do and then be willing to try anything which the other suggests. Lovemaking should be fun! It should be talked about. They should be made to feel that there is nothing they cannot talk over with each other and with you and that they are always welcome.

REFERENCES

Dickinson, R. L.: *Human Sex Anatomy.* The Williams & Wilkins Co., Baltimore, 1949.

Kegel, H.: J. Int. Coll. Surg., **25:** 1956.

Kinsey, A. C., Pomeroy, W. B., and Martin, C. E.: *Sexual Behavior in the Human Male.* W. B. Saunders Co., Philadelphia, 1948.

Oliven, J. F.: *Sexual Hygiene and Pathology.* J. B. Lippincott Co., Philadelphia; 1955.

Silverman, H. L. (Ed): *Marital Therapy.* Charles C Thomas, Springfield, Illinois, 1972.

Appendix

THE AMERICAN ASSOCIATION OF MARRIAGE AND FAMILY
COUNSELORS

What It Is . . .
What It Does

The American Association of Marriage and Family Counselors
(AAMFC) is an organization dedicated to professional marraige counseling and to the field of marriage and family relationships. Over 4500
members throughout the United States and Canada include psychologists, psychiatrists, social workers, ministers, physicians, sociologists,
attorneys, and educators—all of whom are highly trained professional
marriage counselors working to help couples solve their marriage and
family problems. Founded in 1942, AAMFC has national headquarters
in Claremont, California and regional divisions throughout the conti-
nent.

AAMFC performs many functions important to its members, to the
profession of marriage counseling, and to the public. These include
the following.

1. Professional standards—AAMFC sets rigourous membership standards covering specialized academic training and professional experience. These standards not only help elevate the entire profession of
marriage counseling but discourage unqualified practitioners and ensure that skilled, effective counseling will be available to couples who
need it. AAMFC also has a code of professional ethics to which each
member subscribes. AAMFC's goal is to ensure that every person who
practices marriage counseling will meet its professional standards and
observe its code of ethics.

2. Specialized training—AAMFC examines, approves, and encourages training centers in marriage counseling. These centers, located in
major universities and educational institutions, offer advanced training
programs and marriage counseling internships to meet the growing
demand for qualified counseling.

3. Professional publications—The *Journal of Marriage and Family
Counseling* is published quarterly by AAMFC to advance the professional understanding of marriage and family behavior and to improve
the psychotherapeutic treatment of marital and family dysfunction.
The Journal publishes articles on clinical practice, research, and theory
in marriage and family counseling. AAMFC members receive the Journal as a part of their membership benefits. Paid subscriptions are
available to nonmembers and institutions.

4. Professional meetings—AAMFC and its regional divisions conduct
frequent regional, national, and international conferences to provide

members with new ideas, techniques, and developments in the field of marriage and family counseling.

5. Cooperation with other professions—AAMFC maintains vital contact with professional groups in allied fields for exchange of information and cooperation on programs of mutual benefit. AAMFC is working closely with other professional groups to establish and revise state laws pertaining to marriage, divorce, licensing of marriage counselors, and related subjects. AAMFC has held cooperative conferences with the American Academy of Family Physicians, American Association of Obstetricians and Gynecologists, the National Council on Family Relations, the American Bar Association, the American Psychological Association, and many other organizations.

6. Public education—AAMFC carries on intensive educational programs to help people understand more about marriage and family problems, about the role of professional counseling in preventing and solving these problems, and about the dangers of unscrupulous or unqualified persons who pose as marriage counselors. Public education also helps couples learn to solve their own marriage difficulties and build sounder, happer family relationships. AAMFC staff and members provide factual material on marriage and family problems to newspapers, television, radio, and magazines. Members speak to many lay groups and write extensively for periodicals and professional journals.

In a broader sense, the American Association of Marriage and Family Counselors is concerned not just with the profession of marriage and family counseling but also with people and the needs and problems they face in relation to marriage—whether they are now married, will be married, have been married, or may somehow be affected by marriage in our society. AAMFC is also concerned with the institution of marriage itself—its strengths and weaknesses, its changing patterns, and its role in the lives of all people. AAMFC firmly believes that this most important and intimate of human relationships demands increased understanding, research, and education at all levels, and that the professional marriage and family counselor must take the lead to ensure that these needs are met.

For the public, AAMFC provides a nationwide referral service by supplying the names of qualified marriage counselors and general guidelines for seeking their help.

For interested professionals, AAMFC furnishes consultation about membership standards, application procedures, training, conferences, seminars, and related programs.

For any information, contact AAMFC national headquarters. American Association of Marriage and Family Counselors, 225 Yale Avenue, Claremont, California 91711 (714:621–4749).

THE AMERICAN ASSOCIATION OF MARRIAGE AND FAMILY
COUNSELORS

Code of Professional Ethics

PREAMBLE

Members of the AAMFC are professional counselors trained in dealing with marriage and family problems. They are conscious of their special skills and aware of their professional boundaries. They perform their professional duties on the highest levels of integrity and confidentiality and will not hesitate to recommend assistance from other professional disciplines when circumstances dictate. They are committed to protect the public against, and will not hesitate to expose, unethical, incompetent, and dishonorable practices. To maintain these high standards of service, members of the AAMFC have imposed upon themselves the following rules of conduct and will earn highest public confidence.

SECTION I. CODE OF PERSONAL CONDUCT

1. A Counselor provides profesional service to anyone regardless of race, religion, sex, political affiliation, social or economic status, or choice of life style. When a Counselor cannot offer service for any reason, he or she will make a proper referral. Counselors are encouraged to devote a portion of their time to work for which there is little or no financial return.

2. A Counselor will not use his or her counseling relationship to further personal, religious, political, or business interests.

3. A Counselor will neither offer nor accept payment for referrals and will actively seek all significant information from the source of referral.

4. A Counselor will not knowingly offer service to a client who is in treatment with another counseling professional without consultation among the parties involved.

5. A Counselor will not disparage the qualifications of any colleague.

6. Every member of the AAMFC has an obligation to continuing education and professional growth in all possible ways, including active participation in the meetings and affairs of the Association.

7. A Counselor will not attempt to diagnose, prescribe for, treat, or advise on problems outside the recognized boundaries of the Counselor's competence.

8. The Association encourages its members to affiliate with professional groups, clinics, or agencies operating in the field of marriage and family life. Similarly, interdisciplinary contact and cooperation are encouraged.

SECTION II. RELATIONS WITH CLIENTS

1. A Counselor, while offering dignified and reasonable support, is cautious in prognosis and will not exaggerate the efficacy of his or her service.

2. The Counselor recognizes the importance of clear understanding on financial matters with his or her clients. Arrangements for payments are settled at the beginning of a counseling relationship.

3. A Counselor keeps records of each case and stores them in such a way as to ensure safety and confidentiality, in accordance with the highest professional and legal standards.

   a. Information shall be revealed only to professional persons concerned with the case. Written and oral reports should present only data germane to the purpsoes of the inquiry; every effort should be made to avoid undue invasion of privacy.

   b. The Counselor is responsible for informing the client of the limits of confidentiality.

   c. Written permission shall be granted by the clients involved before data may be divulged.

   d. Information is not communicated to others without consent of the client unless there is clear and immediate danger to an individual or society and then only to the appropriate family members, professional workers, or public authorities.

4. A Counselor deals with relationships at varying stages of their history. While respecting at all times the clients' right to make their own decision, the Counselor has a duty to assess the situation according to the highest professional standards. In all circumstances, the Counselor will clearly advise a client that the decision to separate or divorce is the responsibility solely of the client. In such an event, the Counselor has the continuing responsibility to offer support and counsel during the period of readjustment.

SECTION III. RESEARCH AND PUBLICATION

1. The Counselor is obligated to protect the welfare of his or her research subjects. The conditions of the Human Subjects Experimentation shall prevail, as specified by the Department of Health, Education, and Welfare guidelines.

2. Publication credit is assigned to those who have contritubed to a publication, in proportion to the contribution, and in accordance with customary publication practices.

SECTION IV. IMPLEMENTATION

1. In accepting membership in the Association, each member binds himself or herself to accept the judgment of his or her fellow members as to standards of professional ethics, subject to the safeguards provided in this section. Acceptance of membership implies consent to

abide by the acts of discipline herein set forth and as enumerated in the Bylaws of the Association. It is the duty of each member to safeguard these standards of ethical practice. Should a fellow member appear to violate this Code he or she may be cautioned through friendly remonstrance, colleague consultation with the party in question, or formal complaint may be filed in accordance with the following procedure.

   a. Complaint of unethical practice shall be in writing to the Chairperson of the Standing Committee on Ethics and Professional Practices and to the Executive Director. A copy of the complaint shall be furnished to the person or persons against whom it is directed.

   b. Should the Standing Committee decide the complaint warrants investigation, it shall so notify the charged party(ies) in writing. When investigation is indicated, the Standing Committee shall consistute itself an Investigating Committee and shall include in its membership at least one member of the Board and at least two members (other than the charging or charged parties or any possible witnesses) from the local area involved. This Investigating Committee or representatives thereof shall make one or more local visits of investigation of the complaint. After full investigation following due process and offering the charged party(ies) opportunity to defend him or herself, the Committee shall report its findings and recommendations to the Board of Directors for action.

   c. The charged party(ies) shall have free access to all charges and evidence cited against him or her and shall have full freedom to defend him or herself before the Investigating Committee and the Board, including the right to legal counsel.

   d. Recommendation made by the Committee shall be:
      (1) Advice that the charges be dropped as unfounded
      (2) Specified admonishment
      (3) Reprimand
      (4) Dismissal from membership.

2. Should a member of this Association be expelled he or she shall at once surrender his or her membership certificate to the Board of Directors. Failure to do so shall result in such action as legal counsel may recommend.

3. Should a member of this Association be expelled from another recognized professional association or his/her state license be revoked for unethical conduct, the Standing Committee on Ethics shall investigate the matter and, where appropriate, act in the manner provided above respecting charges of unethical conduct.

4. The Committee will also give due consideration to a formal complaint by a nonmember.

SECTION V. PUBLIC INFORMATION AND ADVERTISING

All professional presentations to the public will be governed by the Standards on Public Information and Advertising as follows.

The practice of marriage and family counseling as a mental health profession is in the public interest. Therefore, it is appropriate for the well-trained and qualified practitioner to inform the public of the availability of his/her services. The membership standards of the AAMFC provide the public with the assurance of competence in this field, relieving the individual member of the need to "advertise" his/her services to the public.

However, much needs to be done to educate the public as to the services available from qualified marriage and family counselors. Therefore, the members of the AAMFC have a responsibility to the public to engage in appropriate informational activitie in keeping with the following standards.

I. Telephone Directory Listings

Yellow Pages, All listings should be governed by the principles of dignity, modesty, and uniformity.
   A. Special type (boldface, etc.) and lined boxes or any other technique tending to make one individual or firm's listing stand out from other listings in the directory is a breach of professional ethics.
   B. A proper listing will include no more than the following:
      (1) Name
      (2) Highest earned relevant degree (one only)
      (3) State licensure (including license No.)
      (4) AAMFC clinical membership
      (5) Address
      (6) Telephone number
      (7) Designated specialty
   C. Office hours (or the statement "By Appointment Only") may be listed if permitted by the local telephone company.
   D. Any title including words such as "Institute," "Center," "Clinic," or "Service" is acceptable only if a group practice includes at least three professionals. Other AAMFC members of such a group may choose to be listed under the identifying group practice name as well as separately in the proper alphabetical location.
   E. When titles utilizing the name of a city, county, or state are employed, care should be taken to indicate the private nature of the enterprise.

AAMFC Insignia

A regional division or a chapter of the AAMFC may use the AAMFC insignia to list its members as a group. When all members practicing within a telephone directory district have been invited to list member(s) may do so.

II. Printed Professional Materials

A. *Stationery, Business Cards, and Announcements.* Dignity and good taste should characterize the printed professional materials of an AAMFC member. Select paper stock, type, and composition suitable to the presentation of a professional practice. Imprinting should be limited to a minimum of simple, clearly legible information.

(1) *Name and degree.* Listing more than the highest earned relevant degree rarely adds information and detracts from the dignity. Listing an honorary degree (D.D., D.Sc. etc.) is a violation of professional modesty. Using the title "Dr." in front of one's name in place of or in addition to initials of a doctoral degree following the name is considered improper.

(2) *Type of practice.* The AAMFC member will ordinarily identify himself/herself as a Marriage and Family Counselor. Related professional identification may be included (Licensed Clinical Social Worker, Licensed Psychologist, etc.)

(3) *Specialty.* Should a member wish to emphasize a single specialization within marriage and family practice, he or she may do so provided the designation reflects an exclusive emphasis.

(4) *AAMFC membership.* Persons holding clinical membership in the AAMFC may designate this by the following statement: "Member, American Association of Marriage and Family Counselors."

(5) *Address and telephone.* The location of the professional practice may be designated by appropriate address and telephone number(s).

(6) *Insignia.*

(a) AAMFC Insignia. The AAMFC insignia may NOT be used on printed professional materials of a member, a group of members practicing together, or a training center approved by the AAMFC. It may be used by regional divisions in the course of their bona fide activities as divisions of the AAMFC.

(b) Other Insignia. Professional insignia intended to convey the orientation or focus of professional practice may be proper if the design and content is simple and informational.

B. *Brochures.* The production and distribution of public informational materials are appropriate activities of the marriage and family counselor. The purpose of such material is to inform the public, not to "promote" the individual's practice. Therefore, the emphasis should be on simple statements of services offered, factual presentations of the practitioner's relevant training and experience, and accurate information about contracts and conditions for service.

THE AMERICAN ASSOCIATION OF MARRIAGE AND FAMILY COUNSELORS

Membership Standards

CLINICAL MEMBER

1. Recognized graduate professional education with the minimum of an earned master's degree from an accredited educational institution in Marriage and Family Counseling or a closely related field. In every case the applicant's transcript must establish that a course of study equivalent to a Master's degree in Marriage and Family Counseling has been successfully completed. In addition, the applicant shall satisfactorily complete:

2. (a) 200 h of approved supervision of the practice of marriage and family counseling, ordinarily to be completed in a 2- to 3-year period, of which at least 100 h must be in *individual* supervision. This supervision will occur preferably with more than one supervisor and should include a continuous process of supervision with at least several cases.

   (b) 1000 h of clinical experience in the practice of marriage and family counseling under approved supervision, involving at least 50 different cases.

OR

   (c) 200 h of approved supervision: 150 h in the practice of marriage and family counseling and 50 h in the practice of psychotherapy, ordinarily to be completed in a 2- to 3-year period, of which at least 100 h must be in *individual supervision*. At least 50 h of the individual supervision must be of marriage and family counseling.

   (d) 1000 h of clinical experience: 750 h in the practice of marriage and family counseling under approved supervision involving at least 30 cases; and 250 h in the practice of psychotherapy under approved supervision, involving at least 20 cases.

3. Applicants may be requested to have a screening interview with the national Membership Committee or a regional membership committee or designated representative(s).

4. Demonstrated readiness for the independent practice of marriage and family counseling.

5. Upon completion of the graduate professional degree plus the required supervised clinical experience, the candidate will be expected to have mastered the important theory in the field of marriage and family counseling as defined in the document on supervision: "The Approved Supervisor is responsible for the supervisee's familiarity with the important and relevant literature in developmental psychology, personality theory, human sexuality, behavior pathology, marriage and family studies, and marriage and family therapy."

PERSONAL MATURITY AND INTEGRITY

The applicant shall possess the qualities of character and of personality deemed to be necessary for the task of marriage and family counseling. The Membership Committee shall carry out whatever investigation may be necessary to secure satisfactory evidence of this.

LICENSING

In those states which license marriage and family counselors, an applicant who holds such a licence will ordinarily be deemed qualified for membership. Exception to this will be where state licensing standards do not meet minimum national AAMFC clinical standards. In states which license marriage and family counselors, members of the Association will ordinarily be required to meet the standards for licensing in that state.

CONTINUING PROFESSIONAL EDUCATION

Clinical members of the AAMFC are expected to document their participation annually in some significant continuing professional education experience, with a view to increasing self-awareness and updating professional skills.

OTHER CATEGORIES OF MEMBERSHIP

FELLOW

A minimum of 5 years in good standing as a Member of the Association and significant contributions to the field of marriage and family counseling, as determined by the Board of Directors upon recommendation by the Honors Committee.

STUDENT

The designation "Student" may be given to a person who is currently enrolled in the graduate program of an accredited college or university in an appropriate discipline. The Student category shall ordinarily be for a maximum of 5 years or until satisfactory completion of requirements for Member, whichever shall come first.

ASSOCIATE

The designation "Associate" may be given to a person who has already completed graduate studies and achieved professional competence in an appropriate behavioral science or mental health field and who is now receiving supervision by arrangement with the Membership Committee in order to become qualified as a Member. The Associate category shall ordinarily be for a maximum of 5 years or until satisfactory completion of requirements for Member, whichever shall come first.

DISTINGUISHED AFFILIATE

Upon recommendation of the Honors Committee the Board of Directors may, at its discretion, invite suitable persons to become Affiliates of the Association. Such persons shall be of high standing in a field related to marriage and family counseling and shall be making an outstanding contribution to the field of marriage, the family, or counseling. The total number of Affiliates shall not exceed 2% of the total number of clinical members. All Affiliates shall be subject every 5 years to re-election by the Board of Directors.

HONORARY LIFE MEMBERSHIP

Upon recommendation of the Honors Committee the Board of Directors may, at its discretion, invite suitable persons to become Honorary Life Members of the Association. Such persons shall be of high standing in a field related to marriage and family counseling and shall have made an outstanding contribution to the field of marriage, the family, or counseling. The total number of Honorary Life Members shall not exceed 25.

INDEX

Abortion, 238, 347
Adolescent, as presenting problem, 105
Adoption, 144
Adultery, 276
Affairs, extramarital
  and professional therapy, 60
  as amateur psychotherapy, 50
  as anger, 58
  as emotional separation, 57
  assessed in initial interview, 47
  decision as collusion, 56
  therapeutic intervention, 62, 63
  to seek reassurance, 58
  understanding, 61
  yearning for romance, 59
Aggression, in marriage, 21
Alcoholism and couple counseling, 146
  case study, 154
  interpersonal model, 147
  intrapsychic model, 146
  organismic model, 148
  psychiatric description, 186
  systems perspective, 146
  treatment stages, 157
Allred Interaction Analysis for Counselors, 100
American Association of Marriage and Family Counselors (AAMFC)
  code of Professional Ethics, Appendix
  description of AAMFC, Appendix
  membership standards, Appendix
American Association of Retired Persons, 131
Androgens
  for deficiencies of aging, 287
  for the menopausal woman, 287
Anger, as cover for dependency, 21
Antabuse, 187
Anxiety, 192
Association of Couples for Marriage Enrichment (ACME), 176

Biographical Marital Questionnaire, 170

Child
  as presenting problem, 75, 81
  in the family, 83–86, 88
  modifying behavior, 88
  personality, 92
Childless couple, 134
Climacteric years, in woman, man and family, 283
Clitoris, 352
Co-counselors, 7, 74
Coitus interruptus, 340
Collaborative counseling
  defined, 10

movement to conjoint, 11
  when recommended, 11
Communication, 26
  focused on child, 84
  functional for counselors, 101
Concurrent counseling
  defined, 10
  when recommended, 10
  with psychiatrist, 197, 199
Condom, effectiveness as contraceptive, 342
Conjoint counseling
  advantages of, 8
  and family illness, 164
  defined, 8
  goals, 18, 63
  in divorce counseling, 74
  in initial interview, 35
  in marital counseling, 132
  in parent-adolescent counseling, 107
  in premarital counseling, 300, 307
Contraception and family planning, 340
  coitus interruptus and nonintromission, 340
  condoms, 342
  diaphragms plus cream or jelly, 343, 357
  different modalities of contraception, 340
  douches, foams, creams and jellies, 334, 342
  intrauterine contraceptive device, 346, 357
  oral contraceptives (the pill), 343
  rhythm method, 341
  special situations, 348
    adolescent, 348
    anticipating pregnancy soon, 348
    postpregnancy, 348
    premenopause patients, 349
    special conditions, 349
    woman without prior coitus, 348
  sterilization, 347
Contraceptive, 340
Contract
  in counseling, 14, 30
  in initial interview, 37
Council of Affiliated Marriage Enrichment Organizations (CAMEO), 176
Counseling, marriage
  client configuration in, 6
  compared to therapy, 3, 6, 331
  counselor modeling, 8
  defined, 3
  effectiveness, 8, 12
  forms
    classical psychoanalysis, 5
    collaborative, 10

concurrent, 4, 5, 10
conjoint, 5, 8
conjugal, 6
crisis counseling, 5
group, 4, 5
individual, 4, 5, 11
summarized, 4
tandem, 9
interdisciplinary nature, 4
outcome, 12
the childless couple, 134
training, 19, 100
treatment considerations
co-counselors, 5
contracting, 14
relationship focus, 13
session frequency, 15
session length, 14
structure/control, 13
therapy triangle, 14
treatment modalities
group, 5
individual, 5, 11
Counseling session(s)
frequency, 15, 39
length, 14
relationship focus, 13
visual aids, 39
Counseling, sexual
dysfunctional couples, 250
areas of knowledge, 254
assignments and homework, 255
attitudes toward sex, 252
co-counselors, 255
conceptualizing sexual dysfunction, 251
counselor characteristics, 253
fear of sexual failure, 253
genital pleasuring, description and negative reactions, 261
inadequate sex information, 251
increased awareness of sexuality, 250
individual history taking, 257
medical laboratory reports, 259
physiology and sexual responses, 254
primary and secondary sexual dysfunction, 256
public attitude, 250
roundtable session, 259
secretiveness, 253
self-esteem, 252
sexual problem-oriented examination, 257
systems theory, 251, 255
treatment program, 262
Counselor, marriage
self-awareness, 241
self-confidence, 240
sexual knowledge, 241, 330

training, 9, 170
Counselor, premarital
clergy as, 297, 335
physicians as, 297, 335, 340, 351
Counselor, sex
co-counselors, 255
comfortable feelings, 254
imposing sexual attitudes, 254, 332
talking with clients about sexual problems, 240
Couple interaction patterns, 69
attaching-detaching marriage, 24
child marriage, 29
complementary, 30, 114
half-marriage, 21
neurotic marriage, 30
pseudomarriage, 32
sado-masochistic marriage, 26
symmetrical, 114
therapeutic marriage, 31, 52, 55
Courtship, assessed in initial interview, 41
Creams, effectiveness as contraceptives, 342

Death, 123
Decourting, 76
Dependency
as struggle for intimacy, 24
in courtship, 43
needs in marriage, 21, 27, 47
Depression
counselor's feelings, 77
physical symptoms, 166
psychiatric descriptions, 190
Diaphragm, effectiveness as contraceptive, 343, 357
Divorce
a perspective, 69
a three-generational problem, 70
as treatment method, 275
rarely works, 71
Douche, vaginal effectiveness as contraceptive, 334, 342
Drug abuse, 187

Estrogens
for deficiencies of aging, 286
for the menopausal woman, 286
Ethics, Appendix

Family, climacteric years in, 290
Family council, 95
Family planning, counseling for, 330, 340
Family therapy
and family interaction, 111
compared with marriage counseling, 3, 81
in adolescent-parent problems, 105
in child-parent problems, 81